DEATH AND DYING: UNDERSTANDING AND CARE

DEATH AND DYING

UNDERSTANDING AND CARE

Second Edition

Barbara A. Backer, RN, DSW
Natalie Hannon, PhD
Noreen A. Russell, MSW, ACSW

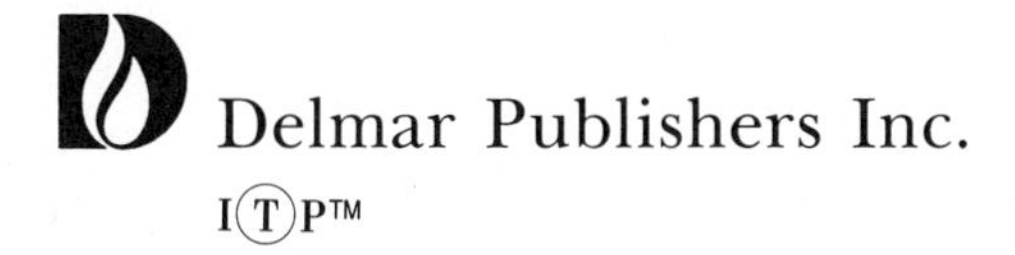

NOTICE TO THE READER

Publisher does not warrant or guarantee any of the products described herein or perform any independent analysis in connection with any of the product information contained herein. Publisher does not assume, and expressly disclaims, any obligation to obtain and include information other than that provided to it by the manufacturer.

The reader is expressly warned to consider and adopt all safety precautions that might be indicated by the activities described herein and to avoid all potential hazards. By following the instructions contained herein, the reader willingly assumes all risks in connection with such instructions.

The publisher makes no representations or warranties of any kind, including but not limited to, the warranties of fitness for particular purpose or merchantability, nor are any such representations implied with respect to the material set forth herein, and the publisher takes no responsibility with respect to such material. The publisher shall not be liable for any special, consequential or exemplary damages resulting, in whole or in part, from the readers' use of, or reliance upon, this material.

Cover graphic courtesy of Satori Artwork © 1990-93 BERKELEY SYSTEMS, INC., from AFTER DARK, the Ultimate Screen Saver. Reproduced under license agreement by Delmar Publishers Inc.
Cover design by Lisa L. Pauley

Delmar Staff
Senior Acquisitions Editor: William Burgower
Senior Editorial Assistant: Debra Flis
Project Editor: Carol Micheli
Production Coordinator: Barbara A. Bullock
Art and Design Manager: Russell Schneck
Art Coordinator: Cheri Plasse
Design Coordinator: Karen Kemp
Electronic Publishing Coordinator: Lisa Santy

For information, address Delmar Publishers Inc.
3 Columbia Circle, Box 15-015
Albany, New York 12212

Printed in the United States of America
Published simultaneously in Canada
by Nelson Canada,
a division of The Thomson Corporation

2 3 4 5 6 7 8 9 10 XXX 00 99 98 97 96 95

Library of Congress Cataloging-in-Publication Data

Backer, Barbara A.
Death and dying : understanding and care / Barabara A. Backer
Natalie Hannon, Noreen A. Russell — 2nd ed.
p. cm.
Includes bibliographical references and index.
ISBN 0-8273-4954-8
1. Terminal care. 2. Death. I. Hannon, Natalie. II. Russell, Noreen A. III. Title.
R726.8.B32 1994
616'.029—dc20 92-42472
CIP

To Charles and Helen Rodkin; and
Rosalie and Edward and Leslie Hannon.

To Otto and Anna Backer; and Tyke.

EAGLE POEM

by Joy Harjo

To pray you open your whole self
To sky, to earth, to sun, to moon
To one whole voice that is you.
And know there is more
That you can't see, can't hear
Can't know except in moments
Steadily growing, and in languages
That aren't always sound but other
Circles of motion.
Like eagle that Sunday morning
Over Salt River. Circled in blue sky
In wind, swept our hearts clean
With sacred wings.
We see you, see ourselves and know
That we must take the utmost care
And kindness in all things.
Breathe in, knowing we are made of
All this, and breathe, knowing
We are truly blessed because we
Were born, and die soon, within a
True circle of motion,
Like eagle rounding out the morning
Inside us.
We pray that it will be done
In beauty.
In beauty.

Contents

Preface

Eleven years have passed since the first edition, *Death and Dying: Individuals and Institutions.* We, the authors, have grown older and have had more personal experience with death, including the deaths of parents, and the deaths of friends with AIDS. Noreen Russell went on to different pursuits and did not participate in this revision.

We started this revision at the beginning of the Persian Gulf War; we watched the television as bombs dropped, killing people in Iraq. We completed the revision as people in Los Angeles expressed their anger about the failure of law and the lack of justice in this country; anger that culminated in death and injury. Daily, we experience how we and our neighbors are potentially faced with death from violence and substance use.

These personal and political events have influenced our writing of this second edition. We have become much more aware of the fragility and tenuousness of our lives and our increasing interdependence with other people—not only on a local and national level but also on a worldwide level. Similarly, we are more cognizant of the need for a unified interdisciplinary approach among caregivers in an increasingly fragmented and cost-effective, outcome-oriented medical system. These events have also helped us to identify what we perceive as a need for the concept of caring when working and living with people who are dying.

Caring, as used in this text, connotes enabling and supporting. It is a concept of empowerment that recognizes the uniqueness of each individual's response to loss, dying, and death. Confronting our own death or coping with the death of a loved one encompasses a complex set of human behaviors and feelings. A caregiver, friend, or significant other is challenged to recognize and to live with these complexities, and to understand and support the person coping with death and dying. The dying person's feelings and thoughts about what is needed to cope are integral components of this concept of care.

Understanding and care should be valued as highly as efficiency and cost-effectiveness in today's high-tech medical system. Indeed, they are vital to balance the effects of the illness-oriented care technocracy, which is considered health care, in America. It is with this belief in mind that we have modified our original text title, and have called this second edition *Death and Dying: Understanding and Care.* We hope for and can offer no less for people who are dying or who are grieving.

The second edition has a number of additional changes besides the title. We recognize the changing demographics of our pluralistic culture as we identify patterns of responses to dying and death in American society, discuss problems related to the termination of life, and examine the structure and process of interaction among the terminally ill, their families, and helping professionals. A new chapter on hospice care is presented, reflecting the proliferation of these programs in the last ten years. The AIDS epidemic has influenced all our lives, and its themes of stigma as well as hope occur in many chapters of the text. A new chapter specifically discussing AIDS has been included. Since no area in death and dying is changing so rapidly as that of ethics, the revised chapter on ethics includes current thinking on euthanasia, living wills, health proxy directives, and organ transplants.

Users of the first edition have commented on the helpfulness of the Learning Exercises and Audiovisual Material at the end of each chapter. These have been updated and remain in the text. Content material is organized into twelve chapters, which should facilitate use of the text for reading assignments throughout a semester. Chapter 1 presents an overview of attitudes toward death and dying in American society, while Chapter 2 discusses individuals' perceptions and feelings concerning dying. How health caregivers are socialized in the care of dying patients is reviewed in Chapter 3. Interaction and communication between caregivers and dying patients are also analyzed. Chapter 4 discusses how hospitals or institutions with cure-oriented goals affect dying patients with care-oriented needs, while Chapter 5 looks at hospice care, or care which is designed to help the dying patient die with dignity. Chapter 6 presents children's perceptions of and reactions to death, and how families respond to the death of children. Chapter 7 is a new chapter on AIDS. Ethical issues surrounding death and dying, such as euthanasia, the right to refuse treatment, and the definition of death, are discussed in Chapter 8. Theories of suicide, suicide prevention, and the impact of suicide are discussed in Chapter 9. Chapter 10 deals with the processes of grief and bereavement, along with suggestions for interventions in these processes. Chapter 11 presents the functions of funerals and the funeral rites of major religions. Chapter 12 views death from a cross-cultural perspective.

We think this book, with its interdisciplinary focus on understanding and care as components of a cognitive and affective humanistic approach to dying people, is unique. It is an important and significant survey text for students in the fields of nursing, social work, sociology, psychology, and medicine. Health care practitioners should find this a valuable text, as will any person interested in learning more about dying, death, and loss.

It would be impossible to thank all of the people who have supported and encouraged us in developing this book. We would like to acknowledge and thank Joseph Reynolds for his encouragement in starting this revision, and Bill Burgower and Debra Flis for their continuous support in development of the manuscript. Thanks go to Serena Nanda, Ph.D., for providing her anthropological perspectives on death and dying; and to Kathleen Nokes, RN, Ph.D., for her insights on AIDS. Thanks also go to Marge Rodkin and Victoria Gilmour who gave up their weekends to type and help edit the book; and to Joann Knowles for her additional typing assistance.

We would also like to express our gratitude and appreciation to our students and patients, who have been continuing sources of motivation and enrichment and who have provided us with the impetus to complete this revision. Finally, we say "thank you" to Jim Peterson and Peter Hannon for their gentleness and humor; and to our parents who, even as we were with them in their dying, were teaching us once again about living.

Barbara Backer
Natalie Hannon

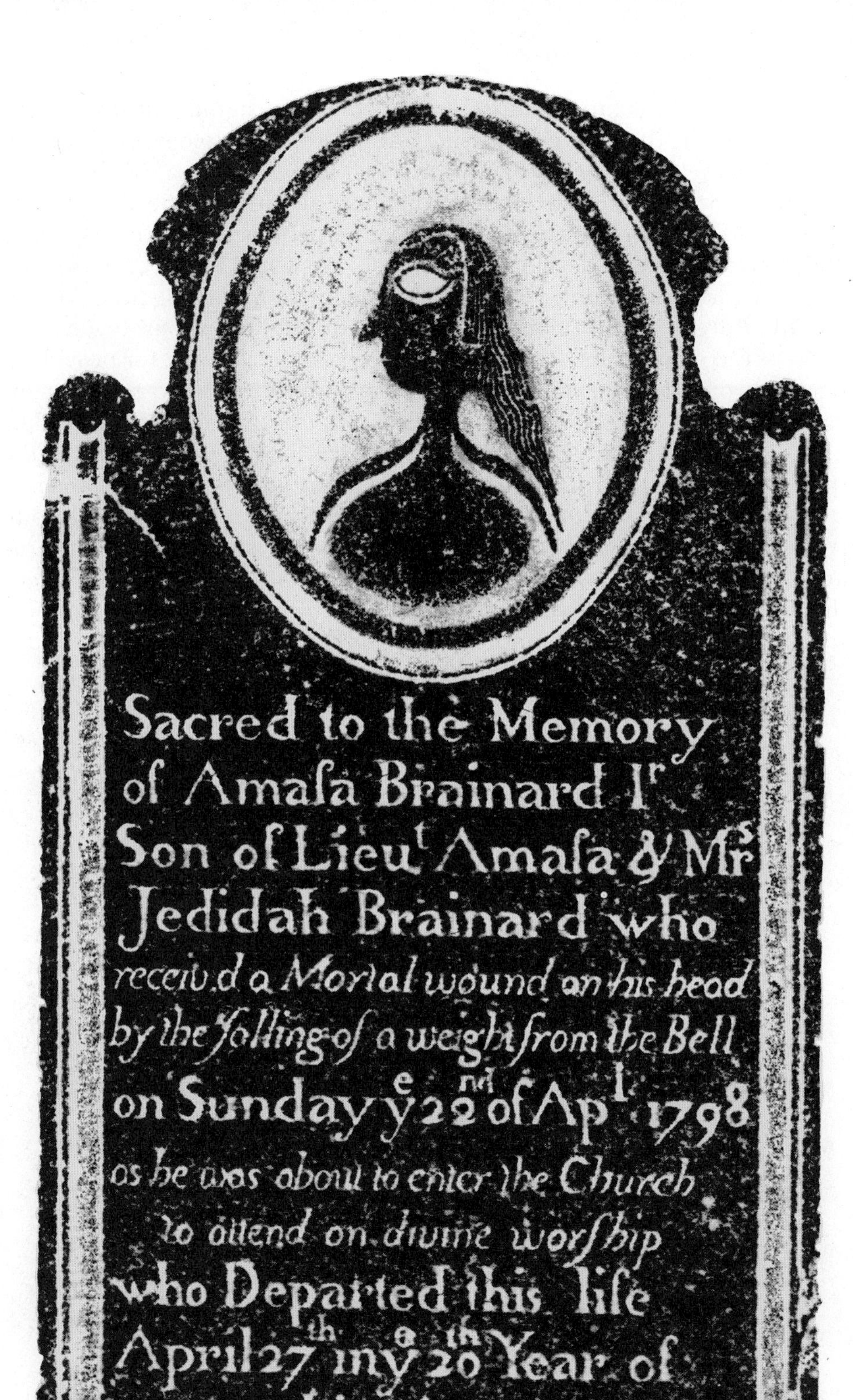
Sacred to the Memory
of Amasa Brainard Jr
Son of Lieut Amasa & Mrs
Jedidah Brainard who
receiv.d a Mortal wound on his head
by the falling of a weight from the Bell
on Sunday ye 22nd of Apl 1798
as he was about to enter the Church
to attend on divine worship
who Departed this life
April 27th in ye 20th Year of
his Age

Chapter 1

Death in American Society

Try talking about dying and death at a party. Watch people's reactions: many people will move away; some people will tell jokes about the subject; and others may just say, "I don't want to talk about such a morbid topic." But there will also be a group of people who will be fascinated by the topic, and a lively conversation may ensue. Most of us do not want to deal with the fact that sooner or later, all of us will die. Yet there is in American society an increased realization that dealing with the subject of death will allow people to live their lives more fully.

Thanatologists, those people who are specialists in studying the various aspects of death and dying, have called the United States a "death-denying" society. Death is considered to have taken the place of sex as pornography (Gorer, 1976) in our society and has taken on the status of a taboo (Rando, 1987). Yet to make the general assumption that all people deny death is too simple. At the same time that most people do not wish to talk about death and dying at a party, Elisabeth Kubler-Ross's *On Death and Dying* and Derek Humphrey's *Final Exit,* a book on how to commit suicide, were best-sellers among trade paperbacks. People may not wear seatbelts, but they carry organ donor cards in their wallets just in case something happens to them. And although the death of a loved one is probably not experienced until adulthood, children view death on television practically every night. It is probably more accurate to say that instead of denial, people are ambivalent in their feelings toward death and dying. How have these attitudes and feelings of ambivalence developed? What helps to explain the attitudes of society toward death and dying?

Photo is courtesy of a private collection

History of Attitudes toward Death and Dying

Attitudes and feelings toward death and dying have changed over time. Phillippe Aries in *Western Attitudes Toward Death* (1974) and *The Hour of Our Death* (1982) traces the cultural attitudes toward death since the Middle Ages.

The traditional attitude towards death was one of resignation and acceptance. It can be summarized by the phrase,"we shall all die" (Aries, 1982, p. 55). Death and life were considered to exist simultaneously. Aries labeled this attitude "tamed death" since death was both "familiar and near, evoking no great fear or awe" (Aries, 1974, p. 13). During the Middle Ages, with the growing importance of religion and the effects of the Black Death, "tamed death" was slightly modified in that people not only resigned themselves to the deaths of others but also to their own deaths.

One could not be isolated from death. In the fourteenth century the Black Death was said to have killed over 25 percent of the population of Europe. In 1603, one-fifth of the population of London was killed by the plague (Thomlinson, 1965, p. 84). People were surrounded by death during this period as shown by the diary entries of the British Admiralty secretary in 1665 (Samuel Pepys, as quoted in Thomlinson, 1965):

> *June 15th, 1665.* The Towne grows very sickly, and people to be afeard of it; there dying this last week of the plague 112, from 43 the week before.
>
> *August 10th, 1665.* By and by to the office, where we sat all the morning; in great trouble to see the Bill this week rise so high, to above 4,000 in all, and of them above 3,000 of the plague. . . . The town growing so unhealthy, that a man cannot depend upon living two days to an end.
>
> *September 20th, 1665.* But, Lord! what a sad time it is to see no boats upon the River; and grass grows all up and down White Hall court, and nobody but poor wretched in the streets! And, which is worst of all, the Duke showed us the number of the plague this week, brought in the last night from the Lord Mayor; that it is encreased from about 600 more than the last, which is quite contrary to all our hopes and expectations, from the coldness of the late season. For the whole general number is 8,297, and of them the plague 7,165 (p. 84).

With the ascendance of Catholicism and then Protestantism, death became viewed as a form of justice. In order to have a good life after death, it was imperative for the dying person to have behaved well. People had to prepare to meet their maker in the proper manner, "In death, man encountered one of the great laws of the species, and he had no thought of escaping it or glorifying it" (Aries, 1974, p. 29). As Jacques Choron (1963) points out:

> The hereafter has become through the efforts of the Church, a source of terror and not consolation. Instead of reward, most people could only expect retribution. In order to secure a blissful existence in the other world. . . . it was necessary to lead such a life in this world as was beyond the endurance of most people, except for a few over-zealous ascetics (p. 91).

True salvation could only be found if all mortal passions were renounced; humanity was only to concentrate on God (Stannard, 1977, p. 21).

Beginning in the eighteenth century, people again became concerned with the death of others, which Aries calls "Thy Death." Death was no longer considered to be banal. Rather than being viewed as part of life, death was seen as a break with life. Death was both frightening and fascinating; it became romanticized. This may seem contradictory, but the contradiction can be explained by Aries's hypothesis that the romanticization of death was a psychological sublimation of the erotic view of death held in the seventeenth century. "Like the sexual act, death was henceforth increasingly thought of as a transgression which tears man from his daily life, from rational society, from monotonous work, in order to make him undergo a paroxysm, plunging him into an irrational, violent, beautiful world" (p. 57). If Aries's hypothesis is accepted, then death can be both frightening and romantic.

The death of another became much more fearful than one's own death. Mourning became exaggerated. Memorials and monuments were built for the dead. The American colonies exemplified this: funerals were extravagant social gatherings wherein hundreds of pounds were spent to mark the death of an individual (Jackson, 1977, p. 9).

In the mid-nineteenth century, the period of "Forbidden Death" began. Death was no longer a dramatic act but rather a technological phenomenon. Important here is the fact that death no longer occurred in the home, but in the hospital, which eliminated any ceremony between the family and the dying person. In addition, funerals came to be held at specialized "parlors," not in the home. Death was no longer a part of everyday life, and it was treated as if it were pornography (Gorer, 1976):

> The natural processes of corruption and decay have become disgusting, as disgusting as the natural processes of birth and copulation were a century ago; preoccupation about such processes is (or was) morbid and unhealthy, to be discouraged and punished in the young. Our great-grandparents were told that babies were found under gooseberry bushes or cabbages; our children are likely to be told that those who

> have passed on are changed into flowers, or be at rest in lovely gardens. The ugly facts are relentlessly hidden; the art of the embalmers is an art of complete denial (p. 74).

Or as Aries (1982) says succinctly, "A heavy silence has fallen over the subject of death" (p. 614).

Yet, people are no longer "silent over the subject of death." Since the 1960s, there has been talk about death. The writings of Elisabeth Kubler-Ross, the hospice movement, ethical issues concerning death, AIDS, and the death education movement have led to "instrumental activism" (Parsons & Lidz, 1967) or to the "containment of death" (Kellehear, 1984, and Moller, 1990). It does not matter whether people have euphemisms concerning death; what is important is that the prolongation of life is valued and that people develop a highly rationalized system for identifying the controllable components of death—the effects of premature death, the physical suffering of dying, and the deliberately imposed death. People need to "contain" death, not deny it. The values and norms of our society are concerned with controlling and managing death and dying. Hence, "the seeming contradiction between America's orientation towards "death-denial and the recent emphasis on death awareness can be readily reconciled" (Moller, 1990, p. 22).

"Containing" Death and Dying

In order to understand why society tries to "contain" death and dying, it is necessary to look at such factors as changing mortality patterns, American values, the institutionalization of dying, the effects of mass death, and family structure.

Changing Mortality Patterns

Calvin Goldschneider (1971, pp. 102–134) points out that in the change from a preindustrial to an industrial society, we have gone from uncontrolled to controlled mortality. Uncontrolled mortality involved three characteristics: mortality was high, it fluctuated over short periods, and it varied widely at any point in time. Under controlled mortality, the opposite conditions prevail: mortality is low, and it does not fluctuate widely either over time or geographic area.

The United States estimated that between the thirteenth and seventeenth centuries, life expectancy ranged from 20 to 40 years (Goldschneider, 1971, p. 107). Table 1.1 shows the expectation of life at birth in eighteenth-century Europe and America (Dublin, Lotka, & Spiegelman, 1949, pp. 35–36). Not only was the life span short, but mortality conditions were such that they could fluctuate to as high as 400 per 1,000 population during times of famine or epidemics. There were smallpox, cholera, and typhus epidemics.

Table 1.1 Expectation of Life at Birth in Eighteenth-Century Europe and America

PERIOD COVERED	AREA	EXPECTATION OF LIFE AT BIRTH
1746	French convents and monasteries	37.5
1735–1780	Northampton, England	30.0
1782, 1788–1790	Part of Philadelphia	25.0
A period before 1789	Massachusetts and New Hampshire	35.5
1772–1792	Montpellier, France	Males 23.4 Females 27.4
A period before 1789	Different parts of France	28.8

in the eighteenth century, 25 percent of all Frenchmen were killed, crippled, or disfigured by smallpox (p. 85).

Famine was also a contributor to high mortality. In Western Europe alone, 450 more or less localized famines were recorded from the years 1000 to 1855 (p. 79). A famine could easily have a severe effect on one area of a country while not affecting an adjacent area because of inadequate transportation. Under uncontrolled mortality, death was random and constantly present. It was, therefore, necessary for society to incorporate it into its ongoing values and structures.

Today, under conditions of controlled mortality, the average life expectancy is 75 years of age, with a death rate of 8.5 per 1,000 population (*World Almanac,* 1992, p. 956). Furthermore, these death rates have hardly fluctuated for the past 20 years.

Another effect of controlled mortality was the change in terms of who died. Prior to controlled mortality, the very young and the middle aged were likely to die. One of the most privileged groups in preindustrial society, the British aristocracy, had an infant mortality rate of 200 per 1,000 live births (Goldschneider, 1971, p. 107). If you lived beyond infancy, you or your spouse were likely to die in the middle of adulthood. Death *had* to be confronted. In the United States in 1991, the infant mortality rate was 9.1 per 1,000 live births (*World Almanac,* 1992, p. 938). (However, the infant mortality rate for African Americans was almost double the rate for whites.) Since it is the elderly who are most likely to die, it is not necessary to incorporate death into our lives before we are old. The expectation is that people will have many years to live in order to accomplish and to achieve their goals. Charles Corr (1979) states that in societies that have controlled mortality:

> It is possible to have lengthy courtship patterns emphasizing romantic love, marriages at a later age, longer marriages, and serial monogamy—divorces and remarriages; to have more energy available for research and therapy aimed at curing disease and further extending life; and to foster future-oriented attitudes of planning, saving and deferred gratification (p. 13).

Clearly, in America, concentration is on prolonging life. Death is no longer relevant.

American Values

Implicit in American values are the notions of innovation, efficiency, and progress (Williams, 1970), and science and technology are central in our values (Moller 1990). Death is approached in the light of these values.

Through science and technology, Americans can maintain the illusion that they can conquer death. This illusion has been strengthened by the fact that the life span has increased by over 20 years since 1900 in the United States. In 1900 the average life span was 47.3 years; today, it is 75.4 (*World Almanac,* 1992, p. 956). Table 1.2 shows the causes of death in 1900 (Lerner, 1970, p. 14) and in 1990. Today, we die of diseases of old age: diseases of the heart, cancer, and stroke cause over 60 percent of our deaths.

Our belief in our ability to conquer death is further shown by the use of life tables. At any given age, one can calculate how much longer one should live and what the probability of death is at any given age. For example, from the life table (Table 1.3) one can see that at age 5, a white female is likely to live 74.6 more years. The chance of death is .23 out of 1,000. For a black female, age 5, the life expectancy is an additional 69.8 years. The chance of death is .40 out of 1,000.

The emphasis on science and technology to control death is seen by the development of a new word, "prolongevity," implying that we have the ability to prolong our lives. Popular magazines have articles with such titles as "How to Live to be 100" (Karras, 1989), "The Search for the Fountain of Youth" (*Newsweek,* 1990) and "Score Three for Longevity" (*U.S. News and World Reports,* 1991). As stated by Elias (1985):

> More than ever before, we can hope today by the skill of doctors, by diet and by medicaments, to postpone death. Never before in the history of humanity have more-or-less scientific methods of prolonging life been discussed so incessantly throughout the whole breadth of society as in our day. The dream of the elixir of life and of the fountain of youth is very ancient. But it is only in our day that it has taken on scientific, or pseudoscientific form. The knowledge that death is inevitable is overlaid by the endeavor to postpone it more and more with the aid of medicine and insurance and by the hope that this might succeed (p. 47).

Table 1.2 The Ten Leading Causes of Death in the United States, 1900 and 1990

RANK	CAUSE OF DEATH	DEATHS PER 100,000 POPULATION	PERCENT OF ALL DEATHS
1900			
1	Influenza and pneumonia	202.2	11.8
2	Tuberculosis	194.4	11.3
3	Gastritis, enteritis, etc.	142.7	8.3
4	Diseases of the heart	137.4	8.0
5	Vascular lesions affecting the central nervous system	106.9	6.2
6	Chronic nephritis	81.0	4.7
7	All accidents	72.3	4.2
8	Malignant neoplasms (cancer)	64.0	3.7
9	Certain diseases of early infancy	62.6	3.6
10	Diphtheria	40.3	2.3
	All other causes	615.3	35.9
1990			
1	Diseases of the heart	289.0	33.5
2	Malignant neoplasms (cancer)	201.7	23.4
3	Cerebrovascular diseases	57.9	6.7
4	Accidents	37.3	4.3
5	Bronchitis, emphysema, and asthma	35.5	4.1
6	Influenza and pneumonia	31.3	3.6
7	Diabetes mellitus	19.5	2.3
8	Suicide	12.3	1.4
9	Homicide	10.2	1.2
10	Chronic liver disease and cirrhosis	10.2	1.2
	All other causes	157.0	18.2

Data for 1990 reprinted with permission from "When, Why and Where People Die" by Monroe Lerner in O. Brim et al. (Eds.), *The Dying Patient,* (Russell Sage Foundation).

Our need to control death is also seen in our reaction to AIDS. AIDS upsets our ideas of containing death. Although we know it is caused by a virus, we cannot predict the course of the virus, nor can we kill the virus. It is not a disease of the elderly, but rather one of the young and middle aged (See Table 1.4). We do not seem to be able to control its spread. Millions of dollars are being spent in research to eliminate the affront of AIDS. AIDS presents us with the reality that death ultimately denies rational analysis. We want answers. We are used to being supplied with answers, and we find it difficult to live with the uncertainties and ambiguities of death from AIDS.

Table 1.3 Expectation of Life and Expected Deaths, by Race, Sex, and Age: 1988

AGE IN 1988 (YEARS)	EXPECTATION OF LIFE IN YEARS					EXPECTED DEATHS PER 1,000 ALIVE AT SPECIFIED AGE[1]				
		White		Black			White		Black	
	Total	Male	Female	Male	Female	Total	Male	Female	Male	Female
At birth	74.9	72.3	78.9	64.9	73.4	9.99	9.55	7.47	19.19	16.26
1	74.7	72.0	78.5	65.2	73.6	0.70	0.73	0.55	1.17	0.88
2	73.8	71.0	77.5	64.3	72.7	0.53	05.3	0.43	0.92	0.73
3	72.8	70.1	76.6	63.3	71.7	0.42	0.41	0.34	0.74	0.60
4	71.8	69.1	75.6	62.4	70.8	0.34	0.34	0.28	0.62	0.49
5	70.8	68.1	74.6	61.4	69.8	0.30	0.30	0.23	0.54	0.40
6	69.9	67.1	73.6	60.4	68.8	0.27	0.28	0.21	0.48	0.32
7	68.9	66.2	72.7	59.5	67.8	0.24	0.26	0.18	0.42	0.28
8	67.9	65.2	71.7	58.5	66.9	0.22	0.23	0.16	0.36	0.25
9	66.9	64.2	70.7	57.5	65.9	0.19	0.20	0.14	0.29	0.24
10	65.9	63.2	69.7	56.5	64.9	0.17	0.17	0.13	0.24	0.25
11	64.9	62.2	68.7	55.5	63.9	0.17	0.18	0.13	0.24	0.27
12	64.0	61.2	67.7	54.5	62.9	0.22	0.25	0.16	0.32	0.30
13	63.0	60.2	66.7	53.6	61.9	0.33	0.40	0.21	0.51	0.32
14	62.0	59.3	65.7	52.6	61.0	0.47	0.61	0.29	0.78	0.35
15	61.0	58.3	64.8	51.6	60.0	0.64	0.85	0.38	1.07	0.38
16	60.1	57.3	63.8	50.7	59.0	0.79	1.07	0.46	1.37	0.43
17	59.1	56.4	62.8	49.8	58.0	0.91	1.25	0.52	1.66	0.48
18	58.2	55.5	61.8	48.8	57.1	1.00	1.37	0.54	1.94	0.55
19	57.2	54.6	60.9	47.9	56.1	1.04	1.44	0.52	2.19	0.63
20	56.3	53.6	59.9	47.0	55.1	1.09	1.51	0.51	2.47	0.72
21	55.3	52.7	58.9	46.2	54.2	1.14	1.58	0.50	2.74	0.80
22	54.4	51.8	58.0	45.3	53.2	1.17	1.61	0.49	2.96	0.89
23	53.5	50.9	57.0	44.4	52.3	1.19	1.62	0.50	3.09	0.97

24	52.5	50.0	56.0	43.5	51.3	1.19	1.60	0.51	3.16	1.05
25	51.6	49.0	55.0	42.7	50.4	1.19	1.57	0.52	3.22	1.13
26	50.6	48.1	54.1	41.8	49.4	1.19	1.54	0.54	3.31	1.21
27	49.7	47.2	53.1	41.0	48.5	1.21	1.53	0.55	3.43	1.30
28	48.8	46.3	52.1	40.1	47.5	1.24	1.56	0.57	3.63	1.39
29	47.8	45.3	51.2	39.2	46.6	1.29	1.62	0.59	3.88	1.49
30	46.9	44.4	50.2	38.4	45.7	1.35	1.69	0.61	4.14	1.58
31	45.9	43.5	49.2	37.5	44.7	1.41	1.75	0.64	4.41	1.69
32	45.0	42.6	48.3	36.7	43.8	1.48	1.82	0.68	4.72	1.82
33	44.1	41.6	47.3	35.9	42.9	1.55	1.89	0.72	5.08	1.96
34	43.1	40.7	46.3	35.1	42.0	1.63	1.97	0.76	5.47	2.12
35	42.2	39.8	45.4	34.3	41.1	1.73	2.05	0.82	5.91	2.30
36	41.3	38.9	44.4	33.5	40.2	1.83	2.15	0.89	6.35	2.48
37	40.4	37.9	43.4	32.7	39.3	1.93	2.25	0.96	6.73	2.66
38	39.4	37.0	42.5	31.9	38.4	2.03	2.36	1.03	7.02	2.84
39	38.5	36.1	41.5	31.1	37.5	2.12	2.47	1.12	7.26	3.02
40	37.6	35.2	40.6	30.3	36.6	2.22	2.60	1.21	7.49	3.22
41	36.7	34.3	39.6	29.6	35.7	2.35	2.76	1.32	7.77	3.44
42	35.8	33.4	38.7	28.8	34.8	2.51	2.94	1.45	8.10	3.66
43	34.9	32.5	37.7	28.0	33.9	2.70	3.14	1.59	8.52	3.89
44	33.9	31.6	36.8	27.2	33.1	2.92	3.38	1.76	9.01	4.13
45	33.0	30.7	35.8	26.5	32.2	3.17	3.65	1.95	9.54	4.39
46	32.1	29.8	34.9	25.7	31.4	3.44	3.96	2.16	10.09	4.69
47	31.3	28.9	34.0	25.0	30.5	3.76	4.32	2.39	10.73	5.04
48	30.4	28.0	33.1	24.3	29.7	4.12	4.74	2.65	11.46	5.46
49	29.5	27.2	32.1	23.5	28.8	4.53	5.21	2.94	12.26	5.95

(table continued on next page)

Table 1.3 Continued

AGE IN 1988 (YEARS)	EXPECTATION OF LIFE IN YEARS					EXPECTED DEATHS PER 1,000 ALIVE AT SPECIFIED AGE[1]				
		White		Black			White		Black	
	Total	Male	Female	Male	Female	Total	Male	Female	Male	Female
50	28.6	26.3	31.2	22.8	28.0	4.98	5.74	3.26	13.16	6.48
51	27.8	25.5	30.3	22.1	27.2	5.47	6.33	3.60	14.11	7.05
52	26.9	24.6	29.5	21.4	26.3	6.01	7.00	3.99	15.03	7,67
53	26.1	23.8	28.6	20.8	25.5	6.61	7.77	4.41	15.90	8.33
54	25.3	23.0	27.7	20.1	24.8	7.26	8.64	4.87	16.76	9.04
55	24.4	22.2	26.8	19.4	24.0	7.96	9.57	5.37	17.62	9.77
56	23.6	21.4	26.0	18.8	23.2	8.72	10.57	5.91	18.59	10.57
57	22.8	20.6	25.1	18.1	22.5	9.56	11.68	6.50	19.82	11.51
58	22.0	19.8	24.3	17.5	21.7	10.49	12.89	7.15	21.39	12.61
59	21.3	19.1	23.5	16.8	21.0	11.50	14.21	7.86	23.26	13.84
60	20.5	18.4	22.6	16.2	20.3	12.61	15.64	8.63	25.31	15.19
61	19.8	17.6	21.8	15.6	19.6	13.78	17.16	9.46	27.42	16.57
62	19.0	16.9	21.0	15.0	18.9	14.97	18.72	10.33	29.49	17.88
63	18.3	16.3	20.2	14.5	18.2	16.18	20.29	11.22	31.44	19.06
64	17.6	15.6	19.5	13.9	17.6	17.42	21.91	12.16	33.32	20.15
65	16.9	14.9	18.7	13.4	16.9	18.72	23.60	13.17	35.26	21.26
70	13.6	11.8	15.0	10.9	13.8	28.19	36.32	20.54	48.13	29.59
75	10.7	9.1	11.7	8.6	10.9	42.46	55.80	32.23	67.66	42.18
80	8.1	6.8	8.7	6.8	8.4	65.54	85.86	52.88	98.61	65.18
85 and over	6.0	5.1	6.3	5.5	6.6	1,000.00	1,000.00	1,000.00	1,000.00	1,000.00

[1]Based on the proportion of the cohort who are alive at the beginning of an indicated age interval who will die before reaching the end of that interval. For example, out of every 1,000 people alive and exactly 50 years old at the beginning of the period, between 4 and 5 (4.98) will die before reaching their 51st birthdays.

Source: U.S. National Center for Health Statistics, *Vital Statistics of the United States,* annual.

Table 1.4 AIDS Deaths, 1990

	NUMBER	RATE PER 100,000
All Ages	24,120	9.6
Under 15	390	0.7
15–24	580	1.6
25–34	8,460	19.3
35–44	9,730	25.7
45–54	3,240	12.7
55 and Older	1,690	3.2
Not Stated	20	—

Source: *World Almanac, 1992*

Another value important in American society is happiness. Our advertising media, with its emphasis on youth, have contributed to our thinking that we must be happy. We are the "Pepsi generation," and happiness is one of our goals. Dying and death interfere with this, and we do not want to accept the interference. As the historian Arnold Toynbee (1968) says: "For Americans, death is unAmerican, and an affront to every citizen's inalienable right to life, liberty and the pursuit of happiness" (p. 131).

The Institutionalization of Dying

With our control over mortality and our belief that death can be avoided, dying has become institutionalized. No longer do people die at home with their families; they die in hospitals. As Quint (1979) points out, the first half of the twentieth century saw the chronic and long-term diseases exceed the communicable diseases. Along with this came greater diagnostic and treatment techniques and the development of scientific medicine. "More and more, hospitals came to be places designed and organized for the purpose of controlling death" (pp. 142–143).

Besides hospitals, after World War II came the development of nursing homes. Although it is a myth that Americans put all their old people in nursing homes (only 6.4 percent of the population between 75 and 84 are in nursing homes), the percentage of people over 85 (the frail elderly) who are in nursing homes is 22 percent (Kearl, 1989, p. 443). In a sense, the population of nursing homes may be defined as dying.

The rise in the percentage of people who die in institutions has been noted by Robert Weir (1989, p. 140). In 1949, 50 percent of all deaths took place in institutions. In the 1950s, it had increased to 61 percent; in the 1970s, to 70 percent, and in the 1980s to almost 80 percent.

Since people die in hospitals, dying has become invisible. We do not have any idea of what dying looks like. Neither the dying patient nor the family is at the center of the ritual of dying—it is the health care professional who is at the center. The difficulty is that hospitals are not set up to deal with dying; rather, they are places to go to be cured. As such, there is very little room for the dying in the rituals of the hospital, and there is very little room for the family to take part in the dying process.

Compare the following account of a woman dying in the 19th century with the picture we have of dying today:

> Mother Drinkwater was critically ill, but some of her family realized the seriousness of her condition. Never having been to a hospital, and without recent contact with a physician, she remained in bed while the rest of the family carried out their regular activities. They took turns caring for her as best they could.
>
> One night while Mary was sitting up with her, Mother Drinkwater "seemed to die in her sleep." Her husband, son and daughter were asleep in other parts of the house (Rosenblatt, 1983, p. 66).

Today, there is an attempt to move dying back into the home with hospice. There are over 1,700 hospices in the United States, with the primary type of hospice care being home care. (See Chapter 5.) Hospice defines the unit of care as not just the dying patient but also the patient's family. It is an attempt to bring the family back into the picture and to make dying visible again.

The Effect of Mass Death

Another reason for our ambivalent attitudes towards death has been the development of the nuclear age. As Lifton (1964) points out, the nuclear age affects our symbolic immortality. In order for us to contemplate our lives and our deaths, we must be sure that we will somehow live on. For example, we have children so that our names will continue; we write books so that the world will know we existed; we have friends so that memories of us will live on.

Seventeen years after the bombing of Hiroshima, Lifton interviewed Japanese people who had possible exposure to significant amounts of radiation at the time of the bombing. Lifton's concern was to explore the psychological elements of what he referred to as the "permanent encounter with death" that the atomic bomb created in those exposed to it. Lifton formulated the premise that:

> We are not absolutely convinced of our immortality, but rather have a need to maintain a sense of immortality in the face of inevitable biological death; and that this need represents not only the inability of the individual unconscious to recognize the possibility of its own demise but also a compelling universal urge to maintain an inner sense of continuous symbolic relationship, over time and space, to the various elements of life (p. 203).

He suggests that this sense of immortality may be achieved through any of several modes:

1. *Biosocially*: We can express our immortality by means of biological reproduction, living on through our sons and daughters, and through their sons and daughters.
2. *Theologically*: We may feel that when we die, we transcend our earthly life for one of a higher existence.
3. *Creatively*: Our writings, art, inventions, and influences upon other people may give us a sense of immortality.
4. *Naturally*: A sense of immortality may be achieved through being survived by nature itself; that is, when we die, we perceive that nature will remain, and that we become part of nature.

However, the concept of nuclear death totally annihilates our sense of immortality. We cannot live on in others since no others would exist. Everything that gave substance to our existence would die with us.

Fulton & Owen (1988) reviewed studies of youths and their concerns about nuclear weapons. The studies showed that youths, whether in grade school or high school, were aware of the annihilating capacity of nuclear weapons. A third of all high school seniors agreed that "nuclear or biological annihilation will probably be the fate of all mankind within my lifetime" (Bachman, 1983, as cited in Fulton & Owen, 1988, p. 391).

One hopes that with the Cold War ending, the threat of nuclear destruction has diminished, and the fears of mass death will also lessen.

Family Structure

The major reason that families are held together in our society is basically for emotional gratification. The emotional dependency within the nuclear family is rarely diffused by other relations. This situation makes separation appear very threatening. The notion of marrying for love developed after industrialization. Before that, marriage was an economic necessity. The roles of the husband and wife were defined in terms of economic production. The extended kinship network also played an important role. With today's emphasis on psychological companionship and the nuclear family, it is more difficult to conceive of a spouse or another loved one dying. One can understand the feelings of the wife on the radio commercial after her husband says he spent his lunch hour shopping for life insurance; the woman does not want to talk about it. To contemplate her husband's death is too painful. In addition, with our emphasis on the nuclear family, rather than the extended family, "great numbers of the elderly must not only live alone, but must die alone as well" (Fulton & Owen, 1988, p. 389).

Death in Society Today

In our society, no one ever dies. We either "pass on," or "rest in peace." Our pets are "put to sleep." Even in hospitals, patients do not die—they expire. Our funeral practices are such that we attempt to make the corpse look as alive as possible. Special fashions and cosmetics are used. We are also concerned with the comfort of the body within the casket. (Chapter 11 looks at funeral practices.)

Hospitals attempt to make the dying invisible. Kubler-Ross (1969) discusses how there suddenly were no dying patients in the hospital in which she worked when she asked to interview a dying patient for a seminar she was giving. Dumont & Foss (1972) provide a quote from a textbook, *Modern Concepts of Hospital Administration,* which they consider highly suggestive of death denial in American hospitals:

> The hospital morgue is best located on the ground floor and placed in an area inaccessible to the general public. It is important that the unit have a suitable exit leading onto a private loading platform which is concealed from the hospital patient and the general public (p. 37).

Another example of death denial occurred in the planning of the renovation of a major medical center in New York City; no space was allocated for the morgue. It was not until the renovation was under way that someone realized the omission. As a result, the morgue is located in a very inconvenient area of the hospital.

In the media, death tends either to be romanticized or depicted as violent. One of the authors at one time did not know that people died with their eyes open since all the movies she had seen showed dying people closing their eyes upon death. Most of us will not die with smiles on our faces, holding hands with our loved ones, or in the violent fashion portrayed in police stories.

Violent death is ubiquitous on television. "By the age of sixteen, according to the National Institute of Mental Health, the typical American has witnessed some eighteen thousand homicides on television." (Kearl, 1989, p. 383).

These issues can lead to three clusters of problems and potentials, as discussed by Lofland (1978, pp. 35–37):

Role problems: The dying role is a new role for people dying from chronic, rather than acute, disease. How is a person supposed to act in this role? Since the dying are generally elderly and isolated in hospitals, we have not seen how people act in this role. We have no experience in dealing with death or dying in our families, and we are not socialized as children into the proper role behaviors for dealing with the dying and the bereaved. As a result, we, as adults, then find it difficult to face either our own deaths or the deaths of others.

Organizational problems: The organization, the hospital, is designed for curing, not caring. As such, it is difficult for hospital personnel to care for the dying properly.

Belief problems: We are without beliefs concerning the meaning of death. We are no longer comforted by knowing a reason for death.

Along with these problems are potentials for solutions: new roles can be developed in which the dying can, if they so choose, talk about their feelings and their dying; new organizations can be designed, such as the hospice, where the care and comfort of the terminally ill are the primary goals; and new meanings to death can be constructed.

Changing Attitudes toward Death

Throughout the 1970s and 1980s people began to talk about death and dying. Americans have become concerned about the various ethical and practical issues that arise from dealing with death as a technological phenomenon. Why this new interest in death and dying?

1. We are becoming an older society. In the 1970s, less than 11 percent of the population was 65 or older. In 2020, the aged are expected to make up almost 16 percent of our population (U.S. Bureau of the Census, 1977, p. 327). This means that dying is becoming relevant to more people.
2. The work of two women: Dr. Elisabeth Kubler-Ross and Dr. Cicely Saunders. The publication of Dr. Kubler-Ross's book, *On Death and Dying* "exposed a sensitive nerve in the health care delivery system of the United States, and crystallized for many not only the problem of the dying patient, but also the issues faced by those whose task it was to deal with the hidden issues of death in a public setting" (Fulton & Owen, 1988, p. 390). Dr. Cicely Saunders was the founder of the modern hospice movement. Her tireless push for hospices in Great Britain and the United States led to a return to a more humane way of treating the dying.
3. The hospice movement forced hospitals to look at how the dying were treated, and led to caring for the dying with respect, dignity and concern for the pain of dying.
4. The development of advanced technology that allows the prolongation of life for those whose quality of life has diminished. Individuals and their families have asked courts to intervene in the decision-making process concerning when a person is allowed to die. The cases of Karen Ann Quinlan and Nancy Cruzan have forced society to look at the ethical issues of dying and living, and to look at how we die.

5. The development of advanced technology that allows us to save more lives; i.e., organ transplants, has forced us to look at how we define death and to change our definition of death to brain death. The traditional definition of death, depending as it did on the heart and lungs, was an obstacle to the successful development of transplants. Transplants allow an individual's death to lead to the prolongation of another's life.
6. AIDS is a new disease with no cure. In the 1970s, we did not know about AIDS; in the 1990s, it is among the top 15 causes of death. AIDS contradicts two widely held myths: (1) that we can contain death; and (2) that death is only for the elderly.

As our attitudes toward death and dying change, Peter Steinfels (1975, pp. 3–4) cautions us how we should proceed. Death must be viewed as a mystery, not as a problem; that is, death should be something we contemplate rather than a problem we must solve. We must be aware that death has an "underside"—that inherent in death are fears and contradictions. Ultimately, though, "discussions of death must be discussions about life." The question must not be, "How should we order our dying?"; but, "How should we order our living?"

SUMMARY ❧

According to Aries, Western civilization has gone from an acceptance of death to the philosophy of "forbidden death" in which death is denied. Yet, given the amount of current writings on death, Americans seem to want to "contain" death more than to "deny" death. The reasons for the current attitudes toward death are a changing mortality pattern, the American value structure, the potential for mass death, and the family structure. American society is changing, though—people are starting to talk about death. One major reason for this is that our society is graying; a larger proportion of the population is becoming elderly. We are prolonging the process of dying, and we are confronting a new incurable disease, AIDS. However, as we as a society come to deal with death, we must realize that "discussions of death must be discussions about life" (Steinfels, 1975, p. 4).

LEARNING EXERCISES ❧

1. Read a newspaper and note the following:
   a. How often is death mentioned?
   b. What deaths are reported?
   c. How is death reported in the obituary column?
   d. How is death reported in the rest of the newspaper?

2. Tell your friends that you are taking a course in death and dying. What are their reactions?
3. Talk about your feelings about death and dying with the person sitting next to you. After five minutes, analyze what has happened in your conversation. What conclusions can you draw from this?
4. Observe how old people are portrayed on television. What do your observations tell you about society's attitudes toward old people? Do the same with dying people.

AUDIOVISUAL MATERIAL ❧

The Nuclear Nightmare: A Forum for Teens Expression, 40 minutes/videocassette/1986. United Learning, 6633 West Howard Street, Niles, Illinois 60648.
Experts on nuclear issues help teens understand their fears and concerns about nuclear war. Comes with an excellent leader's guide.

Fool's Dance, 30 minutes/videocassette/1988. Carle Medical Communications, 110 W. Main Street, Urbana, Illinois 61801.
A new patient in a nursing home instills the joy of life to both staff and residents. In order to live life fully, people in the nursing home learn they must accept death.

We Want to Have It All, 40 minutes/videocassette. Health Sciences Consortium, 201 Silver Cedar Court, Chapel Hill, North Carolina 27514.
The videotape portrays the feelings and thoughts of a terminally ill man, and how his illness has affected his living.

Life, Death and Denial, 43 minutes/videocassette. The Glendon Association, 2049 Century Park East, Los Angeles, California 90067.
College students discuss their attitudes towards death and their attempts to deny their own death.

REFERENCES ❧

Aries, P. (1974). *Western attitudes towards death.* Baltimore: Johns Hopkins University Press.

Aries, P. (1982). *The hour of our death.* New York: Vintage Books.

Choron, J. (1963). *Death and western thought.* New York: Collier Books.

Corr, C. (1979). Reconstructing the changing face of death. In H. Wass (Ed.), *Dying: Facing the facts.* New York: McGraw-Hill.

Dublin, L., Lotka, A., & Spiegelman, M. (1949). *Length of life.* New York: Ronald Press.

Dumont, R., & Foss, D. (1972). *The American view of death: Acceptance or denial.* Cambridge, MA: Schenkman.

Elias, N. (1985). *The loneliness of dying*. New York: Basil Blackwell.

Fulton, R., & Owen, G. (1988). Death and society in twentieth century America. *Omega, 18*, 379–398.

Goldschneider, C. (1971). *Population modernization and social structure.* Boston: Little, Brown.

Gorer, G. (1976). The pornography of death. In E. Shneidman (Ed.), *Death: Current perspectives.* Palo Alto, CA: Mayfield.

Jackson, C. (1977). *Passing*. Westport, CT: Greenwood Press.

Karras, J. (1989). How to live to be 100. *Better Homes and Gardens*, September, *67*, 36–37.

Kearl, M. (1989.) *Endings, A sociology of death and dying*. New York: Oxford University Press.

Kellehear, A. (1984). Are we a death denying society? A sociological review. *Social Science and Medicine, 18*, 717–720.

Kubler-Ross, E. (1969). *On death and dying*. New York: Macmillan.

Lerner, M. (1970). When, why and where people die. In O. Brim & H. Freedman, (Eds.), *The dying patient.* New York: Russell Sage Foundation.

Lifton, R. J. (1964). On death and death symbolism: The Hiroshima disaster. *Psychiatry*, August, *27*, 191–210.

Lofland, L. (1978). *The craft of dying*. Beverly Hills, CA: Sage Publications.

Moller, D. W. (1990). *On death without dignity, The human impact of technical dying*. Amityville, NY: Baywood Publishing.

Newsweek, 3/5/90, *115*, 44–48.

Parsons, T., & Lidz, V. (1967). Death in American society. In E. Shneidman (Ed.), *Essays in self-destruction.* New York: Science House.

Quint, J. (1979). Dying in an institution. In H. Wass (Ed.), *Dying: facing the facts.* Washington, DC: Hemisphere.

Rando, T. (1987). Death and dying are not and should not be taboo topics. In A. Kutscher, A. Carr, & L. Kutscher (Eds.), *Principles of thanatology*. New York: Columbia University Press.

Rosenblatt, P. (1983). *Better, better tears.* Minneapolis: University of Minnesota Press.

Stannard, D. (1977). *The puritan way of death.* Oxford: Oxford University Press.

Steinfels, P. (1975). Introduction. In P. Steinfels & R. Veatch (Eds.), *Death inside out.* New York: Harper & Row.

Thomlinson, R. (1965). *Population dynamics.* New York: Random House.

Toynbee, A. (1968). Changing attitudes toward death in the modern western world. In A. Toynbee, A. K. Man, N. Smart, et al. (Eds.), *Man's concern with death.* New York: McGraw-Hill.

U.S. Bureau of the Census. (1977). *Statistical abstract of the Unites States 1977.* Washington, DC: U.S. Government Printing Office.

U.S. Department of Commerce. (1991). *Statistical abstract of the United States, 1991.* Washington, DC: Government Printing Office.

U.S. News and World Reports, 12/31/90, *109,* 64.

Weir, R. (1989). *Abating treatment with critically ill patients.* New York: Oxford University Press.

Williams, R. (1970). *American society.* New York: Knopf.

World Almanac. (1992). New York: Pharos Books.

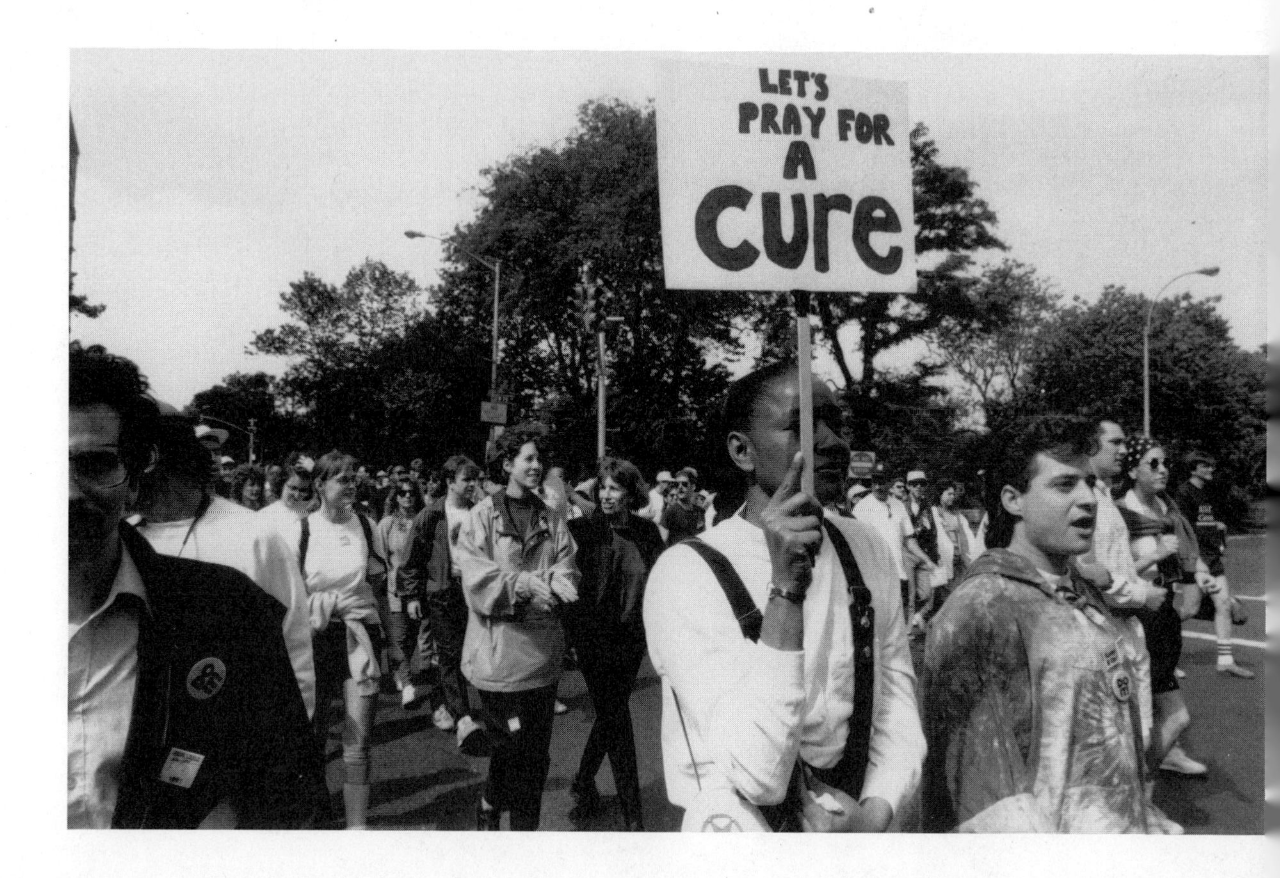
LET'S
PRAY FOR
A
Cure

Chapter 2

Death and the Process of Dying

As noted in Chapter 1, mortality patterns have changed throughout the years and people in the United States are living longer. In addition, many people are dying away from home in institutions separated from family, friends, and pets. These changing patterns can affect the way death is perceived. Increased longevity may support denial of death. The demography of elderly people living in retirement communities and people dying in institutions may support a perception of death as an isolated event, separate from current life-styles. However, urgent social issues such as abortion, euthanasia, AIDS, and capital punishment and such behaviors as alcoholism, drug abuse, and certain acts of violence, involve confrontation in some way with the threat of possible injury or ultimate death to self and others (Feifel, 1990, p. 542).

To facilitate an understanding of the meaning of death and dying in our own lives and in the lives of others, this chapter focuses on perceptions of death as an event, with associated fears and anxieties, and on dying as a process that includes phases and trajectories and may involve stigma, and on coping with death and dying.

Perceptions of Death

Numerous interpretations and perceptions of death have existed throughout history. Jung (1969) saw life and death as part of a continuing process:

> Life is an energy process, like every energy process, it is in principle irreversible and is therefore unequivocally directed towards a goal. That goal is a state of rest. In the long run everything that happens

Photo is courtesy of Sharon Guynup, GMHC

is, as it were, nothing more than the initial disturbance of a perpetual state of rest which forever attempts to reestablish itself (pp. 405–406).

The expression often used when someone dies is "she passed . . . ," which suggests the perception of death as a process or event in which one moves from this life to another. Depending upon the person's religion and/or culture, the next life may be a continuation of the familiar life on earth, may assume more spiritual aspects, or may be one of tribulation.

Cultural and Religious Influences

Related to this perception of continuity is that of perceiving death as a chance for rebirth, or transition between one form of life and another. Hindus, Buddhists, and members of certain other religions believe in reincarnation, in which the embodied self passes through childhood, youth, and old age, and assumes another body after death. The particular form in which the deceased is reincarnated depends upon his or her "karma," or behaviors in previous lives. For the Xhosa people of South Africa, death represents a transition from the mundane world (the world of flesh) to the world of the departed (the world of ancestral spirits) (Gijana, Louw, & Manganyi, 1989–90). There is a strong sense of the presence of the ancestors in the everyday lives of the Xhosa. Other cultures have other perceptions of death, as further discussed in Chapter 12.

Social Influences

Perceptions of death reflect social influences in our lives. Death may be seen as a leveler by some people (Kastenbaum, 1986, p. 31). Despite power, money, or fame, each person will eventually die. When someone wealthy and powerful dies, it once again becomes apparent that "even with all that money, she/he died like everyone else." Kastenbaum also notes that death may be seen as a validator (p. 31). This perception is exemplified in the elaborate funeral arrangements that make one last statement to society about the quality of the person's life and show the esteem felt by the survivors for the dead person. People pay for expensive insurance to ensure themselves a "proper funeral." The elaborateness of the funeral is seen as confirming not only the individual's worth but that of the survivors as well. The survivors have participated in an appropriate rite of passage, approved by society, that validates their status in the community.

Perceptions of death thus may be influenced by culture, religion, and social factors. If death is viewed as a part of the process of living as well as an event, then a closer examination of the influence of human growth and development on death perceptions is warranted. This influence is viewed here within a psychosocial context of American culture. Although individuals have unique responses, age-related tasks can color and shape the "meaning" of death and dying for each person.

Developmental Influences

Under the age of three, illness and death are sources of separation anxiety. The very young child is concerned with physical comfort and the knowledge that the parent/consistent caretaker is available. Children at this age do not understand why a parent has left them and is not protecting them, and they may feel angry and abandoned. The preschooler (three to five) is in a period of struggle with sexually aggressive impulses directed towards parents and siblings. Preschoolers often experience feelings of shame and fear of mutilation and invasion of the body if they become ill. Illness is often viewed as punishment and it impinges on their beginning sense of independence. School-age children (six to ten) react similarly to preschoolers in that they feel responsible for the illness and attribute it to their own bad thoughts and actions. Their major concerns focus on an increased sense of competency and mastery, and illness or death challenges this development. It is essential that parents and caregivers of children in these three age groups provide a constancy of caring to assuage the fears of abandonment. Children should be given every opportunity to gain mastery over their situation. (Chapter 6 has a more detailed discussion of this.)

Adolescence is a time of intense emotional and intellectual preoccupation. The individual is dealing with issues of consolidation of ego identity, emotional separation from the family, and the concomitant greater investment in the peer group (Mufson, 1985). Adolescents can be extremely sensitive about their physical appearance; their self-image is very important. Garfield (1978) asserts that the adolescent does not have a sense of longevity and therefore develops a romantic notion of death. Adolescents are less concerned with the quantity of life and more concerned with quality in that they seek affirmation of their worthiness and sense of self.

Hospitalization and illness impinge on adolescents' growing sense of self. They are very involved in the process of separation from parental authority but now find themselves in a situation where all decisions concerning their bodies are left to their parents. Health care staff, if sensitive enough, may discuss procedures and the like, but parents sign the consent forms. If the adolescent objects, this objection is often met with "You're not old enough to decide yet." The disease and treatment may involve loss of hair, weight, and energy. Garfield (1978) suggests that for caregivers, "the affirmation, confirmation and clarification of an adolescent as a unique and real being may be the most important task" (p. 156).

For the young adult, life is just beginning; developmental tasks for this period include establishing a work identity and intimacy with a loved partner. Marriage and children may be a part of this intimacy. Facing death at this stage of the life cycle is frustrating and disappointing. The young adult feels cheated and speaks about how "unfair" life can be. During this stage of life the individual will often cope with death by expressing rage at the world or by turning the anger inward and becoming depressed. A 22-year-old woman with bone cancer became increasingly depressed and refused to see visitors. When asked to share her feelings, she became outraged and, in an outburst, screamed, "Talking isn't going to help. Unless you can give me back the use of my legs so I can get on with my life, you're useless to me." If the individual has a spouse, a life partner, or children, he or she may worry about who will care for these people when he or she is unable.

The middle years have a deeper interpersonal tone. This is a time of meaningful ongoing relationships, attainment of work goals, and expansion of the self. Energy is directed at establishing and guiding the next generation (Erikson, 1963, p. 267). It is also a time when many middle-aged people experience a parental death, a common form of bereavement during this developmental phase (Dane, 1989). With increased longevity, parents generally do not die until this period in the life cycle of the adult child, and the individual is faced with the double task of incorporating a major loss and facing personal mortality. Shifting economic and employment trends may contribute to the stress and feelings of loss during this developmental age. LeShan (1973) comments:

> The greatest burden we carry into middle age is the burden of our masks. To some degree each of us is an island. We devote enormous amounts of time and energy to keeping up appearances and maintaining a good front while each of us weeps in the privacy of our own souls (p. 188).

People facing death during this phase of life must reconcile themselves to losing the opportunity to enjoy family and life successes, as well as new horizons of growth, and to missing the experience of guiding the next generation. A 50-year-old man hospitalized with leukemia spoke about his sadness in having a terminal illness. He realized he would not see his 15-year-old son finish high school and he would not know his "potential grandchildren." He desperately hoped he would have a year or so of retirement. He explained that since he was a child he had always had to work. Now that he had achieved some financial stability, he wanted to experience what it would be like not to be "on the job 12 hours a day, six days a week. I couldn't allow myself the time then that I really deserved—I always promised myself 'later'."

The older person faces multiple contradictions. This fabled time to sit back and take life easy often is a period of multiple losses: spouse, peers, health, and work. Kastenbaum (1986) calls this a time of bereavement overload (p. 153). This is a period when the individual thinks of death in practical terms. The elderly may fear that they will become burdensome. Institutionalization for the elderly can be a response to increasing infirmity, fragmentation of family life, and inadequate health care supports within the community. The older person may welcome death as an escape from an otherwise unbearable situation. A recently widowed 89-year-old woman was admitted to the hospital because of increasing weakness and periods of dizziness. Prior to her hospitalization, she had lived with her daughter, son-in-law, and five grandchildren. She very much wanted to return there, but said: "I know I can't go back. I feel like such a burden. None of this makes sense anymore. I've outlived my usefulness. Why doesn't God just take me?" Although some people may welcome death, it may also be accompanied by fear and anxiety.

Fear of Death, Dying, and Death Anxiety

The literature about death and dying frequently uses the terms "fear of death" and "death anxiety." The word "fear" ordinarily means that one is afraid of a specific something or someone; for example, a person may fear loud thunder or dogs. Anxiety, on the other hand, conjures up vague, uneasy feelings. The origin of these feelings is often unclear, but the experience of discomfort is very real. Dumont & Foss (1972) suggest that death is sufficiently concrete for fear, sufficiently vague for anxiety (p. 17). Death is specific; it will happen and it may be feared. Yet there are many unknowns associated with death. There is the uncertainty of how, when, and where death will come; of what will happen to survivors; and of what it means to be nonexistent. Such uncertainties can create anxiety. The terms "fear of death" and "death anxiety" thus may be used interchangeably since both feelings may be present together. However, such blending of terms makes interpretation of research study findings in the area of death and dying unclear unless investigators delineate how the terms are used.

Another distinction to be made in use of terms is the difference between fear of death and fear of dying. Research indicates that some people may fear dying more than they fear death, for dying connotes weakness, pain, dependency, loss of control, change in body image, and loss of contact with others (Viney, 1984–85; Thorson & Powell,1990). The expressions of fears of dying may also be seen as a defense against the actual expression of fear of death. Fear of death, with its finality of ceasing to be, may be intensely frightening. Of course, both fears may be present.

There can be potential usefulness in helping people express their actual fears. The fear of death of self, the fear of death of others, and the fear of the dying of others can be different fears with different specific origins. Thus, different avenues can be opened for possible relief. Axelrod (1986–87) discusses the value of "practicing death," an idea based on the assumption that by reflecting on mortality one can overcome a fear of it (p. 51). Talking about death does not so much inform about death as it serves as a reminder about it little by little, again and again, and by doing so, may direct peoples' reasoning to fit the event of death into their lives. Tausch (1988) reports of a person-centered discussion group in which participants contemplated their own deaths; a three month postdiscussion questionnaire indicated that more than 50 percent of the participants said that their fear of death and dying was reduced. While such research supports the idea that a fear of death is prevalent among people in general, other studies question how widespread that phenomenon actually is.

After reviewing the literature on fear of death and death anxiety, Kalish & Reynolds (1981) note that "we can say with certainty that study after study has shown that people *say* they do not fear death" (pp. 34–35). Similarly, Kastenbaum (1986) reports that studies making use of self-report questionnaires in general show low-to-moderate manifest death anxiety. Marks (1986–87), in a study of race and sex difference, high risk, and fear of dying, found groups who were at risk for higher mortality rates did not express more fear of death than groups with lower rates of mortality. In terms of race and sex differences, males and whites were statistically more likely to mention fear of death, but differences were slight. No African-American women in this study expressed a fear of death.

Thus, while people may have some death anxiety, these studies challenge the commonly held assumption that Americans have excessive fear or anxiety regarding death. However, what people say on a questionnaire and what they feel and do in an actual situation may still be very different. Feifel (1990) reports that significant discrepancies exist in many people between their conscious and nonconscious fear of death (p. 539). The idea of fear of death has been extensively researched.

Fear of Death

Kastenbaum & Aisenberg (1972) regard the fear of extinction, annihilation, obliteration, or ceasing to be as the basic fear of death (p. 44). It is their premise that fears about death are not that dissimilar from other fears people have in life. For example, fear of dying often involves feelings of becoming weak and dependent, but people have these feelings in their day-to-day existence. Individuals may be fearful of what may happen to them after death, but often they are fearful in life about what is going to happen tomorrow, or next year. Ceasing to be, however, is a difficult concept to consider.

Just as beliefs in extension or continuation of self beyond one's physical and psychosocial identity may influence how death is perceived, they may also affect fear(s) of death. Among the findings in their study of the relationship between fear of death and the concept of the extended self, Westmann & Canter (1985) report that people indicating fear more frequently described death as final, unnatural, providing no meaning to life, and cold, while people reported less fear and a more extended self if committed to religious life.

However, results of other studies which have empirically examined the relationship between fear of death and religious constructs for Americans have been inconsistent and at times contradictory. Thorson & Powell (1989) and Bristow (1986) found little evidence of a relationship between fear of death and religiosity among their sample populations. Conversely, Koenig's (1988) research showed that people in the study who employed religious behaviors during stressful situations were significantly more likely than "tepid believers" to report low or no fear about death. Religious beliefs thus may affect fear of death in some people, but it is not clear in what direction or whether this is applicable from a cross-cultural perspective. It is important to recognize and acknowledge such diversity and not to impose one's own beliefs upon another.

Along with the fear of extinction, people may be concerned about the loss of things they enjoy in life. When death is contemplated, it is difficult to think about giving up those individuals and aspects of life which bring enjoyment and self-identification. Perhaps there is the fear of what will be missed, of not knowing how life will progress. Many people fear growing old for similar reasons.

Fear of the unknown can be part of the fear of death and dying. What happens after death is simply not known; there is no television camera crew to tape this event. Death evokes a feeling of ultimate powerlessness since, for most people, the time and cause of death are unpredictable. Adding to this feeling of powerlessness is society's emphasis on independence and control of one's own destiny. Loss of consciousness is frightening because this symbolizes loss of self-mastery. Dying may bring with it loss of control of bodily functions such as urination and defecation, and people may fear disrespect and humiliation in needing assistance with such functions.

Such loss of control of bodily functions is also often associated with aging. The question may then be raised as to whether the elderly experience more death fear than other age groups. Research studies in this area suggest that this is not so (Wagner & Lorion, 1984; Given & Range, 1990). Henderson (1990) explored if more specific planning for, and thus more control over, the dying process would decrease anxiety about death among the elderly. Sixty-three residents of a retirement community who had living wills were provided with intervention in the form of counseling and filling out a questionnaire about proxy decision-making, feeding tubes, and other specific life-sustaining treatments. The mean death anxiety score for this experimental group decreased, whereas the control group's mean score did not change significantly. The study results suggest that such discussion and planning facilitate the ultimate goals of a person's wishes about his or her death, lowering death anxiety through planning, and avoiding stressful crisis-oriented decisions at a very sad and painful time (Henderson, 1990).

Another reason for fearing death may be that in death it is no longer possible to achieve. Heuscher (1986) notes that a person senses that death represents the end of opportunities to affirm one's self by means of committed actions. Part of this fear may also lie within America's goal-oriented culture and in the fact that some of people's self-esteem may be related to what they produce, what projects they complete, and how much money they make. G. Booth (personal communication, 1975), hypothesized that when individuals feel they have completed their life's work, they are ready to die.

Fear of death may be related to a dread of isolation or separation. One of the most basic human needs, according to Sullivan (1953), is for intimacy, or relating to other human beings. Death, of course, is the ultimate separation and may be seen as total isolation and aloneness, states of being that are intolerable in life to most people. In Tolstoy's *The Death of Ivan Ilych* (1960), it is possible to sense the anguish of Ivan's fear of the unknown and of separation when he says:

> Yes, life was there and now it is going, going and I cannot stop it. Yes. Why deceive myself? Isn't it obvious to everyone but me that I'm dying, and that it's only a question of weeks, days, . . . it may happen this moment. There was light and now there is darkness. I was here and now I'm going there! Where? (pp. 129–130).

People are often reluctant to make out a will for distribution of their material accumulations, yet they may fear death in terms of what will become of their dependents. Who will take care of the children, the spouse, the elderly parents? Writing a will forces individuals to take an additional step in contemplating their own deaths, and many are reluctant to do this. However, if people enter the medical care system as patients, an assessment is made by caregivers who contemplate their potential for dying at a particular time.

Dying as a Process

Patients entering a medical care institution set into motion a number of immediate responses on the part of professional caregivers. Staff need to determine a diagnosis for the patient, which in turn will help to establish what the projected course of illness will be; what, where, and when interventions can occur; and what the prognosis will be. Rather than rely solely on the medical definition of the course of illness, Strauss, Fagerhaugh, Suczek, & Wiener (1985) use the term trajectory "to refer not only to the physiological unfolding of a patient's disease but to the total organization of work done over that course, plus the impact on those involved with that work and its organization" (p. 8). Thus, in a medical care context, once a physician arrives at a diagnosis of a terminal illness for a patient, the patient will enter a dying trajectory.

> The course of dying—or "dying trajectory"—of each patient has at least two outstanding properties: first, it takes place over time. It has duration. Second, a trajectory has shape. It can be graphed. It plunges straight down, it moves slowly, moving slightly up and down before diving downward radically; it moves slowly down at first, then hits a long plateau, then plunges abruptly to death. Dying trajectories themselves are perceived, rather than the actual course of dying (Glaser & Strauss 1968, pp. 5–6).

There are various types of trajectories:

1. Certain death at a known time. In this trajectory, the time frame for resolving dying issues is quite clear, for example, accidents.
2. Certain death at an unknown time. This trajectory is typical of chronic fatal illness.
3. Uncertain death but a known time when the prognosis will be made. A person may need radical surgery and will need to go through that crisis to obtain a prognosis.
4. Uncertain death and an unknown time when certainty can be known. Examples are genetic diseases, HIV, and multiple sclerosis. People must live with the ambiguity associated with these diagnoses.

Patients themselves may influence their dying trajectories. Cousins (1979) describes how medical personnel had little hope for his recovery from a severe illness, but his own prescription for healing, which included experiencing humor, facilitated his ultimate recovery.

Within the dying trajectory, certain junctures or stages are passed: (a) the patient is defined as dying; (b) staff and family prepare for the patient's death; (c) it is decided that nothing more can be done; (d) the final descent occurs, leading to; (e) the final hours; (f) the death watch; and finally; (g) the death itself (Glaser & Strauss, 1968, p. 7). These junctures may be more easily ascertained during the first and third trajectories. During the second and fourth trajectories, caregivers must be more watchful in determining the critical junctures. If the trajectory goes as it was perceived by the health care professionals, than the caregivers can be prepared for the critical juncture and feel they have done all that was possible. Shneidman (1983) comments on this caregiving function:

> The thanatologist, if he examines his own mind, may very well discover that he is almost constantly aware of the expected "death trajectory"

> of his patient, and he governs the intensity of the sessions, their movement, the climaxes, the protective plateaus, and so on, over the projected time span—just as a skilled psychotherapist tries to control the intensity of the flow of material within any psychotherapeutic hour, trying not to leave the patient disturbed at the end of the session (pp. 8–9).

Holing (1986), in an exploratory study, described the dimensions of the dying trajectory as perceived by the primary caregiver of an adult who died of cancer at home. The trajectory was generally perceived as passing more slowly for the patient than for the caregiver. What, however, is the patient's experience of dying? The research that has been most influential in answering this question has been that done by Elisabeth Kübler-Ross (1969).

Phases of Dying

In her book *On Death and Dying,* Kübler-Ross (1969) describes a process of dying delineated into five phases:

1. *Denial and isolation*: This is the first response Kübler-Ross found once patients were informed that they were dying. They could not believe that the prognosis was true. Kübler-Ross notes that she regards this as a healthy way of dealing with this uncomfortable and painful situation. Denial can function as a buffer after the unexpected news; it allows people to collect themselves and mobilize other defenses. After learning of his diagnosis of inoperable cancer, one patient stated: "I'm relieved that surgery isn't necessary—now I can take my vacation and return to work. Surgery would have interfered with my plans."
2. *Anger*: Denial gives way to feelings of rage, resentment, and envy. Patients ask themselves the question: "Why me?" Anger may be displaced and projected towards the people around them. For example, a 25-year-old patient dying with cancer smashed an IV bottle because a nurse had not responded to her call for help quickly enough.
3. *Bargaining*: Here there is an attempt to postpone death. People may bargain with God in order to gain more time. Usually family events or projects are mentioned. "I've asked God to let me live until my daughter takes her first step." "God knows I have a good book in me. I'm sure this chemotherapy will give me enough time to finish it."
4. *Depression*: When terminally ill patients can no longer deny that they are dying, often because of increasingly severe signs and symptoms of disease such as pain and weight loss, the anger and

rage are replaced by feelings of depression and great loss. It is a phase of anticipatory grief that one may experience in order to prepare for one's death.

5. *Acceptance*: If people have had enough time and have been able to experience the above phases, they may well reach a stage where they can accept their dying. Anger, depression, and loss are no longer powerful feelings to combat; they become distant to the focus of dying. Patients in this phase may turn inward with their thoughts and feelings and their circle of interests diminishes. Families may need more help, support, and understanding than the patients at this time.

Kübler-Ross's work has become an accepted model for the care of the dying. One problem associated with use of the model is that caregivers may view the stages as normative rather than descriptive. At conferences on death and dying, one might hear a caregiver talk about waiting for an angry patient to enter the depression stage. Caregivers may try to fit patients into these stages rather than use the stages as a descriptive tool to understand the dying process. Wasow (1984) notes that the attempt to deal with the anxiety and sadness of death has led to an attempt to make it "prettier" than it is and that this perspective has added to the dying the burden of dying correctly—preferably in stages and with a positive attitude.

Most thanatologists agree that the feeling states described by Kübler-Ross do exist, but suggest they are not always stages that progress in a linear fashion. For example, Shneidman (1983) concluded from his work with patients that the stages of the dying process are not necessarily lived through in any order:

> What I do see is a complicated clustering of intellectual and affective states, some fleeting, lasting for a moment or a day or a week; set, not unexpectedly, against the backdrop of that person's total personality, his "philosophy of life" (whether an essential optimism and gratitude to life or a pervasive pessimism and dour or suspicious orientation to life) (p. 6).

Other critiques about the developmental nature of the sequential stage approach include: (a) stage analysis lacks universality—not all patients show all five types of behavior, and (b) patients may alternate between acceptance and denial, with these and other stage behaviors not being mutually exclusive. Kübler-Ross, to her credit, has emphasized that her theory should not be viewed as a fixed sequence of behavior and feelings.

Charmaz (1980) notes that Kübler-Ross's framework "probably is applicable to the educated, psychiatrically oriented upper middle class although it might not be as useful for persons from other socio-cultural backgrounds" (p. 154). Charmaz questions, for example, if the bargaining stage is a general phenomenon or if it more closely reflects middle-class ideologies wherein negotiation and exchange are part of the cultural assumptions of everyday life (p. 154).

According to Retsinas (1988), Kübler-Ross's stages of dying may not be applicable to the vast majority of people who die, not in middle age as in Kübler-Ross's sample population, but in old age. Retsinas points out that while death of a middle-aged person may be untimely, death of an older person may be timely. In addition, in elderly people "the failure of the body does not begin with the discovery of an encroaching disease . . . but comes instead as an almost inevitable gradual diminution of vitality" (Retsinas, 1988, p. 210). Elderly people make accommodations to such changes and still remain active in their lives.

Further views of the dying process have developed since Kübler-Ross's work. E. Mansell Pattison (1977) sees dying patients going through three clinical phases once they are aware that they are dying: (a) the acute crisis phase, (b) the chronic living–dying phase, and (c) the terminal phase. In the acute crisis phase, the patient will use the defense mechanisms described by Kübler-Ross—denial, anger, and bargaining—because of feelings of anxiety and inadequacy. Once patients begin to deal with their anxieties, they enter a chronic living–dying phase where they must deal with their fears. Patients enter the terminal phase when they begin to withdraw into themselves. At this time, patients' type of hope changes: they move from having *expectational hope* to *desirable hope.* Expectational hope is the expectation that a miracle will happen: a cure will be discovered or a remission will occur. Desirable hope is the feeling that it would be good if one could be cured, but a cure is no longer expected. Pattison does not view these phases as stages but as aids to understanding the dying process.

The psychological autopsy, first developed by Shneidman & Farberow (1961) attempts to reconstruct the patient's dying. It provides insights into why the patient died, how the patient died, and the psychological state of the patient before death. Kastenbaum & Weisman (1972), using the technique of the psychological autopsy, found that the terminally ill did not go through stages or phases of dying. Their study of terminally ill patients in a geriatric hospital indicated that people developed two qualitatively different patterns of adjustment to impending death (Kastenbaum & Weisman, 1972, p. 214). These two patterns were the acceptance of death and the view of death as an interruption. The first pattern generally led to withdrawal from social and recreational life in the institution; people responding with the second pattern remained very involved in these activities. The investigators could not conclude that people either do die or should die in one standardized way (p. 178).

Perhaps one general conclusion to draw about research in phases of dying is that dying may evoke a number of emotions such as anger, sadness, depression, and relief and that these emotions do not occur in any specific order. However, people who are dying must cope not only with their own emotions but also with societal responses to death and dying.

Stigma and the Dying Person

A stigma may be attached to the dying person because that person represents what people fear about their own deaths. This person's confrontation with death shatters people's immortal image of themselves and the plans they have made for the future. The dying patient is a deviant in the medical subculture because death poses a threat to the image of the "physician as healer" (Leming & Dickinson, 1985, p. 59) and to the goals of cure in acute care hospital settings. When a person is labeled deviant, that individual is stigmatized. Goffman's (1963) discussion about stigma seems applicable here:

> By definition, of course, we believe the person with a stigma is not quite human. On this assumption we exercise varieties of discrimination, through which we effectively, if not often unthinkingly, reduce his life chances. We construct a stigma ideology to explain his inferiority and account for the danger he represents, sometimes by rationalizing an animosity based on other differences, such as those of social class (p. 5).

Epley & McCaghey (1977–78), in their study on attitudes toward the terminally ill, found the existence of more negative attitudes toward the dying than are generally found expressed toward the ill or healthy. Values and attitudes that result in isolating people who are dying and not speaking openly about dying support the idea of death as a stigma and the feeling that certain diseases are more feared than others. The stigma of death can thus be transferred to a specific disease entity.

Many people believe that the diagnosis of "cancer" is synonymous with death; that the word cancer is so powerful that a patient's knowledge of this diagnosis can actually hasten death. Relatives and friends may request that a patient not be told this diagnosis because "it will kill her," as if the knowledge and not the disease would be the cause of death. Once patients are told of a diagnosis of cancer, they must cope not only with personal fears but also with those of relatives, friends, health care professionals, and society at large. These fears manifest themselves in a variety of ways, and cancer patients may be confronted with isolation from friends ("I don't know what to say"), loss of employment ("How can a dying person work?"), and neglect or indifference by the medical staff ("There's nothing more to do"). The diagnosis may so alter the image of individuals that they become "different."

On the other hand, the cardiac patient faces none of these dilemmas. It would seem foolish not to inform a patient of a cardiac condition. Family and friends do not worry about what to say to cardiac patients about their disease. To the contrary, what led to the heart attack, course of treatment, and anticipated outcomes are frequent topics of conversation in visits with these patients. Employers often encourage their employees "to take it easy" and arrange for less stressful assignments upon their return to work. Yet cardiovascular diseases claimed 982,574 lives in 1988 while cancer claimed 488,240 lives (American Heart Association, 1991, p. 2). Recent figures provided by the American Cancer Society (1991) indicate that four out of ten patients who get cancer in 1991 will be alive five years after diagnosis (p. 1). Statistics therefore would seem to support our being less cancer phobic and more cardiac phobic. Why is this not so?

Sontag (1979) suggests that the labels, notions, and myths around an illness create a metaphor that transforms the illness and gives it a special meaning. She postulates that cancer lends itself to metaphor because it is "intractable and capricious—that it is a disease not understood—in an era in which medicine's central premise is that all diseases can be cured" (p. 5). Richards (1972) provides a similar description:

> Cancer is one of the most intractable, variable, and incomprehensible forms of cellular derangement. A cancer is a crab as its name indicates. It claws at us, it hides in the sands of our flesh; like a crab it ignores straight walking, progresses sideways both in its refusal to behave in an honest, purposeful manner and in its need to invade neighboring tissues (p. 74).

The crab metaphor will no doubt continue until the cause and cure of cancer are found. Fear of the unknown is universal and takes on special meaning for cancer patients. They have the image of "something" unknown growing in their bodies. They search for a meaning and ask "Why me?" Since the disease appears so irrational, it evokes irrational responses. Patients may view the disease as punishment and experience feelings of guilt, shame, and disgust.

Also concerned with the unknown etiology is a fear of contagion. Although many may consider this American society a sophisticated one, people still worry that being around a cancer patient may be dangerous. One man, a successful, prominent lawyer, spoke about his feelings regarding his mother: "I know this sounds foolish, but I found myself not wanting to touch her. I became worried. We really don't know the cause of cancer. My solution was to hire someone to care for her."

A cancer patient also faces a rigorous treatment regime that may temporarily or permanently affect the body image. Surgery often results in physical disfigurement. Patients with colostomies worry about offensive odors and having "accidents." Postmastectomy patients are reassured that a breast prosthesis or implant will be so lifelike that they will escape detection by the outside world. Such reassurances are a double-edged sword, for the implicit message is that one has something to hide.

Sontag (1979) also notes that we assign a hierarchy to our organs. Cancer frequently occurs in parts of the body—for example, colon, bladder, rectum, breast, prostrate gland—that we are embarrassed to acknowledge. Cancer patients may also fear that they are no longer sexually attractive. Unlike cancer patients, cardiac patients know the etiology of their disease. It is usually organ specific and not the result of "cellular derangement." They can experience more control over the progress and treatment of the disease. A malfunctioning heart may be "fixed" by medication, surgery, diet, and modification of life-style. Cardiac patients rarely are worried that they are no longer sexually attractive. Anxiety is related to the idea that sexual activity may precipitate another attack. The type of death associated with each of these diseases is very different. Cancer is associated with prolonged illness, increasing debilitation and dependency, unrelieved pain, and the knowledge that one is dying. Cardiac death suggests a fast, relatively painless death that comes without warning. The stigma attached to dying may relate not only to fear of death, social attitudes and values, and a specific disease but also to the actual process of dying.

Probably no place else do all these factors gather together so clearly as in the stigma attached to AIDS/HIV infection. AIDS, as opposed to cancer and cardiac disease, is a communicable, sexually transmitted disease associated with terminal illness. The greatest impact of this disease so far has been on already socially stigmatized groups, including gay and bisexual men and intravenous (IV) drug users. The indigent and African American and Latino racial minorities are also disproportionally affected (Jakush, 1987, p. 395).

Women are the forgotten group in the AIDS epidemic. "They are regarded by the public and studied by the medical profession as vectors of transmission to their children and male sexual partners rather than as people with AIDS who are themselves frequently victims of transmission from the men in their lives" (Anastos & Marte, 1989, p. 10). Since AIDS has predominantly affected men, it is identified by signs and symptoms characteristic of male responses. The signs and symptoms of the disease in women have not been as clearly delineated. Women with AIDS may find physicians not especially responsive to their illness, and the disease may be in a fairly advanced stage before it is even diagnosed.

People in these groups are thus in the double bind of being stigmatized individuals with a stigmatized life-threatening illness. It has been suggested that the stigma of AIDS has the emotional impact of leprosy; to be designated as being HIV-infected is to evoke ostracism, calls for quarantine or colonization, and terror of contamination by the most remote interpersonal contact (Geis, Fuller, & Rush, 1986).

Past epidemics in the United States, such as polio and Legionnaire's disease, evoked public mobilization to combat them. The nation's initial response to the AIDS threat was slow in comparison. Casper (1986) suggests:

> Much media coverage has in fact adversely affected motivations to help by instilling the question in people's minds: "What if it spreads to the general population?" This kind of phrasing implies that the syndrome becomes really serious only when it travels beyond the current stigmatized group. It is yet another way of clearly demarcating an "us" and a "them" (pp. 204–205).

Fear of AIDS becomes exaggerated not only because of the obvious and possibly realistic fear of contagion but because of the social and cultural values attached to the transmission of the disease. Human sexuality, and, more specifically, homosexuality and bisexuality, are issues about which many people are uncomfortable and uninformed (Forrester, 1990, p. 613). Also, up until the last few years, AIDS has become synonymous with death, evoking fears of death even among health care providers. That association is now not always made; many people with AIDS/HIV have begun to resist death as an inevitable outcome. This has been facilitated by the advent of new treatment and medication regimens that support living with the disease as a chronic illness for longer periods of time. In addition, people with AIDS/HIV may turn to complementary therapies, such as acupuncture, meditation, massage, guided imagery, and spiritual healing.

The more people can identify with persons with AIDS/HIV the less they will fear them. Research shows social interaction decreases fear of contagion, probably because it increases sensitivity to the concerns of those infected and removes the cultural associations of disgrace (O'Donnell & O'Donnell, 1987). It is important then to get to know persons with AIDS/HIV; to become aware of their values, hopes, and changing dreams for their lives in relation to the disease; and to recognize the shared humanity in all of our experiences. In order to do this, the issue of talking with people about their terminal illnesses and their dying must be considered.

Talking with People about Their Dying

Knowing when and how to talk with dying patients and their families about death-related issues continues to be an area of concern for many health care providers. Benoliel (1987–88) points out that the reasons for such concern are multiple and may include: personal feelings of inadequacy, avoidance of potentially distressing situations, peer pressures against open discussion, and prohibitions by physicians and the family against conversation with the patient concerning the diagnosis and prognosis (p. 345). The judgment, however, about what a dying person should be told is very much connected to deeply rooted social, cultural, and psychological patterns.

Physicians and Disclosure

Physicians have traditionally been the professionals to disclose a diagnosis of terminal illness. Studies done in the 1950s and 1960s regarding physician disclosure indicate physicians' reluctance to tell patients about a terminal prognosis (Fitts & Ravdin, 1953; Oken, 1961). In contrast, Klenow & Youngs (1987) note that studies done in the 1970s and 1980s show that a large majority of physicians apparently inform patients of their dying status. Compatible with these findings is the study by Durand, Dickinson, Sumner, & Lancaster (1990) which indicates that physicians under 50 years of age are more likely to tell a dying patient about his or her terminal prognosis than older, more traditional physicians.

Changes in beliefs and values, in the underlying social structure, and in the health care delivery system may be seen as influencing this trend toward disclosure (Veatch & Tai, 1980). For example, the traditional one-to-one relationship between patient and physician, in which the physician was viewed as a benign but authoritarian figure and the patient's role was one of passive recipient, has changed. Physicians are more willing now to recognize the principles of patient autonomy and self-determination. As this society becomes more consumer oriented and as health care is seen more in terms of disease prevention and self-care, people are becoming more protective of their rights to self-determination.

This right to self-determination has become increasingly evident as technology allows us to survive on life-support machines. People are concerned about their right-to-die and the legal recognition of living wills. Current social values of informed consent require disclosure of the prognosis and the effects of nontreatment in order for the patient to make a knowledgeable decision regarding treatment. Such values are reflected legally. Congress has passed legislation requiring all Medicare and Medicaid providers to inform patients, on admission, of their right to refuse treatment. The move was intended to remind people to make their wishes known by drawing up a living will or by granting a durable power of attorney (Nurses Seek a Voice . . . , 1991, p. 26). Many states have enacted do-not-resuscitate laws, which require physicians to discuss with patients on admission to the hospital their wishes for use of resuscitation if they should experience a life-threatening episode. Patients will increasingly expect the physician and other caregivers to act as technical experts and advisers and to invite and include patient participation in treatment plans.

Communication between Caregivers and Patients

These new roles of patients and caregivers are occurring within a major restructuring of the health care delivery system. Patients receive treatment now within a huge health care bureaucracy involving inpatient, outpatient, and home care with numerous people providing care for one person.

Disclosure of prognosis becomes much more critical as the danger of miscommunication among staff and between staff and the patient can easily occur given the numbers of people involved. The patient is at risk for confusion and distress if mixed messages are received from staff. It is therefore important for caregivers to communicate with other members of the health team concerning what has been told patients about their diagnoses. A team assessment of the patient's need to know about the diagnosis of a terminal illness is helpful.

Fletcher (1960) supports patients' rights to know the medical facts concerning themselves, stating that ". . . as persons, our human, moral quality is taken away from us if we are denied whatever knowledge is available; . . . and that to deny a patient knowledge of the facts as to life and death is to assume responsibilities which cannot be carried out by anyone but the patient, with his own knowledge of his own affairs" (pp. 60–61). However, nurses, physicians, and social workers are expected by patients and society to use judgment and discretion in the disclosure of information.

Patients' Needs for Disclosure

Patients will vary in their need to be aware of their dying and in their ability to cope with that knowledge. It is important to assess very carefully the patients' and their families' understanding of the disease, their ways of dealing with stress and crises in the past, their cultural orientation to death and grieving, and their support systems. For example, Morgan (1986) reports that in China aggressive treatment is maintained right to the moment of death, and while the family is informed if the patient's disease is terminal, the patient seemingly is not. Takahashi (1990) suggests that the vast majority of physicians in Japan still avoid informing a patient of a malignant illness. He relates this not only to physicians' own fears but also to the Japanese culture's emphasis on interdependence; to be labeled as having a malignant illness means not only that the person is dying but also that the important relationship of interdependence is destroyed (Takahashi, 1990, p. 88).

There seems to be no set rules about what and how much patients should be told about their diagnoses of terminal illness. In practice, listening to patients talk about their illness and their knowledge of the outcome will reveal a great deal. If patients say they feel upset, they can be encouraged to talk about that feeling, or if statements are offered such as "well, I don't think I'll need this medicine much longer," they need to be encouraged to clarify that. Hinton (1980) proposes that if caregivers provide careful listening and attentive responses, there is little for them to actually "tell."

In keeping with this approach of careful listening, Shneidman (1983) points out that *how* people know is the core issue: "though they are capable of knowing the fact that they are dying, they will modulate it in a number of ways, consciously and unconsciously, with wide variations in insight, repression, denial, understanding, terror, and equanimity" (p. 30). Thus, it becomes important for caregivers to provide people with information at the pace at which they desire it. People who are dying do not allow themselves to hear more than they are ready to accept at that moment. People deserve thorough assessments of their needs and of their abilities to cope with the knowledge of dying.

Coping with Death and Dying

How persons cope with their dying will be very individual. Coping strategies utilized with a life-threatening illness or death threat may vary from those strategies used to deal with nonlife-threatening situations such as loss of a job, or competition. According to Feifel (1990), "differences noted in these situations suggest not so much the employment of new coping strategies as modifications in the patterning or configuration of an individual's more usual coping modes" (p. 539). While keeping in mind that coping strategies used in dying can be both individual and situational, it is also possible to use research findings that provide a base from which assistance in coping may be provided to the dying person.

A Coping Framework

Arblaster, Brooks, Hudson, & Petty (1990) conducted a study on terminally ill patients' expectations of nurses. Five factors resulting from the study findings are used to provide a framework for understanding what assistance individuals need to cope with dying. The factors of normalcy, empowerment, and autonomy focus on individual needs. The factors of support and partnership focus primarily on family needs. Concepts similar to these five factors have been discussed in the literature on coping with dying (Weisman, 1980; Moller,1986; Feifel, 1990).

Normalcy. For many people, coping with dying may involve an emphasis on "keeping things normal." Support and care are needed to maintain the status quo as much as possible within the individual's life and within the family unit. One person stated:

> I feel like people are seeing me differently—I have another dimension now. I don't feel differently towards them. They feel like I'm having a mystical experience. With my family, I plan on normalcy—on the living—not the dying.

Of course, dying persons want freedom from pain and odors, but they also express the desire to be able to see, to be able to talk, to be able to think clearly, to be able to love, and to be loved in return (Martocchio, 1986, p. 17). Dying persons also have agendas—plans for the future.

Empowerment. Important here are the concepts of sharing and equality among dying persons and caregivers in decision making and of people wanting to have control over their lives. The dying person is not perceived as subordinate by caregivers, but as a person able to choose a course of action that feels comfortable. Identification of each person's agenda in regard to dying is vital. The person must be supported in asking her or himself, "What would I still like to do?" Empowerment enhances the person's decision-making abilities.

Autonomy. It is important that people are involved in their own care to the extent that they desire. Many dying people may be physically unable to participate in their care, but they are able to participate in decision making. For example, a person may choose to deal with pain quite differently at its inception than several months later. Weisman (1980) states that "It is reasonable to assume that . . . the dying want to be as autonomous as possible for as long as possible and then to be cared for in ways that do not corrupt or degrade their individuality" (p. 64). When people are recognized and appreciated for their integrity and their input in decision making about their treatment process, there is reduced depression and diminished feelings of guilt and inadequacy, not only in themselves but also in their caregivers and family (Feifel, 1990).

Support. People may request help in coping with their illness. Sources of support often come from family and friends. Caregivers need to recognize that often many issues are best dealt with by the dying person and the family. It is the role of the caregiver not to intrude in these issues unless invited. An example of this was a frail elderly woman, caring for her dying husband at home, who politely but adamantly refused the home health aide who was sent by the hospital to provide respite care for her. The woman later explained that she felt her capabilities and the control of her own home were being challenged.

Partnership. The idea of partnership is a culmination of the other factors already discussed. Partnership conveys that there be a sensitive approach to the sharing of care between health professionals, the dying persons, and the families. It connotes "working with" rather than "doing to" (Arblaster, Brooks, Hudson, & Petty, 1990). Open and honest communication is an important component of this factor. Partnership, as with all four factors in this coping framework, must be assessed in terms of the individual and family situation, including patient autonomy, family involvement, issues of family dynamics, and coping mechanisms. Focus of care may vary; some families may not be able to be involved, and some dying people may not want their families involved. Coping behaviors of terminally ill people may differ markedly depending on their individual circumstances.

This is only one framework for helping people cope with dying. It is based on responsiveness to the individual's needs and to the uniqueness of each person's life and death. Careful ongoing assessment of the person's experience, always asking what is appropriate for this person at this time, can facilitate coping with dying.

SUMMARY ❧

Perceptions of death vary among individuals and cultures. Affecting these perceptions are religious beliefs, psychosocial influences, and developmental stages through the life cycle. Death, which symbolizes the unknown, loss of control over living, and mortality, may consciously and unconsciously be associated with fear and anxiety. Some diseases, such as cancer and HIV/AIDS, are associated with dying and are also feared because of the stigma attached to them.

Dying today usually occurs within some type of health care institution. Just when a person who is terminally ill enters the dying process is difficult to say, but once in an institution, a person's dying trajectory is established. The dying process may also include a series of phases which the person experiences. E. Kübler-Ross and E. Mansell Pattison are researchers who have formulated theories about these phases that should be considered descriptive of the dying process rather than normative.

Recognition of people's individual ways of experiencing life and death is an important beginning in assisting them in coping with their dying. People may be able to experience comfortable dying and dying with dignity if they can be supported in identifying their agendas for their remaining life and helped to implement them. Such support may provide dying people with the opportunity to bring closure to their lives.

LEARNING EXERCISES ❧

1. Discuss with your family and friends the idea of making a will and having life insurance. What does the discussion indicate about their thoughts and feelings about dying and death?
2. Visit a cemetery. By reading the epitaphs, can you make any inferences about people's ideas and feelings about death?
3. Read *The Death of Ivan Ilych* by Leo Tolstoy. Describe Ivan Ilych's process of dying. Did he accept death at the end?
4. Do you agree with Dr. Elisabeth Kübler-Ross's stages of dying? Why or why not?

AUDIOVISUAL MATERIAL ❧

To Live Until You Die. 57 minutes/videocassette/1983. Ambrose Video Publishing, Inc. 1290 Avenue of the Americas, New York, NY, 10104 This video portrays Dr. Elisabeth Kübler-Ross in her work with dying patients.

Coping with Death. 30 minutes/videocassette. PBS Video, 1320 Braddock Place, Alexandria, VA, 22314–1698.
Six high school students share their personal stories about the death of a loved one, and how they have learned to cope with their loss.

Death, Dying, and Recreation. 15 minutes/videocassette/1981. National Audiovisual Center, 8700 Edgeworth Drive, Capitol Heights, MD, 20743–3071.
This video discusses some of the needs of dying people, for example, alleviation of pain, maintenance of independence, and assurances of one's past existence. It also depicts the positive and negative aspects of stress associated with dying.

From Tragedy to Grace: Stages in the Process of Dying and The Experience of Dying: A Guided Meditation. 2 pts. 52 minutes/videocassette/1984. Original Face Video, 6116 Merced Avenue, No. 165, Oakland, CA, 94611.
The stages of dying are presented, as well as the mind states that come and go as death approaches. Personal experiences are shared by participants.

Why Me? 10 minutes/videocassette/1979. Pyramid Film and Video, P.O. Box 1048, Santa Monica, CA, 90406.
This unique, animated dialogue explores with insight, humor, and understanding the full range of human responses to imminent death.

REFERENCES ❧

American Cancer Society. (1991). *Cancer Facts and Figures–1991.*

American Heart Association. (1991). *1991 Heart and Stroke Facts.*

Anastos, K., & Marte, C. (1989). Women—the missing persons in the AIDS epidemic. *Health/Pac Bulletin. Winter,* 6–13.

Arblaster, G., Brooks, D., Hudson, R., & Petty, M. (1990). Terminally ill patients' expectations of nurses. *Australian Journal of Advanced Nursing.* 7 (3), 34–43.

Axelrod, C. (1986–87). Reflections on the fear of death. *Omega: Journal of Death and Dying. 17* (1), 51–64.

Becker, E. (1973). *The denial of death.* New York: The Free Press.

Benoliel, J. Q. (1987–88). Health care providers and dying patients: Critical issues in terminal care. *Omega: Journal of Death and Dying. 18* (4), 341–363.

Bristow, T. A. (1986). Death concern and Roman Catholic worship attendance. *Journal of Psychology and Christianity. 5* (1), 46–49.

Brody, A. (1985). Death is forever: Living is now. *The Psychotherapy Patient. 2* (1), 135–138.

Casper, V. (1986). AIDS: A psychosocial perspective. In D. A. Feldman & T. M. Johnson (Eds.), *The social dimensions of AIDS: Method and theory* (pp. 197–209). New York: Praeger.

Charmaz, K. (1980). *The social reality of death.* Reading, MA: Addison-Wesley.

Cousins, N. (1979). *Anatomy of an illness as perceived by the patient: Reflections on healing.* New York: Norton.

Dane, B. O. (1989). Middle-aged adults mourning the death of a parent. *Journal of Gerontological Social Work. 14* (3–4, 75–85.

Dumont, R. G., & Foss, D. C. (1972). *The American view of death: Acceptance or denial?* Cambridge, MA: Schenkman.

Durand, R. P., Dickinson, G. E., Sumner, E. D., & Lancaster, C. J. (1990). Family physicians' attitudes toward death and the terminally ill patient. *Family Practice Research Journal. 9* (2), 123–129.

Epley, R. J., & McCaghey, C. H. (1977–78). The stigma of dying: Attitudes toward the terminally ill. *Omega: Journal of Death and Dying. 8* (4), 379–393.

Erikson, E. (1963). *Childhood and society.* New York: Norton.

Feifel, H. (1990). Psychology and death: Meaningful recovery. *American Psychologist. 45* (4), 537–543.

Fitts, W. T., Jr., & Ravdin, I. S. (1953). What Philadelphia physicians tell patients with cancer. *Journal of The American Medical Association. 153,* 901–904.

Fletcher, J. (1960). *Morals and medicine.* Boston: Beacon Press.

Forrester, D. A. (1990). AIDS in the 1990's: An ethical challenge. In J. McCloskey & H. Grace (Eds.), *Current issues in nursing* (pp. 612–617, 3rd edition). St. Louis: Mosby.

Freud, S. (1961). Thoughts for the times on war and death. In J. Strachey (Ed. & Trans.), *The standard edition of the complete psychological works of Sigmund Freud* (Vol. 14, 2nd ed., pp. 273–302). London: Hogarth Press and The Institute of Psychoanalysis.

Garfield, C. (1978). *Psychosocial care of the dying patient.* New York: McGraw-Hill.

Geis, S. B., Fuller, R. L., & Rush, J. (1986). Lovers of AIDS victims: Psychosocial stresses and counseling needs. *Death Studies. 10* (1), 43–53.

Gijana, E. W. M., Louw, J., & Manganyi, N. C. (1989–90). Thoughts about death and dying in an African sample. *Omega: The Journal of Death and Dying. 20* (3), 245–258.

Given, J. R., & Range, L. M. (1990). Life satisfaction and death anxiety in elderly nursing home and public housing residents. *Journal of Applied Gerontology. 9* (2), 224–229.

Glaser, B., & Strauss, A. (1968). *Time for dying.* Chicago: Aldine.

Goffman, E. (1963). *Stigma.* Englewood Cliffs, NJ: Prentice-Hall.

Gray, R. E. (1988). Meaning of death: Implications for bereavement theory. *Death Studies. 12* (4), 309–317.

Henderson, M. (1990). Beyond the living will. *Gerontologist. 30* (4), 480–485.

Heuscher, J. E. (1986). Death and authenticity. *American Journal of Psychoanalysis. 46* (4), 310–317.

Hinton, J. (1980). Speaking of death with the dying. In E. S. Shneidman (Ed.), *Death: Current perspectives* (2nd ed., pp. 187–196). Palo Alto, CA: Mayfield.

Holing, E. V. (1986). The primary caregiver's perception of the dying trajectory. *Cancer Nursing. 9* (1), 29–37.

Jakush, J. (1987). AIDS: The disease and its implications for dentistry. *Journal of The American Dental Association. 115*, 395.

Jung, C. (1969). The soul and death. In H. Read, M. Fordham, G. Adler, & W. McGuire (Eds.), & R. F. C. Hull (Trans.), *Collected works: The structure and dynamics of the psyche* (Vol. 8, 2nd Ed., pp. 404–415). Ballingen Series 20. Princeton, NJ: Princeton University Press.

Kalish, R. A., & Reynolds, D. K. (1981). *Death and ethnicity: A psychocultural study.* Farmingdale, NY: Baywood.

Kastenbaum, R. (1986). *Death, society, and human experience.* (3rd ed.) Columbus, OH: C. E. Merrill.

Kastenbaum, R., & Aisenberg, R. (1972). *The psychology of death.* New York: Springer.

Kastenbaum, R., & Weisman, A. (1972). The psychological autopsy as a research procedure in gerontology. In D. Kent, R. Kastenbaum, & S. Sherwood (Eds.), *Research, planning and action for the elderly* (pp. 210–217). New York: Behavioral Publications.

Klenow, D. J., & Youngs, G. A., Jr. (1987). Changes in doctor/patient communication of a terminal prognosis: A selective review and critique. *Death Studies. 11* (4), 263–277.

Koenig, H. G. (1988). Religious behaviors and death anxiety in later life. *Hospice Journal: Physical, Psychosocial, and Pastoral Care of the Dying. 4* (1), 3–24.

Kübler-Ross, E. (1969). *On death and dying*. New York: Macmillan.

Leming, M. R., & Dickinson, G. E. (1985). *Understanding dying, death, and bereavement*. New York: Holt, Rinehart, and Winston.

Leshan, E. (1973). *The wonderful crisis of middle age*. New York: D. McKay.

Mantocchio, B. C. (1986). Agendas for quality of life. *Hospice Journal: Physical, Psychosocial, and Pastoral Care of the Dying. 2* (1), 11–21.

Marks, A. (1986–87). Race and sex differences and fear of dying: A test of two hypothesis: High risk or social loss? *Omega: Journal of Death and Dying. 17* (3), 229–236.

Moller, D. W. (1986–87). On the value of suffering in the shadow of death. *Loss, Grief, and Care. 1*, Fall, 127–136.

Morgan, J. D. (1986). Death, dying and bereavement in China and Japan: A brief glimpse. *Death Studies. 10* (3), 265–272.

Mufson, T. (1985). Issues surrounding sibling death during adolescence. *Child and Adolescent Social Work Journal. 2* (4), 204–218.

Nurses Seek A Voice in Right-To-Die Cases. (1991). *American Journal of Nursing. 91* (3), 26.

O'Donnell, L., & O'Donnell, C. R. (1987). Hospital workers and AIDS: Effect of in-service education on knowledge and perceived risks and stresses. *New York State Journal of Medicine. 87*, 278–280.

Oken, D. (1961). What to tell cancer patients. *Journal of the American Medical Association. 175* (April), 1120–28.

Pattison, E. M. (1977). The experience of dying. In E. M. Pattison (Ed.), *The experience of dying* (pp. 43–60). Englewood Cliffs, NJ: Prentice-Hall.

Retsinas, J. (1988). A theoretical reassessment of the applicability of Kübler-Ross's stages of dying. *Death Studies. 12* (3), 207–216.

Richards, V. (1972). *Cancer: The wayward cell*. Berkeley, CA: University of California Press.

Shneidman, E., & Farberow, N. (1961). *The cry for help*. New York: McGraw-Hill.

Shneidman, E. (1983). *Deaths of man*. New York: Jason Aronson, Inc.

Sontag, S. (1979). *Illness as a metaphor*. New York: Vintage Books.

Strauss, A., Fagerhaugh, S., Suczek, B., & Weiner, C. (1985). *Social organization of medical work*. Chicago: University of Chicago Press.

Sullivan, H. S. (1953). *The interpersonal theory of psychiatry*. New York: Norton.

Takahashi, Y. (1990). Informing a patient of malignant illness: Commentary from a cross-cultural perspective. *Death Studies. 14* (1), 83–91.

Tausch, R. (1988). Reappraisal of death and dying after person-centered behavior workshop. *Person-centered Review. 3* (2), 213–228.

Thorson, J. A., & Powell, F. C. (1989). Death anxiety and religion in an older male sample. *Psychological Reports. 64* (3), 985–986.

Thorson, J. A., & Powell, F. C. (1990). Meanings of death and intrinsic religiosity. *Journal of Clinical Psychology. 46* (4), 379–391.

Tolstoy, L. (1960). *The death of Ivan Ilych and other stories.* New York: New American Library.

Veatch, R. M., & Tai, E. (1980). Talking about death: Patterns of lay and professional change. *Annals of the American Academy of Political and Social Science. 447*, 29–43.

Viney, L. (1984–85). Loss of life and loss of bodily integrity: Two different sources of threat for people who are ill. *Omega: Journal of Death and Dying. 15* (3), 207–222.

Wagner, K. D., & Lorion, R. P. (1984). Correlates of death anxieties in elderly persons. *Journal of Clinical Psychology. 40* (5), 1235–1241.

Wasow, M. (1984). Get out of my potato patch: A biased view of death and dying. *Social Work. 9* (4), 261–267.

Weisman, A. D. (1980). What do elderly, dying patients want, anyway? *Journal of Geriatric Psychiatry. 13* (1), 63–67.

Westman, A. S., & Canter, F. M. (1985). Fear of death and the concept of extended self. *Psychological Reports. 56* (2), 419–425.

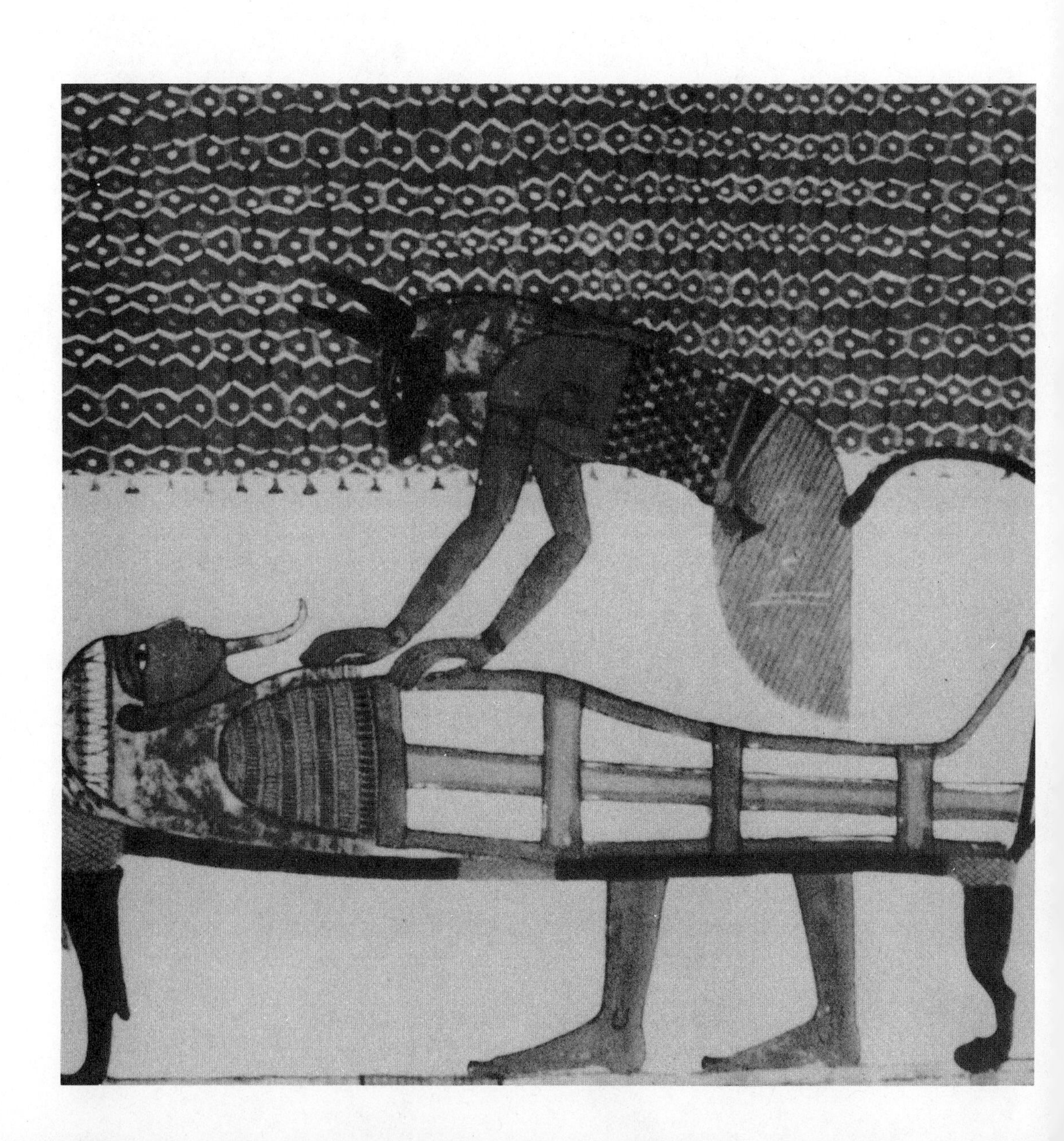

Chapter 3

The Helping Professions and the Terminally Ill

The challenges involved in caring for people who are terminally ill can be immense, but the rewards are fulfilling and worthwhile. The experience, if the caregiver is open to it, can evoke a spectrum of human emotions:

> . . . confusion, grief, helplessness, fear, anger, draining, loneliness, inadequacy, ambivalence, nameless feelings, intimacy, love, pity, needing appreciation, guilt, increased commitment, entrapment, needing release, superiority, lacking knowledge, intrusiveness, threatening, disintegration, wanting the person to live, wanting the person to die, protectiveness, abandonment, avoidance, alienation, lacking authenticity, intolerance, distance, and vulnerability (Barton, 1977, p. 72).

Caring for dying people can promote learning for caregivers that goes beyond simple intellectual development; it can offer them new perspectives that may allow for exploration of their own lives and what it means to be human.

The challenges involved in caring for people who are terminally ill may also result in burn-out, or exhaustion, and may even cause caregivers to change careers. The work will never be easy. In some ways, a part of the caregiver dies with each dying patient. The struggle to find a balance and harmony in the continuation of one's own personal and professional life while being involved with another person's exiting life can be difficult. The struggle can be compounded by its taking place within institutions, the medical system, and a society where the value of caring is given scant recognition and the process of dying is preferably kept out of sight.

Photo courtesy of Gary C. Croland, Photographer

How do caregivers respond to these challenges, and how do these responses bring results as varied as rewards and exhaustion? This chapter explores nurses' and physicians' responses to terminally ill patients and how these caregivers are educationally prepared to provide terminal care. The importance of communication between the two groups of caregivers is discussed as a major contributing factor in provision of quality nursing, medical, and interdisciplinary care for terminally ill patients.

Nurses

Nurses are the professional caregivers who are in continuous contact with dying patients in institutions and at home and who provide them with the most direct care. Nurses face their own fears, anxieties, and concerns about death each time they are involved in providing the technological, emotional, and psychosocial skills required in the holistic care that facilitates a patient's dying in dignity and peace. This first section of the chapter discusses how nurses learn to provide this care; their interactions with dying patients and families; and the effects of experience, nursing specialty, and institutional practices on their nursing care.

Nursing Education in Death and Dying

The landmark works of Quint (1967) and Kübler-Ross (1969) encouraged nurse educators to begin to recognize the importance of specifically including death education in the nursing curriculum. A further review of the nursing literature through the 1960s, 1970s, and 1980s indicates that although nursing educators have begun the teaching of death content, curricula in this area are still being developed and advanced.

The study of a random stratified sample of nursing schools by Thrush, Paulus, & Thrush (1979) revealed that only 5.4 percent of the 205 responding schools included a formal course of death and dying in their curricula. Additionally, 11.7 percent offered elective courses on the subject, yet relatively few students enrolled in them. Ninety-two percent of the institutions surveyed indicated they integrated concepts and issues concerning death and dying into a number of courses in their curriculum, most in modular form. The amount of time devoted to the subject, when handled in modular form, was reported to range from two to three hours to three weeks (p. 136).

In a 1984–85 study, Dickinson, Sumner, & Durand (1987) received responses to a curriculum death content questionnaire from 332 schools of nursing. Fifteen percent offered complete courses in death education, while 80 percent reported integrating their death and dying offerings into other courses.

The above two survey studies indicate that almost 20 years after Quint's (1967) proposal that nursing education include systematic death education with planned clinical assignments for students, there are still proportionately few such required courses in the curriculum. Degner & Gow (1988a) note that three current approaches to death education are presented in the literature: (a) integrating material throughout the curriculum, (b) offering an elective course, and (c) requiring a course. Most schools of nursing use an integrated approach without systematic assignment of students to dying patients. The educational value of such an approach can be questioned if students have no opportunity to use their learning in clinical practice. There have been, however, research studies indicating that specific death education courses reduce nursing students' death anxieties and improve their attitudes in providing care to patients who are terminally ill (Lev, 1986; Degner & Gow, 1988b; Lockard, 1989).

A study done by Hare & Pratt (1989) raises many questions regarding the effects of experience and education on nurses' responses to dying patients. It is a significant study because the sampling includes paraprofessional nurses (CNAs, or certified nursing assistants) as well as professional registered nurses. The study examined differences in nurses' fear of death and level of comfort with patients having a poor prognosis for survival as a function of the nurses' occupational level, work setting, and level of exposure to such patients. Nurses with high and moderate exposure to patients having a poor prognosis for survival were found to be significantly more comfortable with such patients than were nurses with low exposure.

Compared to professional nurses, CNAs were significantly less comfortable with patients having a poor prognosis for survival. Because 94 percent of the CNAs in this sample worked in nursing homes, this difference in level of comfort may be particularly important because the number of patients dying in these facilities is greater than in hospitals (Hare & Pratt, 1989). CNAs provide most of the nursing care for patients in nursing homes and are increasingly providing the basic nursing care for patients at home. The significance of research that evaluates the effects of death education for this group of nurses becomes apparent, and further studies are urgently needed.

Jinadu & Adediran (1982) pointed out that many studies on the effects of death education in the nursing curriculum have been conducted in developed countries under socioeconomic and cultural environments different from developing countries. In view of the fact that there is a paucity of similar studies in developing countries, these researchers conducted a study to research the effects of nursing education on attitudes of nursing students toward dying patients in the Nigerian sociocultural environment. The null hypothesis formulated to guide the study was: there will be no significant difference between the attitudes of Preliminary Nursing Students (PNS) and Final Year Nursing Students (FYNS) toward the dying patients, as measured by the Attitude Towards Dying Patients Questionnaire (p. 22). The study findings supported the null hypothesis. The authors offer several reasons for this. One reason might be that the curriculum included no more than two hours on the physical care of the dead with emphasis on the "task" aspect of that care. Another reason offered was that, in Nigeria, dying and death is still a family affair, and the majority of people still die in their homes. All the students in the study had experience with dying people before entering nursing; the majority with blood relatives. This suggests that experience and culture, as well as education, can affect caregivers' responses and attitudes toward death and dying.

These studies indicate support of specific and required death education in the nursing curriculum, although the question may be raised as to the effects a change in death attitudes or death anxiety in nursing students will actually have on delivery of their care to terminally ill patients. Waltman (1990) found in her research that death anxiety in nurses was not predictive of their behavioral intentions toward the dying.

Degner and Gow (1988a) suggest that three central nursing research issues—focusing on how much death education is needed, use of longitudinal experimental designs with sufficient sampling to detect significant effects, and measurement of care results—need to be addressed if the profession is to determine the most appropriate method to prepare nurses to care for dying people. An additional suggestion is that research and education may not necessarily need to look at how to change students' attitudes about death but, perhaps more realistically, to look at how to prepare students to meet the death of a significant other in a more positive manner (Hopper, 1977, p. 447).

Further research on the inclusion of death education in the nursing curriculum is certainly indicated at a time when nurse educators are confronted with cramming more and more material into already tightly packed curricula. Faculty must have a belief system that values care of terminally ill patients. They need to feel comfortable in caring for dying patients and be able to support and sustain students' experiences in this care area. With the pressures of current faculty assignments, which can include teaching, practice, and research, this is often a difficult responsibility to assume. Faculty themselves may need support and guidance in teaching students. Mentoring, peer supervision, and faculty development programs are approaches that can be used to facilitate faculty learning and practice.

As one possible first step in the development of nursing students' self-awareness related to death and dying, Lambrecht (1990) suggests the use of interactive, computer-assisted instruction. Such programs on death education provide for immediate feedback for some of the student's concerns and fears. The development of this self-awareness forms a significant basis of nurses' interactions with terminally ill patients.

Nurse/Patient Interaction

All nurses are familiar with assessment, the first step of the nursing process used to collaborate with patients in initiating, planning, and evaluating their nursing care. In caring for dying patients, nurses need to assess their own feelings and responses about death as well as those of their patients. Without this self-awareness, nurses are in danger of imposing their own beliefs and judgments about death upon patients, a function of paternalism rather than of advocacy. This becomes especially important when faced with moral dilemmas in the care of dying people such as the continuation of life-support systems. Gadow (1980) suggests that understanding death at the philosophical, the clinical, and the personal levels is vital to making ethical decisions. (See Chapter 8 for further discussion of ethical issues.)

Values clarification may be needed as part of developing self-awareness in terms of identifying responses to dying patients whose life-styles are different from those of caregivers. Nurses care for patients who are dying from AIDS, from drug overdoses, from chronic and acute illnesses, from accidents, and from gunshot and stab wounds. Obtaining some clarity about one's personal values and feelings toward patients is necessary to begin to understand what professional responses are required for providing care.

Bartnof (1988) recommends that health care professionals be involved in continuing education that involves recognition of the phobias surrounding AIDS, including the phobia of death and dying. Preliminary findings from the first comprehensive national survey of the knowledge, attitudes, and practices of physicians and nurses concerning AIDS indicate that given the choice, a larger percentage of physicians and nurses would rather provide care to homosexual men than to intravenous drug users (*Research Activities*, 1991, p. 2). The physicians and nurses also reported that since the appearance of AIDS they had become more negative in their feelings about intravenous drug users. If caregivers can recognize and discuss these feelings, it becomes possible to see how they may affect patient care and to plan how care may be optimally provided. This study also indicated that despite the commonly held belief that AIDS is discouraging young people from entering the health professions, few of the physicians and nurses surveyed said they were leaving patient care because of AIDS. Nurses ranked AIDS far behind job stress, salary, lack of autonomy, and lack of career mobility as a reason for leaving patient care (p. 2).

Self-awareness becomes important as nurses face conflicts of both personal and professional identity in caring for dying patients. Personal death anxieties may surface. Defending against these anxieties may take the energy and focus away from the dying patient's needs. A discussion of death with a patient can evoke fear, sadness, and anger about one's own mortality and powerlessness. These are uncomfortable feelings in a society and a profession where keeping one's emotions in control is emphasized. Given the highly technological and scientific emphasis of this society, death can represent both existential and personal failure (Holman, 1990, p. 17). Feelings of professional failure may occur since nurses are educated to anticipate any untoward events that may place patients at risk and to plan appropriate interventions for prevention.

People who are dying may increasingly become dependent upon nurses for assistance in activities of daily living such as personal hygiene, nutrition and elimination, exercise, and socialization. How nurses provide this assistance is critically important for the patient, not only for basic physiologic survival but also because nursing care can convey basic respect or disrespect for the patient as a human being.

Conveyance of respect begins as nurses collaborate with patients in planning nursing care. Even if patients are totally dependent on staff for this care, they may still take part in decision making in such matters as when they will have a bath, dressings changed, pain medication, or whether or not they want visitors that day. One nurse asks her patients each morning, "What are your plans for today?" She then works with each patient to decide how to schedule activities, rest, treatments, and visitors throughout the day.

The actual touching involved in providing physical care may also be critical. Krieger (1979) has developed the concept of "therapeutic touch" that emphasizes the nurse's laying hands on or close to the body of an ill person for the purpose of helping or healing. A nurse researcher is currently investigating the actual physiological changes occurring in premature infants in response to their being touched by nurses who are giving them care (M. Wetzel, personal communication, September 4, 1991). Patients often need this direct expression of human contact. A child in pain in a hospital once said to a nurse, "Touch me where it hurts." Adults in American culture may find it difficult to ask to be held or touched. It is far easier and acceptable to ask for medication, perhaps not only for pain but also for recognition of one's self and one's existence. Dying people, besides often experiencing pain, may feel unclean or repulsive, believing that there is an unpleasant odor about them that will keep people away. People with AIDS may feel that others do not want to touch them because of fear of contagion. Therefore, how nurses touch patients when providing nursing care can convey acceptance, respect, and caring.

Caring for patients who are dying and who are dependent on others is a challenging part of nursing. The day-to-day physical care and emotional and psychological support required continually taps into nurses' personal resources and energy levels. Nurses do not have the same mobility on hospital units as physicians and social workers do; they cannot come and go throughout the day, evening, or night. Nurses remain on the unit with the patients. Although this can be problematic at times in terms of nurses' need to obtain some distance from the situation even for a short time, it also provides them with a unique experience—being present when patients need someone and sharing that moment with them. One patient, dying in a hospital, asked a night nurse when she made her hourly check on patients to stop and hold his hand for a few minutes even if he were asleep. He simply said, "I don't want to be alone."

Nurses coordinate the care and decisions made by the various people involved in caring for the dying person. They serve as the patient's advocate if necessary in supporting the individual's right to make decisions about how he or she wishes to live and die. Nurses' provision of comfort to dying patients involves not only physical and psychological care but also collaboration with the patients in deciding upon their plan of care; facilitating their decisions about day-to-day living; encouraging open communication between them and those close to them; and sustaining them in the maintenance of their dignity, self-worth, and self-respect throughout their dying (Benoliel, 1977, p. 135).

In a study of nurses' accounts of nursing the terminally ill on a coronary care unit, Field (1989) found that nurses did not report any severe coping difficulties associated with their care of dying patients. Their most severe difficulties were those related to telling relatives about a patient's death. Unit organizational structure that facilitates positive coping responses includes high staff–patient ratio, low staff turnover, good, supportive relationships among staff, and the policy of open and honest communication about prognosis (Field, 1989, p. 114). Studies by Thompson (1985–86) and Power & Sharp (1988) also indicate that organizational structure and goals, as well as nursing specialty, can influence nurses' responses to dying patients.

As discussed earlier in this chapter, nurses may experience feelings of powerlessness and of personal and professional failure when caring for dying patients. They may use a variety of coping strategies to deal with these conflicts and anxieties. Benoliel (1987–88), in her review of the research literature on health care providers and dying patients, notes that there is some evidence that avoidance is a preferred coping strategy among nurses relating to dying patients. Behaviors that nurses may use to avoid interacting with patients include evading conversation, briskness and efficiency in providing physical care, speaking only when spoken to by the patient, and talking about topics that are comfortable for the nurse. One nurse checked out her avoidance techniques in relation to dying patients and found herself saying "I'm too busy," "Someone else can profit more from my care," "He needs the rest," or "She prefers to be alone" (Speer, 1974, p. 70). On realization of this avoidance, she discovered that she could indeed schedule 20 to 30 minutes of each working day to be with a dying patient.

Homer (1984) studied the organizational defenses and defensive strategies that were employed by staff members of a hospital for the chronically ill. Strategies that were used by staff members working with terminally ill patients included denial, splitting, idealization, and psychiatric labeling (pp. 148–152). Use of avoidance as a coping strategy by nurses was seen in two defenses: (a) staff might be assigned different patients each day, and (b) routine everyday work had to be done before nurses could spend time talking with patients.

However, given the nursing care needs of acutely ill patients, nursing staff must frequently triage their patients. A priority assessment must be made as to which patients require professional nursing care. Nursing staff, often coping with a shortage of registered professional nurses, may delegate care of terminally ill patients to nurses' aides or "float" nurses (assigned to that unit for just one day) because of the acute care needs of other patients.

Decisions in triaging are difficult to make and, once again, self-awareness becomes an important factor in what is decided. If a patient has a "Do Not Resuscitate" order, do nurses assign that patient to someone else for care based on priorities of need of all the patients on the unit? Or is avoidance occurring here, rationalized by thinking that the patient is going to die anyway regardless of who provides the care? Peace & Vincent (1988) question if the acuity levels of the conditions of the other patients affect the frequencies with which nurses interact with dying patients, and if so, should dying patients be admitted to hospital units that include acutely ill patients? (p. 344)

These are a few of the many questions that indicate need for further research on interactions between nurses and dying patients. Individual characteristics of nurses such as age, nursing experience, personal experiences with dying people, and death anxiety may contribute to degree and quality of patient interaction, as may organizational structures of specialty units, goals, numbers of nursing staff, and interdisciplinary staff relationships. The interaction of these factors also influence nurses' responses and their behavior with dying patients' families.

Nurse/Family Interaction

The concept of the patient and family as the unit of care is a significant one in working with dying patients (Parry & Smith, 1985). Based on systems theory, the concept of the family as a unit is used to facilitate understanding about how the health or illness of one member can influence the well-being of other members and affect the total functioning of the family group. Spouses of patients who are critically ill may experience intense feelings of impending loss. Hospitalization of the patient may enhance these feelings of loss as the spouse experiences interruption to all daily routines, including sleep and meal patterns; forced autonomy; a drastic reversal of roles; possible loss of financial support; and interruption of an interpersonal reward system (Youll, 1989). If the patient has been chronically ill, the family's physical and emotional resources may be already depleted, with little reserve left over for family members to cope with impending death. Nurses using the conceptual framework of the patient and family as the unit of care focus on collaborating with all family members, including the patient, in assessing and planning what care is needed by that unit. Families of dying patients have identified nursing care that they have perceived as supportive or helpful to them as well as to the patient.

The 121 family caregivers in a home-based hospice program who responded to a survey questionnaire reported their caregiving needs as: (a) communication with professionals, (b) assistance with patient care, (c) legal matters, (d) religious concerns, and (e) household tasks (Garland, Bass, & Otto, 1984). Nugent (1988) found that the social support requirements of family caregivers of terminal cancer patients also included provision of information about patients' conditions or care from health care providers.

Freihofer and Felton (1976) conducted a study to identify those nursing behaviors that provided the most support and comfort to loved ones of a fatally ill, hospitalized adult patient (p. 333). Spouses, relatives, or close friends of a dying patient ranked nursing behaviors that progressed on a continuum from caring for the physical needs of patients, to caring for their emotional needs, to caring for the physical and emotional needs of the bereaved. The data analysis of the total group sample indicated the four most desired behaviors (in order of ranking) as: (a) keep the patients well-groomed, (b) allow the patients to do as much for themselves as possible, (c) give the pain medication as often as possible (as indicated by physician's orders), and (d) keep the patients physically comfortable. The four least desired behaviors (in order of ranking) were (a) encourage me to cry, (b) hold my hand, (c) cry with me, and (d) remind me that the patient's suffering will be over soon. The convenience sample of 25 interviews limits the findings of this study.

Studies by Welch (1981) of family members of hospitalized adult cancer patients and by Skorupka & Bohnet (1982) of family caregivers in home hospice care also investigated family members' perceptions of helpful nursing behaviors. These studies similarly suggest that grieving family members may need nursing behaviors to be directed toward the comfort, support, and easing of suffering of the dying patient rather than toward themselves. Kristjanson's (1989) study of families' identification of salient indicators of quality terminal care indicated that relief of the patient's pain was most important to family members. The most important family care need identified in this study was the need for information: families wanted honest answers to their questions and specific information that might help them in caring for the patient. These research studies suggest that health caregivers consider the needs of families to be involved in the decision making, planning, and implementing of care for their loved ones who are dying. Consideration is also given to family needs for support.

Martinson, Adams, Deck, Folta, & Bates (1988) identify one of the myths about dying and bereavement as that of the extended family always meeting the emotional needs and providing the necessary support for the dying and their survivors. Other people can be helpful when family is not available or cannot offer this care and support. The International Work Group in

Death, Dying, and Bereavement recommends that family members have the opportunity to talk about dying, death, and related emotional needs with staff (Qvanstrom, 1988). Research on the needs of family members suggests that families prioritize the care given to the ill patient as primary but also identify their own needs for caregiver support and communication as important. Nursing care approaches have been developed to respond to these needs (Logan, 1988; Kirschling, 1986; Youll, 1989; Woolley, 1990).

Woolley (1990) describes four categories of family needs to aid nurses in assessing and planning care with families of critically ill patients: (1) initial anxieties and informational concerns, (2) emotional support and interfamily contact, (3) involvement with care, and (4) personal needs.

Initial Anxieties and Informational Concerns. It is important to remember that family members may be in a crisis state of disequilibrium when first confronted with a loved one's diagnosis of terminal illness or the possibility of her or his impending death. Information needs to be presented clearly and simply, with the recognition that it may have to be repeated later. Family members can be encouraged to remain with the patient as much as possible and comfortable for them to do so.

Emotional Support and Interfamily Contact. Open communication, both of medical information and of personal concerns, is the key to emotional support. When patients and families sense permission in the hospital environment to acknowledge their emotional stress and pain, they are able to release the tension that accompanies these feelings: accepting and showing their pain, they feel less isolated and less threatened by fears of going crazy (Dugan, 1987a, pp. 28–29). Nurses and family members may explore together coping strategies previously used by the family in past crises and if these strategies should be continued. New strategies may need to be developed.

Nurses are involved in keeping communication open and clear between the patient, family, staff, and friends. Kathleen MacInnis (1992), a hospice nurse, writes to a dying person about making good-byes:

> Get a confessor. Early on, find someone with whom you can talk "dirty." A friend, nurse, physician, or family member who will allow you to say words like "dead, kick the bucket, croak, tumor, cancer." All those things you—and your loved ones—are thinking but are too polite to say out loud. Say them. It won't hurt and you'll feel better (p. 120).

This kind of open communication is not without its problems. The dying patient may at a given time want to talk about impending death. The listener, a family member or friend, may feel at this time that the discussion is unbearably painful. One husband responded to his wife's talking about her dying by stating, "I feel I'm a victim of terminal candor" (Jaffee & Jaffee, 1976, p. 1938).

Nurses also encourage family members and friends to keep in close contact with each other if this is possible. Maintaining existing support systems can improve a person's psychological well-being (Woolley, 1990). Farrell (1989) suggests that nurses need to find out from relatives how they want to be notified if they are not there when the patient dies: it is difficult for a relative to be informed of death when alone, and every effort should be made to contact other family members and friends so that they can comfort each other at this time.

Involvement with Care. If the patient is in the hospital, families can be offered the opportunity to participate in the nursing care where circumstances permit (Coutler, 1989). Participation in care may help family members cope with feelings of helplessness and powerlessness in that they are "doing" for their loved one. However, family members may show great variation in their desire and ability to do this, and this needs to be respected by staff. Family roles may change, such as switching from being a caregiver to being a care recipient. It is also important that patients participate in this decision, as both patients and family members may be apprehensive about the actual safety and technical aspects of providing care. These latter concerns become more prominent if the patient is at home. As identified in the previously cited research studies, family members need nurses to help them care for the patient, teach them what to do, and provide them with support and encouragement as they administer this care.

Personal Needs. Family members assisting in the care of their relatives may need to be reminded of their own needs for rest, relaxation, and some time of their own. If family members are to remain an effective means of support, both to the patient and to each other, they must receive adequate rest, sleep, and nutrition themselves (Woolley, 1990, p. 1406). A wife who is with her dying husband in the hospital every day may need a nurse to talk with her and suggest: "We'll be here with him and call you if you're needed—why don't you go home and try to relax for a while?" Family members who are caring for patients at home may need to know what alternatives are available when they feel they need some respite. They may also need support in not feeling they have failed as caregivers if they do ask for help.

Patients who are critically or terminally ill and their families require nursing care that includes both high technology skills and competence as well as high touch compassion and support. While often the technology skills are those most valued, the art of high touch must not be devalued. As Thomas (1975) notes:

> It consists of what is sometimes called "supportive" therapy. It tides patients over through diseases that are not, by and large, understood.

> It is what is meant by the phases "caring for" and "standing by." It is indispensable (p. 36).

As nurses collaborate with dying patients and their families in providing ongoing high tech and high touch care, they themselves may need to be "cared for," to grieve, and to accept support.

Nurses and Grieving

One perspective associated in the past with being a professional nurse included such admonitions as: "Don't get emotionally involved with your patients"; "Don't get too close to the patients;" "You'll never make a good nurse if you can't control your feelings." Fulton (1987) puts these admonitions to rest, stating that "if the traditional kinship network falters or if family members disengage from their dying relative, nurses and other caregivers find themselves participating in the social and emotional support of patients under their care. Emotional bonds are established and the health care team members find they are the grievers when the patient dies" (pp. 252–253). Similarly, nurses using a holistic nursing care approach may establish deep and profound emotional bonds with patients that arc painfully severed when the patients die.

There are many occasions when grief is just as normal a response for staff as it is for patients and family members (Parkes, 1986). Nurses may need to go through a grieving process when a person who has been a patient and a friend dies. Chapter 2 noted that patients often fear the process of dying—the loneliness, the isolation, the loss of dignity—more than death itself. Sonstegard, Hansen, Zillman, & Johnston (1976) suggest that nurses working with dying patients fear the same isolation and wonder who will be available to them to share their feelings of joy and sorrow, anger and acceptance, when patients die (p. 1490). Young staff nurses may need to discuss their feelings about dying patients, particularly if the patient is another young adult of the same age. Older nurses who may be trying to come to a realistic acceptance of their own mortality may also need to talk about death and dying, especially if, for example, they are seeing themselves in each dying patient.

In a workshop held for nursing staff who work with chronically and terminally ill patients, Mandel (1981) asked the participants to list in order of priority the issues that bother them the most in providing nursing care to this group of people. The following responses were given: (a) anger and guilt, (b) anxiety, (c) lack of skills, (d) overidentification, (e) depression and sadness, and (f) role confusion. Shanfield (1981) discovered while teaching a seminar on the health professional as a survivor that the students did experience mourning and loss when patients died. Small, Engler, & Rushton (1991) describe that in pediatric intensive care units there are times in which multiple deaths or other traumatic events occur in rapid succession,

". . . allowing little opportunity for caregivers to process their feelings before they are expected to provide highly challenging and potentially lifesaving care to another patient" (pp. 103–104).

The literature reflects nurses' needs for support and to grieve. It is important that nurses accept these needs as a part of caring for terminally ill patients. Herrle & Robinson (1987) suggest seven ways that nurses can be encouraged to care for themselves, and by doing so, facilitate their provision of quality care to patients and families (Table 3.1).

While development of personal coping mechanisms for grieving is important, nurses can also provide support for each other through sharing their feelings and responses about caring for terminally ill patients with each other. According to Parkes (1986), "no seriously ill person should be cared for in circumstances that do not allow the patient and family to share their feelings with staff and staff to share their feelings with each other" (p. 6). Nurses working in an area where patient deaths are frequent may want to organize a monthly support group. Encouragement of informal peer support such as giving each other "strokes," especially in times of stress, can be helpful at all levels of nursing. Educational experiences such as conferences and workshops on death and dying to facilitate cognitive, affective, and personal learning can be requested.

Consideration of unit and organizational system changes is important. Nurses who are caring for dying patients may need some time during the day for themselves to examine their own feelings, time to think and to feel about this experience. If a patient dies, they may need some time to come to terms with their own feelings and to center themselves to prepare to care for the next patient. Building in a formal system of dealing with stress might involve taking time off for conferences, rotating different responsibilities on the unit, and utilizing mental health days. Mandel (1981) suggests "ventilation rooms," where nursing staff can express powerful emotions in privacy, and special compensation for those involved with the dying. As part of a bereavement and loss program, one intensive care unit set up a follow-up plan that allows staff to maintain contact with bereaved families in the months following the death (Small, Engler, & Rushton, 1991).

Table 3.1 Nursing Care for Nurses

*Explore your feelings concerning your own losses.
*Identify those losses you are still struggling to overcome.
*Identify resources that can help you deal with loss.
*Think about your idea of life after death.
*Recognize your own personal limitations.
*Actively deal with a patient's death.
*Reduce your own stress by practicing a positive attitude, exercising, and relaxing.

Reprinted with permission from "Helping Staff Cope with Grief" by S.M. Herrle and B. Robinson, in *Nursing Management,* Vol. 18, No. 9, September 1987, p. 33–34.

Nurses, in collaboration with other health caregivers, patients, and families, need to take the initiative in making the changes in the current disease-oriented, highly technological medical system that will recognize and provide for humanistic care for dying patients. By "being with" patients, by listening, touching, and providing pain medication, nurses may help people maintain integrity, self-esteem, and control while dying. The interdependent functions of nurses and physicians contribute significantly to holistic care of terminally ill patients. The remaining parts of this chapter look at physicians' responses to dying patients and the vital role communication between nurses and physicians assumes in patient care.

Physicians

Physicians' roles are primarily as healers of the sick. They are supposed to cure, while having "presence of mind . . . clearness of judgment in moments of grave peril. The physician who has the misfortune to be without it (imperturbability), who betrays indecision and worry and shows that he is flustered and flurried . . . loses rapidly the confidence of his patients." (Osler, as cited in Hendin, 1974, p. 106)

The physician should not show uncertainty, since there is the belief that by showing certainty, the doctor maintains the power and control in the doctor–patient relationship (Katz, 1984). Yet, what happens to the doctor's role if the patient is dying; the physician is not curing nor can certainty be professed in treatment. As Benoliel points out (1974), the dying may represent a loss of power and the ability to control, especially as the medical care becomes more and more precarious.

Weisman (1974) discusses the four major goals of the physician vis-à-vis patient care: (1) diagnosis, (2) treatment, (3) relief, and (4) safe conduct. Although the goal of diagnosis is the same for the terminal and nonterminal patients, the other three goals take on different meanings for the care of the dying patient.

Treatment. Treatment is usually considered to lead to curing. When the patient cannot be cured, however, the goal of the treatment changes: it may be to increase the length of the life of the patient; it may be to help to relieve the symptoms of the patient's illness; or it may be to satisfy the physician that he or she did everything that was possible. Clinical pathology conferences, or "death rounds" where the medical staff involved discusses all the alternatives that should have been used to avoid death, may lead to treatment for treatment's sake. "At stake is not only the patient's life, but also the clinician's reputation and self-esteem" (Coombs & Powers, 1975, p. 25). This was further confirmed by Benoliel's review of the literature on the care of the dying (1988). "Caregiving practices were also influenced by the expansion of biomedical and intensive care activity" (p. 350).

Noyes & Clancy (1977) make the point that one of the major difficulties for physicians in caring for the dying is that they have confused the dying role with the sick role. A person in the sick role wants to get well and cooperates with the physician in order to achieve the end of getting better. The duty of dying persons is to desire to live as long as possible; they must also cooperate with their caretakers. Sick people, for the limited time they are sick, are allowed to be dependent, whereas the dying are encouraged to be more independent, to remain active, and to care for themselves as much as possible. The physician may view the patient as if he or she were sick, rather than dying, and both the physician and patient must act as if the patient were improving. One manifestation of this is the continual and active treatment given the patient by the physician.

Relief. As stated by Weisman (1974): "Adequate relief to pain is mandatory; almost everything is secondary to pain relief." Control of pain for the terminally ill should be the primary goal of treatment. However, the primary goal for many physicians is to extend the patient's life.

Diana Crane (1975), in her extensive study of physicians, found that 43 percent of 660 internists studied were willing to increase their prescription of narcotics even if there was a high risk of respiratory arrest. However, only 29 percent of 750 residents in internal medicine would increase the dosage under the same circumstances. As Crane interprets the findings: for the older physician, the important use of narcotics is to control pain; however, younger physicians are afraid that their superiors will perceive their actions as hastening death instead of controlling pain.

In addition, medical personnel are not necessarily cognizant of new methods of pain control for the terminally ill (Benoliel, 1988). (For further discussion of pain management, see Chapter 5.)

Safe Conduct. For a patient who recovers, the guarantee of safe conduct is unnecessary. However, for those patients who are dying, who may have to yield control to others, there is a need for safe conduct. Such patients must trust that they will be taken care of with concern and dignity. Patients must feel that they are safe; that they can communicate their fears and their feelings; and that their questions will be answered honestly. (Bruhn & Fuentes, 1987)

Physicians find this particularly hard to do since death may be conceived as a failure of the physician's skills (Krant & Sheldon, 1971). Since nothing can be done to cure the patient, the physician feels a loss of mastery. The doctor's fantasy of being able to guarantee eternal life to all patients is shattered (White, 1977).

Responses of Physicians to Dying Patients

As a result of the difficulties in achieving their goals when dealing with the terminally ill, physicians will generally respond in one of three ways to the dying patient (Moller, 1990): The physician will try to employ all his technical skills to save the patient at all costs; or the physician will practice avoidance-neglect, or the physician will exhibit detached-sympathetic support.

The first approach is exemplified by the following from *The Death of Ivan Ilych* (Tolstoy, 1960):

> The doctor said that so-and-so indicated that there was so-and-so inside the patient, but if the investigation of so-and-so did not confirm this, then he must assume that and that. If he assumed that and that, then . . . and so on. To Ivan Ilych only one question was important: was his case serious or not? But the doctor ignored that inappropriate question. From his point of view it was not the one under consideration. The real question was to decide between a floating kidney, chronic catarrh, or appendicitis. It was not a question of Ivan Ilych's life or death, but one between a floating kidney and appendicitis (p. 121).

The second approach, avoidance-neglect, develops as the "caring" aspect overshadows the "curing" aspect of treatment. There are few rewards in terms of status and prestige for providing that care and fulfilling the patient's needs. The physician uses the rationalization of medical prioritizing to avoid the patient, since, as said so often by physicians, "Nothing more can be done to save the patient."

The physician who shows detached-sympathetic support will interact well with the dying and be aware of the needs of the dying. But, as Moller points out, these physicians are the mavericks "in that there is little formal, structural sanctioning and support of their non-technical activities" (p. 35).

Communication with the Terminally Ill Patient

There has been increasing openness in telling terminally ill patients their prognoses. According to Stevenson (1987), we have gone through three distinct phases:

1. Until the 1970s, doctors hid the fact that patients were dying. The doctor felt that patients' knowing they were dying would lead to undue emotional suffering. This began changing when studies such as those by Glaser & Strauss (1968) and Kübler-Ross (1969) showed that patients knew they were dying and wanted to talk about their dying.
2. In the 1970s and 1980s, "full disclosure" became the key words. Physicians now believed that denial was hurtful and that patients should know the whole truth. This was further supported by the report on informed consent issued by the President's Commission

for the Study of Ethical Problems in Medicine and Biomedical and Behavioral Research (1983):

> The Commission finds that patients who have the capacity to make decisions about their care must be permitted to do so voluntarily and must have all relevant information regarding their condition . . . (p. 2).

3. Phase three is the recognition that neither withholding the truth nor always telling the truth is beneficial; patients should be told that they are dying, but they have the right to deny this information.

Although there is currently recognition that we need a "dynamic process of communication between physician and patient" (Stevenson, 1987, p. 157), it is very difficult to achieve since this involves *mutual* communication between the patient and the physician. "Knowing when and how to talk with them (dying patients) about death related issues continues to be a problem for many" (Benoliel, 1988, p. 345). As pointed out in the preceding section, those who can communicate with the dying are the "mavericks."

Socialization

The process of socialization is the means by which persons acquire the knowledge and skills to perform in various roles. Medical school education is a primary component in the socialization process of physicians. The form of medical education has basically remained the same since 1910. As pointed out by Tosteson (1990):

> Its (medical education) principal features are a clear separation between the basic and clinical sciences, with the basic sciences taught in the first year or two and the clinical subjects taught in the last two or three years; the heavy use of didactic instruction in the form of lectures to large groups of students; an emphasis on the teacher's role as an expert; relatively independent and poorly coordinated courses; the heavy use of residents as teachers during clinical clerkships; and the domination of the third and fourth years by concern over choice of residency. (p. 235)

Studies of the effects of medical education also show its unchanging nature over time.

In 1958, Samuel Bloom discussed the three effects of medical education:

1. There is a dehumanization effect implicit in the first two years of medical school (the preclinical years), since the student has no contact with patients while working on cadavers in pathology.

2. There is a compartmentalization or segmentation effect implicit in the whole medical curriculum. During the preclinical years, the students study localized pathology; dissection is stressed, which reduces the whole to its parts. During the clinical years, patients are viewed as disease entities rather than people. Throughout training, the student is overwhelmed by the amount of knowledge that must be learned, which heightens the need for specialization.
3. There is an institutionalization effect implicit in the training in modern hospitals where students are taught to see patients as hospital cases. The functioning of the institution becomes more important than the individual patient.

These three effects of a medical education lead to a highly technically trained physician who is able to deal with a diseased kidney or liver, but who may not be able to deal with the person containing these diseased organs.

In 1979, Renee Fox (as cited in Moller, 1990) found that one of the key elements in the education of second-year medical students, the autopsy, led to the same results as was found by Bloom; for example:

> Now when I see a lung, for example, I concentrate on its structure . . . I don't picture its being someone who was once living, breathing, and talking (p. 27).

In 1984, a study by the Association of American Medical Colleges (Culliton) found that the likelihood of medical education producing compassionate doctors was slim.

Medical education is beginning to change. There are some pioneer program that are patient centered such as New Pathways at Harvard Medical School; however, they remain in the minority.

For dying patients, when caring is more important than curing, the effects of medical education are dysfunctional in terms of how patients should be treated. Only recently has medical education begun to institute programs that are "patient centered." (For example, see Wallace [1986].)

Coombs & Powers (1975) studied the specific stages medical students go through in terms of their socialization for dealing with death. They conducted 229 interviews of a class that entered medical school in 1967 and graduated in 1971. (These findings are still valid since medical education has changed little in the past twenty years.) They saw medical students going through developmental stages:

Stage 1 Idealizing the Doctor's Role: Freshmen saw the physician as protecting patients from death; they were upset with physicians who did not show compassion over death.

Stage II Desensitizing Death Symbols: In the preclinical years, the students are immediately introduced to a cadaver, which is generally met with initial shock and nausea. They come to cope with their anxieties by losing themselves in the technical details of the work such as memorizing the scientific names of the bones. In the second year, the students must perform an autopsy. Again, to cope, the students become involved in the technical aspects. A detached scientific attitude is developed, which is reinforced in the basic science courses where illness is discussed on an intellectual, not an emotional, basis.

Stage III Objectifying and Combating Death: When the student begins to work with patients in the third year, "early experiences with dying patients make clear the necessity of detaching oneself from the emotional trauma of death" (p. 22). In order to do this, the students begin to define patients as scientific entities, and to deal with the pieces of the organism. (These effects are similar to the effects discussed by Bloom.)

The following example from Krant & Sheldon (1971) demonstrates this view of the patient.

> A 64-year-old woman died of gastrointestinal carcinoma. Her dying had been slow and in many ways difficult because of confusional periods, severe bed sores that were difficult to control and marked nausea. But, through the six weeks that she was a patient on the unit, she was uncomplaining and warm, and several of the nurses involved in her care developed strong positive feelings for her. Immediately after the patient was pronounced dead, the fourth-year medical student who was involved with her care went to the nursing station and asked for an endotracheal tube because he wished to practice endotracheal tube placement. The nurse at the station, who had been on the unit for five years, refused to give him the tube and in the ensuing argument, accused the student of being inhuman, of using the patient as his plaything. The medical student, a sensible and capable young man, retreated, bewildered by the outburst (pp. 17–18).

During this stage, death also comes to be viewed as the enemy.

Coombs & Powers see some physicians, after they graduate and gain more experience, as going through two more stages.

Stage IV Questioning the Medical Model: Physicians may question the glorification of the science of medicine (a knowledge of the disease processes) at the expense of the art of medicine (the interpersonal abilities.) They may also come to question whether death is the enemy, especially after seeing the extremes to which some physicians may go in keeping someone alive.

If the physician does not go through this stage, Coombs & Powers hypothesize that the individual will develop a "God complex" and try to control death by demonstrating clinical mastery over it.

Stage V Dealing with Personal Feelings: This stage comes when physicians realize that in order to deal with patients' feelings, they must begin to deal with their own feelings. However, little evidence exists that physicians are likely to reach this stage. Much of the evidence would lead to the opposite conclusion (Schulz & Aderman, 1980).

Death education could help medical students reach the last developmental stages. Those physicians who have taken courses in death and dying have been found to have more positive attitudes towards the dying and relate better to the dying than those who have not taken such a course (Dickinson & Pearson, 1981). Medical schools are likely to include some death education in their curricula (96 percent), but very few (13 percent) offer a complete course in death education (Dickinson et al., 1987). Although it is encouraging that medical schools are recognizing the need for some death education, the majority of physicians are still not being adequately prepared to deal with death and dying.

Personality Factors

Another reason why physicians have difficulty dealing with the terminally ill has been attributed to the personality characteristics of physicians. They tend to have more fears and anxieties concerning death than others in the population. (See Benoliel, 1988.) It has been hypothesized that persons decide to become physicians because of these fears, that by becoming physicians they hope to control death and thereby lessen their fears.

C. W. Wahl (1959) sees the choice of medicine as representing a defense against death, a reaction formation against a fear that could not be conquered in childhood. Supporting this, Feifel et al. (1967) found that physicians were more likely to have had to deal with a threat of death before the age of five, compared with the laypeople studied, who did not face a similar threat until after the age of six. Toufexis & Castronaro (1983) reported that physicians often had to deal with death or serious illness in their childhood.

Feifel et al. (1967) studied 81 physicians and compared them with control groups of 95 healthy laypersons and 92 critically ill patients (40 of whom were terminally ill). The physicians were less likely to think about death, but they were more likely to be afraid of death. They showed greater negative imagery concerning death and had more difficulty in answering the questions than did the comparable group.

Livingston & Zimet (1965) studied death anxiety and the authoritarian personality in 114 medical students. The authoritarian personality has repressed certain impulses that have never been integrated into the conscious self-image. The defense mechanisms of reaction formation and compensation are used "to deal with pre- or unconscious tendencies of fear, weakness, passivity, sexuality or aggression" (p. 222). Livingston & Zimet found that there was an inverse relationship between authoritarianism and death anxiety: the higher the authoritarianism, the lower the death anxiety. This finding was expected since a person higher in authoritarianism would be better defended against her unconscious. Those students who chose surgery as their specialty were lowest in death anxiety; psychiatrists were highest.

One would have assumed that surgeons, a type of physician likely to deal with death, would have high death anxiety. However, Livingston & Zimet were measuring overt death anxiety. Because of the relationship between death anxiety and authoritarianism, the students choosing surgery were probably highly defended against death anxiety, which would lead to lower death anxiety on Livingston & Zimet's measure.

A further finding by Livingston & Zimet is that although death anxiety increases as the student progresses, it is largely determined before the student enters medical school.

A study of internists, surgeons, and psychiatrists in the New York City area found that death anxiety varied inversely with age and experience. Older physicians with more experience had lower death anxiety than younger physicians (Kane & Hogan, 1985). This may have been related to the fact that the younger physicians, interns and residents, more frequently confronted death.

A family physician, quoted by Hendin (1974), succinctly states the result of death anxiety in doctors:

> I must admit that when the anxiety, the fear provoked within me as the physician becomes too great, it's very, very comfortable to deal with the dying process on a technical level. Because then there is no real involvement. There have been times when I haven't been able to cope with an individual patient in a terminal situation, and in a cowardly way, I have run to the stereotyped role of myself as a scientist and technical expert, who doesn't concern himself with people's feelings. Certainly, depending upon the individual physician, some may find the anxiety so great that they always deal with it in this way. (p. 116–117)

What Must Be Done

Since there is a recognition of the factors that contribute to the withdrawal of physicians from the dying, these must be examined to see where they could be changed. Although one would not recommend intensive psychoanalysis for all physicians, it is certainly important for medical education to be cognizant of the personality factors that may affect physicians' care of the dying. We must also question our "deep-seated cultural values that give primacy to lifesaving activity, high technology medical care, and physician dominance in patient care decisions" (Benoliel, 1988, p. 355).

Interdisciplinary Concern: Communication

Communication between nurses and physicians literally can be a matter of life or death. Research of treatment courses and outcomes of patients in intensive care units at 13 hospitals indicated that the involvement and interaction of critical care personnel can directly influence the outcome of intensive care (Knaus, Draper, Wagner, & Zimmerman, 1986). In comparing actual and predicted death rates using group rates as a standard, this study found that one hospital had significantly fewer deaths than another, which had more deaths than expected. The researchers state that these differences were related more to the interaction and coordination of each hospital's intensive care unit staff than to specific treatment modalities. If communication between physicians and nurses can be so important as to affect patient mortality rates, it becomes crucial to look at how such communication may be improved in order to enhance patient care.

Role Expectations

Nursing and medical students generally receive their professional education in separate schools. They may graduate without having much interaction with each other's professions and may have stereotyped versions of each other's roles. Mechanic & Aiken (1982) suggest that "probably the most important factor contributing to poor physician–nurse relationships is a lack of understanding between both groups about the kinds of problems each faces" (p. 750).

This lack of understanding of each other's roles, problems, and orientation to patient care can be a significant factor in the difficulty physicians and nurses, along with other caregivers, have in working together to provide care to terminally ill patients. A team approach is often used in this care, yet Vachon (1987) found that most of the stress that hospice caregivers reported in their work with dying patients was related to difficulties with colleagues and within institutional hierarchies. Teamwork evolves through an often painful and ongoing process of team members assessing their own intergroup dynamics.

Six characteristics influence and delineate team functioning: (a) goals or tasks, (b) role expectations, (c) decision making, (d) communication patterns, (e) leadership, and (f) norms (Plovnick, Fry, & Rubin, 1977; Rubin & Beckhard, 1972). An exploration of all of these characteristics by Kahn (1974) revealed little congruence between the professional norms, goals, and perceptions of physicians, nurses, and social workers:

- Nurses felt that physicians tended to take charge and give orders despite the official emphasis on collegial team relations.
- Social workers insisted on the confidential nature of their records.
- Physicians sought "quick solutions."
- Nurses felt they were willing to do dirty work; whereas social workers offered nothing "tangible" and stirred up feelings.
- Social workers felt nurses sought quick heroic solutions and did not deal with their feelings.
- There is overlapping in nurse–social worker activity.
- Nurses, social workers, and doctors have different social class backgrounds, different educational status, different social distance from clientele, with resulting conflicts in perceptions and relationships (p. 19).

Working at group dynamics becomes an important team function when such lack of congruence in expectations of each other's roles is present.

Another difficulty in team care arises from the assumption that caregivers from different professions can automatically function as a team because they have the apparent mutual goal of caring for the patient. A health care team needs training to function as a team, but this is consistently overlooked. Rubin, (cited in Wise, Beckhard, Rubin, & Kyte, 1974) remarked that:

> . . . it is naive to bring together a highly diverse group of people and expect that by calling them a team they will in fact behave as one. It is ironic indeed to realize that a football team spends 40 hours a week practicing teamwork for the 2 hours on Sunday afternoon when their teamwork really counts. Teams in organizations seldom spend 2 hours per year practicing when their ability to function as a team counts 40 hours per week (p. xviii).

Part of a health team's training in order to function as a team involves practice in communication. Team communication stressors identified by hospice caregivers included: difficulty developing trust within an interdisciplinary team; difficulty with communicating information; power struggles;

handling conflict; "incest" on the health care team; and ensuring longevity beyond the life of the original team (Vachon, 1987, p. 88). Lack of mutual respect among team members may also leave the patient a victim in a battle for professional turf.

Status and Personality Factors

Professional status differences, as well as respect, may influence communication. In her study on interpersonal distance of hospital staff on two medical and two surgical units, Kerr (1986) hypothesized that more frequent and closer interpersonal interaction between nurses and physicians should be seen as professional status and social roles become less distinct. The study did not support this hypothesis. Physicians interacted with physicians, nurses interacted with nurses, and there was limited interaction between physicians and nurses. A variable to consider, however, is that the nurses practiced functional nursing, doing specific tasks, while the head nurse coordinated all nursing activities. Physicians might presume that the head nurse was the only nurse able to provide reliable information. The study could be repeated in a setting where nurses practiced primary nursing, a type of care which designates one nurse to have total responsibility and accountability for a particular group of patients. Study results might be different in this type of setting.

While the above research indicates that the variable of situational context may influence nurse–physician communication, another influencing variable could be the personal characteristics of the participants in the interaction. A research project conducted by Baldwin, Welches, Walker, & Eliastam (1987) investigated the relationship between nurses' self-esteem and their views of and willingness to collaborate with physicians and hospital administrators. Nurses in this study sample reported high self-esteem. The study demonstrated statistically significant—although weak—correlations between nurse self-esteem and collaboration with physicians. Further research is indicated to study the relationship between the personal characteristics of physicians, as well as nurses, to interdisciplinary collaboration.

True collaboration involves an appreciation of each individual's skills and a continual openness on the part of each individual to role renegotiation and redefinition. Political skills, such as compromise and the use of trade-offs, are also involved here. Davis (1986) points out that in collaborative practice, the practice activities of one collaborator often begin to resemble those of the co-collaborator (p. 206). Nurses collaborating with physicians in care of dying patients may become extremely competent in titrating pain medication, while physicians may develop increasing skills in listening to patients discuss their concerns. This type of professional role diffusion also extends to the diffusion of leadership in health care teams that are functioning therapeutically. "In a team, no one has the ultimate answer and everyone has a partial answer, while all are seeking a holistic pattern of answers that no particular profession is prepared to formulate" (Pruyser, 1984, p. 366).

Improving Communications

While there may be no definitive answers as to how to facilitate and enhance communication between nurses and physicians, there are some possibilities to consider. The coordination of basic education might be a way to enhance communication among members of the health team. The National Commission on Nursing (1981) recommended that health care professional education include curricula and socialization processes that facilitate collaborative approaches to planning, implementing, and evaluating patient care. If students in nursing and medicine could participate together in the core courses of their professional education, they might develop an appreciation of one another's ideas, approaches, values, and goals. Ideally this appreciation and understanding would continue as they assumed responsibility for patient care. A related curriculum approach might involve student fieldwork experience with the other profession. One medical and nursing school developed an innovative nursing rotation for first year medical students to familiarize the students with nurses' roles (Ziegfeld & Jones, 1987). Each medical student was assigned to a nurse preceptor and spent several days working with that nurse as she/he cared for patients. Socialization experiences such as these could enhance students' development as future health care team members.

However, as mentioned earlier, team development is ongoing hard work. Benoliel (1990) suggests moving beyond the team approach to create caring work environments: "Activities to foster the shift of work environments from the current patriarchal, superior–subordinate team orientation toward a view of work as a communal effort is no easy task" (p. 7). She suggests that one approach to this change might be to find ways of incorporating alternative principles of power into the current working relationships. Such principles of power include power sharing, orientation to human processes as much as to outcomes of activities, and use of decision making by consensus (Wheeler & Chinn, 1989).

The principle of power sharing encompasses patients also. Dugan (1987b) writes of advocating for patients' rights—"rights to autonomy, to informed consent, to beneficent, non-maleficent medical treatment, to truth-telling and fidelity" (p. 139). A shift from the dominant model of power grabbing, or power-over in the traditional medical setting to one of power sharing is a dramatic one that is consistent with the egalitarian concept of health care teams.

Another concept vital to the functioning of health care teams is that of mutual aid. Members of a team form a community of caring among each other as well as with patients, and only when a team provides love and nurturing to its members can it provide adequate help to patients (Pruyser, 1984). This need for mutual aid becomes evident when a patient cared for by the team dies. Nurses' and physicians' responses to patients' deaths have been discussed earlier in this chapter. With the current emphasis in this "New Age" on health promotion and disease prevention, both family and staff may feel guilt as well as grief that the death occurred.

Leibenluft, Green, & Giese (1988) describe and conceptualize a specific staff's reaction to the death of a patient from metastatic carcinoma in terms of the stages of normal bereavement: denial, anger, depression, and resolution. These authors stress the need for staff to meet in an ongoing process group to facilitate necessary grief work required by a patient's death. Caregivers need a variety of supports to cope with grief, but most of the time it is the working group, or unit team that should support each other. Regular meetings at which staff are encouraged to talk about the problems that arise and their own feelings will often provide this support (Parkes, 1986), but such interdisciplinary communication can be difficult.

> Intellectually, it seems obvious that an atmosphere of open communication relieves emotional stress, enables people to endure suffering more humanely, and facilitates the resolution of ethical dilemmas. The difficulty, in each context, is managing the emotional discomfort and pain that accompanies experiencing losses and talking of them (Dugan, 1987a, p. 29).

Acknowledgment of our own humanity as caregivers is necessary to communicate caring. We may often come to an impasse in sharing our feelings and reactions with each other; it is almost as if we negate the human aspect of our beings. Perhaps we feel that because we have not cured dying patients, we have failed not only them but also ourselves and our colleagues. Perhaps our own fears of death are so frightening that we cannot share these feelings. The creation of a caring work environment may give us the permission to feel and, therefore, to grieve the loss of a patient. As staff members become more comfortable with sharing feelings of grief, they in turn may become more comfortable with helping clients and families experience their losses. Our emotional vulnerability can be an asset in our caring; it allows us to be open and receptive to what people are feeling and trying to express. If we realize we have the support of colleagues, this vulnerability need not be feared, but it can be used as a vehicle for our own growth as well as for that of our patients.

SUMMARY ❧

Caregivers and patients share the very human fears and anxieties associated with death in the American culture. Professional education that facilitates nurses' and physicians' awareness and exploration of attitudes and feelings about death may be influential in enhancing the appropriate care of dying patients and their families. However, death and dying content in both nursing and medical schools is primarily integrated into other courses in the curriculum and further research is needed to determine what and how much actual content and experience is needed to affect patient care outcomes.

Although delivery of care to terminally ill patients is often provided by interdisciplinary teams, caregivers generally do not have the knowledge or experience of how to work together in such teams. Communication between nurses and physicians has been identified as important to patient care outcomes as well as to staff morale, yet this also can be problematic. Attention may need to be focused on the creation of a caring work environment that allows for the development of mutual aid, loving, and nurturing among staff and that allows staff to grieve the loss of a patient. Caregivers may then be able to use their own humanity as a resource in caring for dying patients, knowing that this resource in turn will be cared for and replenished by and with their colleagues.

LEARNING EXERCISES ❧

1. If someone in your family were dying, what are three important needs you would want a nurse to meet for this person? For a physician to meet? What are the three least important needs for each of these caregivers to meet?
2. Imagine that a family member or a close friend has just died. How would you like to be notified of this person's death? Who would you like to tell you? Who would you like to be with you when you are notified?
3. In interdisciplinary team rounds concerning the care of a dying patient, who should lead the discussion? Describe your thinking in reaching this decision.
4. If some nurses and physicians have difficulty in caring for dying patients, do you think another profession should be developed to do this? If so, what would you expect this professional person to do?

AUDIOVISUAL MATERIAL ❧

The Artistry of Medicine. 19 minutes/videocassette/1983. Distribution Department, Health Services Consortium, 201 Silver Cedar Court, Chapel Hill, NC, 27514.
This videotape focuses on the medical field's preoccupation with technology. Norman Cousins and patients discuss how this

preoccupation can actually exclude patients from participating in their own care. It is a helpful tape for physicians and medical students to become more aware of the importance of communicating with patients.

Why Won't They talk To Me? How To Break Bad News. 5 videocassettes/30 minutes each/1986. For sale only. International Tele-Film Enterprises Ltd., 47 Densley Avenue, Toronto, Canada, M6M 5AB. Two British physicians offer for all health care professionals a series of presentations on effective communication of "bad news"—any news that significantly alters the patient's view of the future.

The Cancer Patient. 18 minutes/videocassette/1986. Distribution Department, Health Sciences Consortium, 201 Silver Cedar Court, Chapel Hill, NC, 27514.
Patients with cancer talk about their reactions and responses to this disease. Doctors, nurses, and clergy discuss how they react to the patients and their needs at different stages of the disease.

Caring For The Dying Patient. 28 minutes/videocassette/1985. Distribution Department, Health Sciences Consortium, 201 Silver Cedar Court, Chapel Hill, NC, 27514.
This roundtable discussion includes two nurse oncologists, a medical oncologist, a medical social worker with a special interest in cancer, and a patient who has recovered from Hodgkin's disease. The focus is on the pivotal role of the nurse in helping the patient to accept death. It also supports health professionals working together as a team.

REFERENCES ❧

Baldwin, A., Welches, L., Walker, D., & Eliastam, M. (1987). Nurse self-esteem and collaboration with physicians. *Western Journal of Nursing Research, 9* (1), 107–114.

Bartnof, H. S. (1988). Health care professional education and AIDS. *Death Studies. 12* (4), 547–562.

Barton, D. (1977). The caregiver. In D. Barton (Ed.), *Dying and death* (pp. 72–86). Baltimore, MD: Waverly.

Benoliel, J. Q. (1974). Anticipatory grief in physicians and nurses. In B. Schoenberg, A. Carr, A. Kutscher, D. Peretz, I. Goldberg (Eds.), *Anticipatory grief.* New York: Columbia University Press.

Benoliel, J. Q. (1977). Nurses and the human experience of dying. In H. Feifel (Ed.), *New meanings of death* (pp. 123–142). New York: McGraw-Hill.

Benoliel, J. Q. (1987–1988). Health care providers and dying patients: Critical issues in terminal care. *Omega: Journal of Death and Dying. 18* (4), 341–363.

Benoliel, J. Q. (1990, September 13). *Undervalued caregiving: A major issue for the thanatology community.* Paper presented at the First National Congress on Thanatology, Columbia-Presbyterian Medical Center, New York City.

Bloom, S. (1958). Some implications of studies in the professionalization of the physician. In E. G. Jaco (Ed.), *Patients, physicians and illness.* New York: Free Press.

Bruhn, J., & Fuentes, R. (1987). Education and patient care in thanatology: A multidisciplinary approach. In A. Kutscher, A. Carr, & L. Kutscher (Eds.), *Principles of thanatology.* New York: Columbia University Press.

Coutler, M. A. (1989). The needs of family members in intensive care units. *Intensive Care Nursing. 5* (1), 4–10.

Coombs, R., & Powers, P. (1975). Socialization for death: the physician's role. In L. Lofland (Ed.), *Toward a sociology of death and dying.* Beverly Hills, CA: Sage Publications.

Crane, D. (1975). *The sanctity of social life: Physician's treatment of critically ill patients.* New York: Russell Sage Foundation.

Culliton, B. (1984). Medical education under fire. *Science. 226,* 419–420.

Davis, L. L. (1986). The politics of interdisciplinary collaboration in professional practice. *Journal of Professional Nursing. 2* (4), 206, 266.

Degner, L. F., & Gow, C. M. (1988a). Evaluations of death education in nursing: A critical review. *Cancer Nursing. 11* (3), 151–159.

Degner, L. F., & Gow, C. M. (1988b). Preparing nurses for care of the dying: A longitudinal study. *Cancer Nursing. 11* (3), 160–169.

Dickinson, G. & Pearson, A. (1981). Death education and physician's attitudes toward dying patients. *Omega: Journal of Death and Dying, 11,* 167–174.

Dickinson, G., Sumner, E., & Durand, R. (1987). Death education in U.S. professional colleges: Medical, nursing, and pharmacy. *Death Studies. 11* (1), 57–61.

Dugan, D. O. (1987a). Death and Dying: Emotional, spiritual, and ethical support for patients and families. *Journal of Psychosocial Nursing and Mental Health Services. 25* (7), 21, 25–29.

Dugan, D. O. (1987b). Masculine and feminine voices: Making ethical decisions in the care of the dying. *The Journal of Medical Humanities and Bioethics. 8* (2), 129–140.

Farrell, M. (1989). Dying and bereavement: The role of the critical care nurse. *Intensive Care Nursing. 5* (1), 39–45.

Feifel, H., Hanson, S., Jones, R. & Edwards, L. (1967). *Physicians consider death. Proceedings of the 75th Annual Convention of the American Psychological Association.* Washington, DC: American Psychological Association.

Field, D. (1989). Nurses' accounts of nursing the terminally ill on a coronary care unit. *Intensive Care Nursing. 5* (3), 114–122.

Freihofer, P., & Felton, G. (1976). Nursing behaviors in bereavement: An exploratory study. *Nursing Research. 25* (5), 332–337.

Fulton, R. (1987). The many faces of grief. *Death Studies. 11* (4), 243–256.

Gadow, S. (1980). Caring for the dying: Advocacy or paternalism. *Death Education. 3* (4), 387–398.

Garland, J. N., Bass, D. M., & Otto, M. E. (1984). The needs of patients and primary caregivers: A comparison of primary caregivers' and hospice nurses' perceptions. *The American Journal of Hospice Care. 1* (3), 40–45.

Glaser, B., & Strauss, A. (1968). *Time for dying.* Chicago: Aldine.

Hare, J., & Pratt, C. C. (1989). Nurses' fear of death and comfort level with dying patients. *Death Studies. 13* (4), 349–360.

Hendin, D. (1974). *Death as a fact of life.* New York: Warner Paperbacks.

Herrle, S. M., & Robinson, B. (1987). Helping staff cope with grief. *Nursing Management. 18* (9), 33, 34.

Holman, E. A. (1990). Death and the health professional: Organization and defense in health care. *Death Studies. 14* (1), 13–24.

Homer, L. E. (1984). Organizational defenses against the anxiety of terminal illness: A case study. *Death Education. 8* (2–3), 137–154.

Hopper, B. L. (1977). Nursing students' attitudes towards death. *Nursing Research. 26* (6), 443–447.

Jaffee, L., & Jaffee, A. (1976). Terminal candor and the coda syndrome. *American Journal of Nursing. 76* (12), 1938–1940.

Jinadu, M. K., & Adediran, S. O. (1982). Effects of nursing education on attitudes of nursing students toward dying patients in the Nigerian sociocultural environment. *International Journal of Nursing Studies. 19* (1), 21–27.

Kahn, A. (1974). Institutional constraints in interprofessional practice. In H. Rehr (Ed.), *Medicine and social work* (pp. 14–25). New York: Prodist.

Kane, A., & Hogan, J. (1985). Death anxiety in physicians: defensive style, medical specialty, and exposure to death. *Omega: Journal of Death and Dying, 16,* 11–22.

Katz, J. (1984). Why doctors don't disclose uncertainty. *Hastings Center Report, 14,* 35–44.

Kerr, J. A. C. (1986). Interpersonal distance of hospital staff. *Western Journal of Nursing Research. 8* (3), 350–364.

Kirschling, J. M. (1986). The experience of terminal illness on adult family members. *Hospice Journal: Physical, Psychosocial, and Pastoral Care of the Dying. 2* (1), 121–138.

Knaus, W. A., Draper, E. A., Wagner, D. P., & Zimmerman, J. E. (1986). An evaluation of outcome from intensive care in major medical centers. *Annals of Internal Medicine. 104,* 410–418.

Krant, M., & Sheldon, A. (1971). The dying patient: Medicine's responsibility. *Journal of Thanatology, 1,* 1-21.

Krieger, D. (1979). *The therapeutic touch: How to use your hands to help or to heal.* New York: Prentice-Hall, Inc.

Kristjanson, L. J. (1989). Quality of terminal care: Salient indicators identified by families. *Journal of Palliative Care. 5* (1), 21–30.

Kübler-Ross, E. (1969). *On death and dying.* New York: Macmillan.

Lambrecht, M. E. (1990). The value of computer-assisted instruction in death education. *Loss, Grief, and Care. 4* (1–2), 67–70.

Leibenluft, E., Green, S. A., & Giese, M. D. (1988). Mourning and milieu: Staff reaction to the death of an inpatient. *The Psychiatric Hospital. 19* (4), 169–173.

Lev, E. L. (1986). Effects of course in hospice nursing: Attitudes and behaviors of baccalaureate school of nursing undergraduates and graduates. *Psychological Reports. 59* (2, pt. 2), 847–858.

Livingston, P., & Zimet, C. (1965). Death anxiety, authoritarianism and choice of specialty in medical students. *Journal of Nervous and Mental Disease. 140,* 222–230.

Lockard, B. E. (1989). Immediate, residual, and long-term effects of a death education instructional unit on the death anxiety level of nursing students. *Death Studies. 13* (2), 137–159.

Logan, M. (1988). Care of the terminally ill includes the family. *Canadian Nurse. 84* (5), 30–32.

MacInnis, K. (1992). Making goodbyes. *American Journal of Nursing. 92* (3), 120.

Mandel, H. R., (1981). Nurses' feelings about working with the dying. *American Journal of Nursing. 81* (6), 1194–1197.

Martinson, I., Adams, D. W., Deck, E., Folta, J., & Bates, T. (1988). Statement on care of the dying and bereaved in developing countries. *Death Studies. 12* (4), 353–358.

Mechanic, D., & Aiken, L. (1982). A cooperative agenda for medicine & nursing. *New England Journal of Medicine. 307*, 747–750.

Moller, D. W. (1990). *On death without dignity, the human impact of technical dying.* Amityville, NY: Baywood Publishing.

National Commission on Nursing. (1981). *Initial report and preliminary recommendations.* Chicago, IL.

Noyes, R., & Clancy, J. (1977). The dying role: Its relevance to improved patient care. *Psychiatry*, February, *40*, 41–47.

Nugent, L. S. (1988). The social support requirements of family caregivers of terminal cancer patients. *The Canadian Journal of Nursing Research. 20* (3), 45–58.

Parkes, C. M. (1986). The caregiver's griefs. *Journal of Palliative Care. 1* (2), 5–7.

Parry, J. K., & Smith, M. J. (1985). *The hospice: Physical, psychosocial, and pastoral care of the dying. 1* (3), 37–49.

Peace, H. G., & Vincent, P. A. (1988). Death Anxiety: Does education make a difference? *Death Studies. 12* (4), 337–344.

Plovnick, M., Fry, R., & Rubin, I. (1977). *Managing health care delivery: A training program for primary care physicians.* Cambridge, MA: Bellinger.

Power, K. G., & Sharp, G. R. (1988). A comparison of sources of nursing stress and job satisfaction among mental handicap and hospice nursing staff. *Journal of Advanced Nursing. 13* (6), 726–732.

President's Commission for the Study of Ethical Problems in Medicine and Biomedical and Behavioral Research. (1983). *Making health care decisions: The ethical and legal implications of informed consent in the patient–practitioner relationship.* Washington, DC: Government Printing Office.

Pruyser, P. W. (1984). Existential impact of professional exposure to life-threatening or terminal illness. *Bulletin of the Menninger Clinic. 48* (4), 357–367.

Quint, J. C. (1967). *The nurse and the dying patient.* New York: Macmillan.

Qvarnstrom, U. (1988). International standards provide guidelines for curriculum content. *Journal of Palliative Care. 4* (1–2), 38–40.

Research Activities (1991). Physicians, nurses and AIDS: Preliminary findings from a national study. June, No. 142, 2–3. Rockville, MD: Agency for Health Care Policy and Research Publications and Information Branch.

Rubin, I. M., & Beckhard. R. (1972). Factors influencing the effectiveness of health teams. *Milbank Memorial Fund Quarterly, 50,* 317–335.

Schultz, R., & Aderman, D. (1980). How the medical staff copes with dying patients: A critical review. In R. Kalish (Ed.), *Caring relationships: The dying and bereaved.* Amityville, NY: Baywood.

Shanfield, S. B. (1981). The mourning of the health care professional: An important element in education about death and loss. *Death Education. 4* (4), 385–395.

Skorupka, P., & Bohnet, N. (1982). Primary caregivers perceptions of nursing behaviors that best meet their needs in a homecare hospice setting. *Cancer Nursing. 5* (5), 371–374.

Small, M., Engler, A. J., & Rushton, C. H. (1991). Saying goodbye in the intensive care unit: Helping caregivers grieve. *Pediatric Nursing. 17* (1), 103–105.

Sonstegard, L., Hansen, N., Zillman, L., & Johnston, M. K. (1976). The grieving nurse. *American Journal of Nursing. 76* (9), 1490–1492.

Speer, G. M. (1974). Learning about death. *Perspectives in Psychiatric Nursing. 12* (2), 70–73.

Stevenson, R. (1987). Death in a context of open communication. In A Kutscher, A. Carr, & L. Kutscher (Eds.), *Principles of Thanatology.* New York: Columbia University Press.

Thomas, L. (1975). The technology of medicine. In L. Thomas (Ed.), *The lives of a cell: Notes of a biology watcher* (pp. 35–42). New York: Bantam Books.

Thompson, E. H. (1985–86). Palliative and curative care nurses' attitudes toward dying and death in the hospital setting. *Omega: Journal of Death and Dying. 16* (3), 233–242.

Thrush, J., Paulus, G., & Thrush, P. (1979). The availability of education on death and dying: A survey of U.S. Nursing Schools. *Death Education. 3* (2), 131–142.

Tolstoy, L. (1960). *The death of Ivan Ilych.* New York: New American Library.

Tosteson, D. (1990). New pathways in general medical education. *The New England Journal of Medicine. 322* (4), 234–238.

Toufexis, A., & Castronaro, V. (1983). Turning illness into a way of life. *Time,* April 18, p. 69.

Vachon, M. L. S. (1987). Team stress in palliative/hospice care. *Hospice Journal: Physical, psychosocial, and pastoral care of the dying. 3* (2/3), 75–103.

Wahl, C. (1959). The fear of death. In H. Feifel (Ed.), *The meaning of death.* New York: McGraw Hill.

Wallace, A. (1986). Teaching the human touch. *New York Times Magazine,* December 21, p. 22.

Waltman, N. L. (1990). Attitudes, subjective norms, and behavioral intentions of nurses toward dying patients and their families. *Oncology Nursing Forum. 17* (3), 55–62.

Welch, D. (1981). Planning nursing interventions for family members of adult cancer patients. *Cancer Nursing. 4* (5), 365–370.

Wheeler, C. E., & Chinn, P. L. (1989). *Peace and power: A handbook of feminist process* (2nd ed.). New York: National League for Nursing.

Weisman, A. (1974). Care and comfort for the dying. In S. Troup & W. Green (Eds.), *The patient, death and the family.* New York: Scribner's.

White, L. (1977). Death and physicians. In H. Feifel (Ed.), *New Meanings of Death.* New York: McGraw Hill.

Wise, H., Beckhard, R., Rubin, I., & Kyte, C. (1974). *Making health teams work.* Cambridge, MA: Ballinger.

Woolley, N. (1990). Crisis theory: A paradigm of effective intervention with families of critically ill people. *Journal of Advanced Nursing. 15* (12), 1402–1408.

Youll, J. W. (1989). The bridge beyond: Strengthening nursing practice in attitudes towards death, dying, and the terminally ill, and helping the spouses of critically ill patients. *Intensive Care Nursing. 5* (2), 88–94.

Ziegfeld, C., & Jones, S. (1987). An innovative strategy to facilitate nurse-physician interaction. *Journal of Continuing Education in Nursing. 18* (2), 47–50.

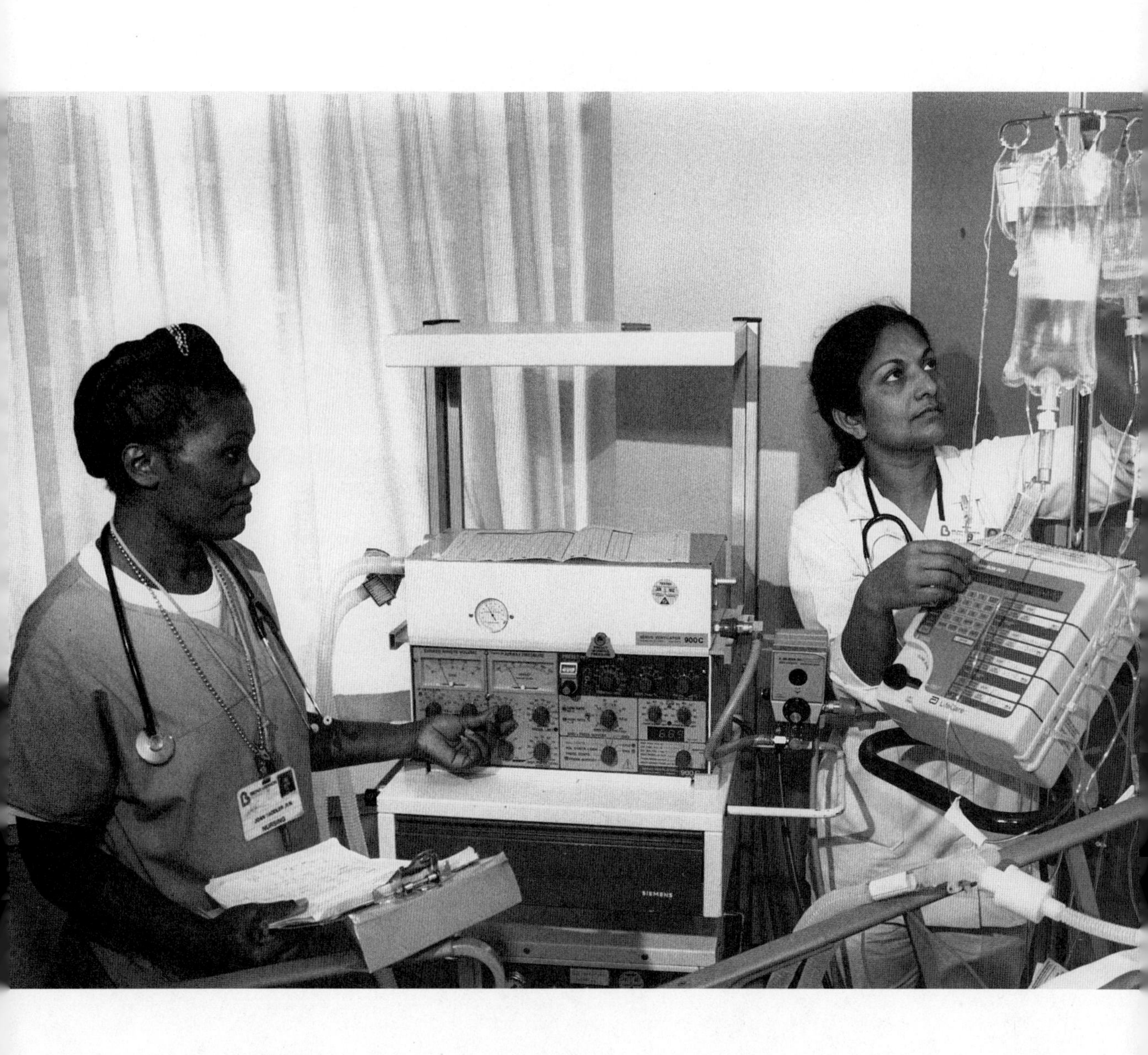
SERVO VENTILATOR 900C
SIEMENS

Chapter 4

Hospitals and Dying Patients

Most Americans will die in some type of health care or health-related institution. The absence of multigenerational and extended family units, coupled with high technology and beliefs of controlling mortality, have contributed to this institutionalization of dying in the United States. In addition, the medicalization of major human transition experiences, such as birth, old age, and death, has led to more people seeking help in coping with these experiences from experts frequently practicing in institutions.

Califano (1986) states that "America is at the dawn of the first four-generation society in the history of the world; we will soon become a society in which it will be common to have two generations of the same family in retirement, on Social Security, on Medicare, in the hospital" (p. 177). The implications of these social and demographic changes are immense in terms of restructuring the health care system, allocating resources within it, and perhaps in ultimately answering the question of who lives and who dies. Although these health policy issues will significantly affect all our lives, what becomes an immediate priority when dying patients enter institutions is the care they want and need.

This chapter discusses the influences affecting the provision of that care. It includes the interactions of health care providers among patients and families and among themselves, and the effects of cultural beliefs, organizational structure, and institutional values on caregiving. Challenges for changes in policy affecting the care of dying patients are offered. It is recognized that hospitals, nursing homes, and hospices all provide significant caregiving for dying patients; however, since most patients enter acute care hospitals as their initial experience in institutions, the discussion is centered on the hospital.

Photo courtesy of Bronx-Lebanon Hospital Center

Evolution of Hospital Care

The earliest hospitals existed as the healing temples of ancient Egypt, followed by the public hospitals of Buddhist India and the Muslim East. The modern hospital of the Western world has evolved from European medieval institutions with the same name but different functions (Burling, Lentz, & Wilson, 1956). In their origin, these hospitals did not have patient cure as their primary goal; in actuality, they were not concerned with the care of the sick at all. During the religious pilgrimages in the Age of Faith, many travelers were in need of overnight lodgings, but there were no commercial inns or hotels. Religious organizations, supported by the gifts of wealthy parishioners, met this need by establishing inns and lodging houses called *hospitals*, a name derived from the Latin *hospes*, meaning "host." Gradually these hospitals began to take in the homeless and the poor within the cities and provide more permanent lodging for them. The original hospitals, then, were not for the practice of medicine nor were they even concerned with the care of the sick. However, as many of the poor and homeless seeking refuge in the hospitals were physically ill, some kind of nursing care, and eventually medical care, was provided. The provision of such care was minimal and haphazard, and the hospitals were crowded and unsanitary. The hazards to health were usually greater in the hospital than in the home, and admission to these institutions was frequently regarded as a disgrace (Commission on Hospital Care, 1957, p. 424). Religion and religious orders continued to have an influence on the development of hospital care. Wars also contributed to this development, as care was needed for those who became sick or wounded in battle.

In the eighteenth century, there were still many people who believed that the only possible place for recovery from disease was in the natural environment of social life, the family. The ill person at home was freely exposed to all the natural curative and caring aspects of family life—the benevolence, the comfort, the consolation. Physicians made home visits and family members nursed the ill person. Added benefits of this "home care" were that the cost of sickness to the nation was reduced to a minimum, and the risk of the disease spreading to a large hospital population was avoided. Current "modern" ideas of home care and the hospice movement (see Chapter 5) were already being practiced 200 years ago.

> Generally speaking, it might be said that up to the end of the eighteenth century medicine related much more to health than to normality; it did not begin by analyzing a "regular" functioning of the organism and go on to seek where it had deviated, what it was disturbed by, and how it could be brought back into normal working order; it referred, rather, to qualities of vigor, suppleness, and fluidity, which were lost in illness and which it was the task of medicine to

> restore. To this extent, medical practice could accord an important place to regimen and diet, in short, to a whole rule of life and nutrition that the subject had imposed upon himself. This privileged relation between medicine and health involved the possibility of being one's own physician (Foucault, 1973, p. 35).

Nineteenth-century medicine, on the other hand, was regulated more in accordance with normality than with health (Foucault, 1973, p. 35). Pathological anatomy—utilization of autopsies to ascertain the focal point of disease—and scientific and technological advances focused the experience of medicine on pathological reactions, physiological knowledge, and on diagnosis and intervention. Florence Nightingale's recognition of the relationship between filth and hospital death rates, Pasteur's work with bacteria, Lister's work with antisepsis, and the popularity of "trained nurses" and their use of aseptic techniques were among the major factors that helped the hospital to become a safer place.

By 1890 most hospitals had established schools for nurses, recognizing that the apprenticeship system of nursing education in which student nurses cared for patients in exchange for clinical experience provided an almost cost-free labor force (Ashley, 1976). At that time medical students did not have access to such clinical experience, but with the growth and development of medicine as a science, medical educators became acutely aware of the need to use the hospital as a laboratory for the study of disease.

During the last few years of the nineteenth century, a new medicine and teaching developed, based on careful observation of patients and broader theoretical teaching. For the clinical experience of medical students and for the advancement of medical and scientific knowledge, it was necessary for hospitals to reorganize their structure to include teaching and research functions. This reorganization, however, did not affect the nursing apprentice system, which was continued. Having a school of nursing remained a popular and inexpensive means of providing patient care. It was not until much later that the nursing profession established its own educational system in academic settings away from the hospitals and the apprentice system. The focus of nursing, however, continued to be the care of patients.

Foucault (1973) suggests that the turning point in medical knowledge that influenced the goals of the hospital came during the last years of the eighteenth century. The new philosophy of medicine could be demonstrated by the difference in a basic question: "What is the matter with you?" was what the eighteenth-century doctor asked the patient; it was now replaced by the other question: "Where does it hurt?" (Foucault, 1973, p. xviii). The latter question focuses on the idea of a cause-and-effect relationship of disease, with the implication that once these are determined, intervention can proceed. The "cure" orientation for medicine and hospitals was established. Hospitals thus have evolved from being providers of lodging for travelers—and a last resort for the poor, helpless, and dying—to being centers that serve communities for both minor and major illnesses. They also serve as sources of private initiative, teaching, research, and for many communities, employment.

What then, are the structures, values, and norms of a health care institution with a cure orientation, and how does a dying person, someone who cannot be "cured," receive care within such an institution? In answering these questions, it is helpful to look at the determinants of the type of care dying patients receive in institutions. These determinants include hospital goals and structure, role expectations, caregivers' responses to dying patients, patients' social class and status, and dying trajectories.

Hospital Goals and Structures

According to Goss (1978), the goal that all hospitals share is the provision of medical services aimed at cure, amelioration, and prevention of disease in individuals (p. 277). The curing goal of hospital care today reflects the American culture's contemporary concepts of illness. There is a general belief that health and physical well-being are ends worth pursuing, and that they are possible to attain (Mumford, 1967, p. 32). Illness is regarded as a mishap, something that can be overcome, and health care professionals are expected to help people get well when illness occurs. As a people, Americans believe that there should be a new and better way for doing everything, and that there must be a way to solve each problem. Ambiguity is not well tolerated; there is a certainty that an answer can be found to conflicting situations. These beliefs about life, health, and illness have stimulated many people in the United States to concentrate their energies and attention on the healing arts and sciences, and they are reflected in the consistent emergence of significant technological and scientific knowledge. Hospitals, as organizations of people in this culture, also reflect these beliefs and values.

Hospitals as Bureaucracies

Many hospitals, because of their increase in size as well as the quantity and quality of services offered, high client turnover, and tendencies toward increased specialization, have become formal bureaucracies. Merton (1969) describes bureaucracy in terms of organizational goals and structure as "a formal, rationally organized social structure involving clearly defined patterns of activity in which, ideally, every series of actions is functionally related to the purposes of the organization" (p. 47). A bureaucracy is an organization that is set up so that its goals will be met efficiently.

Professional caregivers working within a hospital bureaucratic system are involved in two dimensions of authority—professional and bureaucratic

—both of which are important to the hospital's functioning but which may also lead to conflicts for caregivers. Professional authority lies within the person who has the freedom and responsibility to make assessments and decisions about patient care based on professional skill and knowledge.

Bureaucratic authority emphasizes adherence to procedures, tasks, and rules, and these processes may assume more value than patient care. Caregivers working within such a structure may encounter conflicts between what they professionally assess is necessary for the quality of their patients' care and what hospital policy dictates. A physician may want to keep a terminally ill patient in the hospital for treatment longer than rules and payment policies dictate. A nurse, allowing a dying woman's young children on the unit to visit, is acting against a hospital visiting policy. The conflict and frustration in such situations are real; the solutions not often easily found.

If the goal of the hospital bureaucracy is to cure people, then what happens to those patients who cannot be cured? Mauksch (1975) points out:

> The dying patient represents a series of human events where the needs of the patient cease to be translatable into routines and rituals. It is in this fundamental sense that the dying patient threatens the hospital and its personnel. The routine orders, the predictable activities, when applied to the dying patient, cease to be meaningful, cease to be effective, and above all, cease to be satisfying either to the people doing them or to the patients who receive them. (pp. 9–10).

Professional caregivers and hospital administrators can work together to establish a structure that will support both organizational and professional goals and provide the important flexibility needed for dying patients to receive the individualized care they need. The multiple lines of authority within the hospital, traditionally maintained by the bureaucratic concept of power-over, might be melded by the concept of power sharing. Power sharing involves the sharing of responsibility for decision making and for acting on those decisions in a lateral network rather than in a hierarchical one.

It is possible now to begin to understand some of the conflicts and problems that develop for hospitalized dying patients and for the people who provide care for them. Within a bureaucratic organization with cultural beliefs that something can be done about illness and with expectations that the modern hospital, with all its advanced knowledge, can diagnose and cure, staff and dying patients are now confronted with the uncomfortable ambiguity of death.

Care and Cure Work

There frequently are no definitive answers to offer dying patients about the time and manner of their death, what it will be like, and why this is happening to them. Caregivers, who are used to providing answers, may find this vagueness unacceptable to their professional identities. Caregivers may also feel that they have failed because perhaps they did not do enough for the patient. They may ask themselves whether they explored every possible treatment for this person. They may carefully review everything they did with the patient, for there can often be a haunting doubt that an error was committed that may have contributed to the death (Mauksch, 1975). Caregivers may also grieve, and as discussed in Chapter 3, it is important to remember that there are many occasions when grief is just as normal a reaction for staff as it is for patients and relatives.

Patients may feel angry because their expectations for help and for care are not being met. At a time when they are reaching out for acknowledgement of their uncertainty and fear, patients are often confronted with a myriad of tests they may not understand and an army of caregivers, none of whom they may see more than once or twice. Much of the care that dying patients require falls into categories of comfort work and sentimental work (Strauss, Fagerhaugh, Suczek, & Wiener, 1985). Comfort work is directed toward alleviating the aches, pains, nausea, and other physical discomforts associated with terminal illness. Sentimental work provides recognition of the person as a sentient human being.

This type of caring work is not valued as highly as medical or technological work. In the achievement-oriented culture of the United States, not much prestige is associated with the task per se of *caring* for patients (Coser, 1963). Caring is perhaps also undervalued because it is associated with "women's work." People who are entering nursing, a predominantly women's profession with care as its foundation, often are asked, "Why are you doing that? A smart person like you should be a doctor!"

The question reflects the values and status of care vs. cure. The cure orientation of health care practice is demonstrated in a study done by Mumma & Benoliel (1984–85). These researchers investigated the relationship of the cause of dying, length of hospital stay, and age to medical treatment orientation and the amount of work expended. The study findings show that the medical treatment orientation was overwhelmingly toward the cure end of the care–cure continuum, despite the fact that the majority of patients had conditions labeled by their physicians as terminal and had been designated to receive no CPR (cardiopulmonary resuscitation). Cassell (1976) noted that:

> the dying patient in the modern hospital is in an environment ideally suited for the pursuit of knowledge and cure, but representing in its technology and idealized representative—the young doctor—technical values virtually antithetical to the holistic concept of person. This does not imply that the most personal and humane care cannot be and is not given in such hospitals, but rather that those who do give such

> care must struggle against their technical depersonalized thinking about the body, and against the structure of the hospital that such thought has produced (pp. 459–460).

However, the differences in value emphasis between care work and cure work may be not only those of ethics and technology but also those of financial reimbursement to the institution for services provided to patients. Diagnosis-Related Groups (DRGs) were adopted by Congress in 1983 to deal with spiraling health care costs. DRGs were devised to provide incentives for cost containment. Hospitals are paid a predetermined price for their services, a price based on the average cost of treating a patient with a particular diagnosis (Dolenc & Dougherty, 1985). They cannot charge what they want, not even what their services cost, and are reimbursed only for what the DRGs allow. Prospective payment financing introduces the question of whether patient diagnosis, treatment, and discharge are influenced by considerations other than provision of quality care. Benoliel (1987–88) suggests that the initiation of predetermined reimbursement for health care based on established diagnostic categories (DRGs) has fostered profit-oriented corporate hospital care, which emphasizes efficiency of operation and a patient-as-product orientation to services (p. 355).

There are no DRGs for comfort and sentimental work. Indeed, such work may not be seen as professional work at all but as the duty of the family. Financial rewards for the institution and organizational rewards for the staff come from effectiveness and efficiency in the technological work directed towards a cure. With this emphasis, the human experience of dying becomes subsumed by the technological order in which it occurs (Charmaz, 1980, p. 104).

Care and cure in health care institutions need not be mutually exclusive, but as long as cure assumes higher priority, status, and rewards, it will remain the primary emphasis and goal for the staff and the organization. However, dying patients and their families may have different perspectives from the staff in regard to treatment goals and trajectories. Staff may also have various expectations for patients and for each other. Such differences in expectations and perspectives within an institution can affect patient care.

Role Expectations

For each position (patient, nurse, doctor, aide, social worker) in a social organization such as a hospital, there are some expectations about what the person in that position is supposed to do. "These include the rights and privileges that go with the position and also the obligations and duties" (Mumford, 1967, p. 57). The combination of expectations about what one is supposed to do in such a position is called the *role*. Examples of role expectations in a hospital setting are: patients follow doctors' orders, nurses administer medications, aides make beds, social workers talk to families and assist in aftercare planning. Conflicts may arise among people when their ideas of fulfilling their roles do not coincide; patients may disagree with doctors' orders, and nurses may ask patients to administer their own medications. Such conflicts can lead to further clarification, understanding, and development of roles, or they can result in an impasse among participants, with a possible detriment to patient care.

The Sick Role

Society has created a special role for sick people. Role expectations for the ill include the right to be dependent, to accept help from strangers, and to expect to be helped. People who are ill in a hospital are expected to conform to the rules and regulations of its bureaucratic structure. In their study of a large medical center's functioning, Duff & Hollingshead (1968) state:

> Between admission to and discharge from the hospital, the patients were subject to the orders of the staff. They were separated from their families. Their street clothes were shed. They were assigned to beds, given numbers, and dressed in bedroom apparel. They had to permit strangers access to the most intimate parts of their bodies. Their diet was controlled, as were the hours of their days and nights, the people they saw, and the times they saw them. They were bathed, fed, and questioned; they were ordered or forbidden to do specified things. As long as they were in the hospital they were not considered self-sufficient adults (p. 269).

Although the dying role is less frequently discussed than the sick role, it has been reviewed in the professional literature in regard to behavioral expectations of the dying. Noyes & Clancy (1977) define the dying role as including the expectations that the dying person will continue to wish to live, make use of available supportive measures and persons, decrease dependence upon the physician, accept loss of freedom and privileges, cooperate with the rules and routines of caregivers, and maintain independent functioning to the limit of abilities. Rights of dying patients include their right to be cared for in an appropriate setting by personnel who regard their needs as having high priority (p. 45).

However, Thompson (1984) asserts that for many people the phenomenon of dying in a sterile, institutionalized hospital setting attached to life-support machines has obscured the boundaries between death, personhood, and individual rights. This situation relegates the dying person to a secondary role in her own death; the control shifts from the person to the outside environment. Ill or dying people who are at home still have some control over their environment. They may decide when they will eat and sleep and may be responsible for taking their own medicine. They may still retain their family roles of parent, child, grandparent, and so on, and are still usually included in family decision making and planning.

Once people enter the hospital as patients, they lose their normal social roles and must learn to interact in a totally alien environment. Patients need to learn what questions to ask of whom; in order to do this, they must understand the division of labor in the hospital and the staff status hierarchy. Questions about prognosis will most likely be answered by doctors; nurses will respond to questions about hospital policy and rules; and nurses' aides are people who will give the most realistic information about the ward routine and how things really get done! Patients will need to learn the jargon of the hospital before they can comprehend what is expected of them in this new role. If a patient is simply told that he may have pain medication "prn," the patient may have no idea that this means pain medication is available as needed.

Patients from countries other than the United States may well have their own cultural role behaviors associated with illness and have no idea what role expectations are in this country. Caregivers who expect patients to conform to established sick and dying role behaviors may consider them complainers, noncompliant, or attention seekers. Patients who have English as a second language may be at particular risk for misunderstanding established treatment protocols and for being misunderstood by caregivers. However, as one patient explained to a nurse, "Just because I'm from a foreign country and have an accent, doesn't mean that I'm dumb!"

Role Perceptions Related to Bureaucracy

Role expectations may also be related to perceptions of where and how people "fit" in the hospital hierarchy and may influence how care is given and received. Do caregivers perceive patients as being at the top of the totem pole, as important people for whom mobilization of professional resources are needed to assist them physically and emotionally? Or are patients seen at the bottom of the system's hierarchy, as people who should do as they are told and who will receive services as directed by staff? Coser (1962) points out that "as an ideology, hospital staff adhere to the belief that concern for the Patient (with a capital "P") as a total person is the mainstay of their practice but that in reality, the individual patient tends to remain an object or a case" (p. 34). With this latter orientation, the patient is seen, not as a person in a strange environment who is ill and frequently in a state of physical and mental powerlessness, struggling to maintain autonomy, identity, and respect, but as someone to be "managed"—as one would manage a thing rather than a human being.

Excerpts from a letter written by a patient to hospital staff summarize the preceding statements quite candidly.

2:00 A.M.

12 December 79

To all who care about patients:

1979, for me, was a year filled with much pain and agony, trauma and shock, sadness and hurt, setbacks, recoveries, happiness, and hope. I've overdone my time here at the hospital . . . I was admitted with lower body pains and as a result of an overactive spinal tumor and many complications I'm now a paraplegic. I spent a wonderful month of October at home for the first time since November '78 only to have to return to the hospital again. Hopefully I'll be honorably and permanently discharged next week and with some home physical therapy and outpatient chemotherapy, I aim to stay there for a while.

Enough history, though I hope just the right amount to sufficiently prove that I've had ample experience in the role of patient. Speaking medically, I was well taken care of by many competent doctors and outstanding nurses, though many isolated incidents irreparably tarnished the view of doctor as omnipotent and patient (me) as blind obeyer. I started asking many questions, getting unsatisfactory or evasive answers, and then finally learning the truth, which generally was not pleasant. . . .

I still question; I still complain; and I grieve over what I think is one of the **WORST** problems in this hospital and probably in other large institutions . . . that patients are looked at and treated by many just as Case #16, Disease #12, Temperature 38. Do you know what it feels like to wake up to 12 pairs of eyes (rounds) staring at you in the morning, or one pair shaking you awake at 2:00 A.M. and in both cases, "and how are you today?" In one case, I don't know yet as I was sleeping; in the other, it had taken me an hour to finally fall asleep and what am I supposed to say now?! Ever have a hematoma (black and blue in street language) on your arm, a foot long, and they still insist on taking blood from the same place? Ever been emotionally upset, drained, about surgery, and then going through ups and downs of rescheduling and canceling? not to mention the anxiety of the families too? It's all happened, that and more, again and again, to me!! There's a problem here that many forget, that **PATIENTS ARE PEOPLE, TOO!** . . . like any other people, except we're suffering in some way and that makes us oversensitive and less tolerant. We've no privacy of body or soul; closed curtains don't often stop the uninvited from entering. How many patients know that there is a document stating patient rights? How about some compassion; a smile? Just sacrifice some mechanical performance and call me by my name! Show concern for me and not just for my liver!

Staff and patients may also have different perceptions of the purposes of the hospital, which can cause different expectations about their roles and hospital functions. In her study of physician–client relationships in a medical center, Roberts (1977) found that medical students, interns, and residents felt that the first purpose for their being in that setting was education; patients, on the other hand, felt that since this was a hospital, its obvious purpose was to provide for their care and treatment (pp. 45–46). Such differences in perceptions of purposes may result, for example, in patients expecting one physician (intern or resident) to care for them throughout their hospital stay, while the reality may be that in order to acquire learning, several physicians may be involved in their care.

Negotiating Roles

However, although the hospital purposes and bureaucratic rules and regulations may be different from patients' expectations, there is some leeway in how policies are interpreted. Staff and patients are involved in ongoing negotiation processes within the hospital structure. For example, physicians seeking hospital admission for their patients may be told by admissions personnel that no beds are available. The physicians may then negotiate: if they discharge one of their patients the next morning, the new patient may be admitted. A physician and a nurse may negotiate regarding treatment plans for a particular patient, each having a different plan and both trying to arrive at a unified approach.

Patients enter the negotiating process also; they may negotiate for information that is important to their own understanding of their illness or for a treatment that fits their life-style. Ideally, any treatment plan is made by caregivers in collaboration with patients. However, dying patients and their families may have to negotiate a great deal with staff in order to receive the care and treatment they desire. Why does this occur?

Caregivers' Responses to Dying Patients

In the hospital the idea of dying may label a patient and place a frame of interpretation around a person (Sudnow, 1967). Dying patients may be assigned a private room at the end of the corridor, away from other patients and the nurses' station. This is ostensibly for the patient's peace, quiet, and privacy, but a closer analysis could indicate the staff's unwillingness to be in contact with that patient. Once the patient is admitted, staff may find many reasons not to go into that room at the end of the hall unless absolutely necessary. These reasons may be that they are "Too busy," or

"Other clients are more sick," or "I'll spend time there tomorrow." "We speak often of the loneliness of dying patients and they are indeed lonely, for not only are they going where no one wants to follow but also the people around them prefer to pretend that the journey is not really going to happen" (Morison, 1973, p. 57).

In working with dying patients, staff must often function within a network of ambiguous definitions of what might be done, what should be done, what must be done (Duff & Hollingshead, 1968, p. 307). As discussed in Chapter 2, caregivers consider conflicting questions as to what extent evasions, misrepresentations, or untruths should be used to "protect" the patient and the family, and to what extent a disease should be treated. Patients also deal with conflicting questions such as: "Is the physician telling me all I need to know, or should I ask about my illness? If I ask, will I be realistically answered? If I get an answer, should I tell my family? Will the physician tell my family?" Family members may ask the physician not to disclose information to the patient for fear of emotional upset. Pretenses about the fatality of an illness are not so easy to maintain as the illness advances in severity. Patients begin to question the more frequent, longer visits of their families and their increased kindness and solicitude. Patients ask more questions about their illnesses that often evoke even greater pretenses on the part of family and staff. Eventually patients may tire of trying to get answers, and they live out the rest of their lives without discussing their impending death with any other person. The result of such situations is the isolation of all the people involved, and the most isolated person is the patient.

Effects of Who Knows What

Whether or not patients have been told about their dying, and who knows what about the matter, has a definite effect on the interactions between staff and patients in hospitals. In their book *Awareness of Dying,* Glaser & Strauss (1965) discuss "awareness context," a term that "refers to who, in the dying situation, knows what about the probabilities of death for the dying patient" (p. ix). Their research suggests that, depending upon who knows what, there are discernible and predictable patterns of interaction between dying patients, families, and staff. Glaser & Strauss identified four typical awareness contexts: (a) closed, (b) suspected, (c) mutual pretense, and (d) open (p. 11).

In **closed awareness**, patients do not know they are going to die, even though everyone else does. Staff interactional patterns in this awareness context are based on a fictitious approach to patients in that patients must be led to believe that their illnesses are not fatal and that things will turn out "all right."

In **suspected awareness**, the patient suspects what others know and tries to confirm or negate that suspicion. Patients in this awareness context seem always to be on the offensive in trying to get realistic information from a defensive staff. This is a very uncomfortable and unstable state for patients as there is no consensual validation of their perceptions with staff and vagueness and insecurity persist.

The **mutual pretense** context exists when all people involved know that the patient is dying but all in some way tacitly agree to act as if this is not so. There are various rules to follow in playing the mutual pretense game. Dangerous topics, such as the patient's death, are avoided. Safe topics are permissible for discussion; these may include chatter about the events on the ward, sleeping and eating habits, the weather, social and political events. Safe topics are those that signify that life is proceeding as usual.

The context of **open awareness** exists when all people involved acknowledge openly their knowledge that the patient is dying. Staff and patients may have different expectations of each other in terms of the dying process, but one of the positive aspects of open awareness is that these discrepancies can be discussed. Awareness of impending death gives patients a chance to close their lives with some control. They can plan for their family, finish projects, say farewell to friends. They can play a part in managing their own deaths. However, caregivers themselves may have difficulty in participating in open awareness and in caring relationships with patients.

Attitudes and Coping Responses

To understand the difficulty some caregivers may have in providing care rather than cure and in not informing patients of their dying, it becomes important once again to go back to the cultural expectations of the helping professions and of hospitals in the United States. Treatment of disease is expected; caregivers are expected "to do" something. Miracles are looked for instead of death. Knight & Field (1981) observed that failure to inform dying patients that they are dying persists for a number of reasons: physicians and nurses claim that not telling protects the patient from depression and anxiety. In addition, there may be genuine uncertainty with regard to both outcome and time of death. As discussed in Chapter 3, health caregivers own orientations to death are also important determining factors in their provision of care.

Caregivers must understand that they are a part of a society that does not readily recognize death. Unless they make a conscious effort to look at their own attitudes toward death and dying, they may be unaware of how these attitudes influence their care of dying patients. Caregivers' responses to dying patients, the goals and structure of the hospital, role expectations, and whether or not staff discuss diagnoses with patients will all influence patient care. Patients' social class and status may also influence not only their care but also how and when they die.

Determinants of the Care of Dying Patients

Sudnow (1967) discusses the rather strong relationship between the age, social background, and perceived moral character of patients brought into an emergency room and the amount of effort that is made to attempt revival when "clinical death signs" are detected (p. 103). Once patients arrive at the hospital, the older they are the more likely it is that tentative death will be accepted without resuscitation. Sudnow's study at a county hospital revealed that efforts at revival of patients brought into the emergency room were admittedly superficial with the exception of attempts to revive the very young or occasional wealthy patients who by some accident were brought to the county emergency room (p. 103). Sudnow also found that at private, wealthier hospitals, the overall attention given to patients who were initially dead was greater than that given to patients in the public county hospital.

The shift from retrospective to prospective reimbursement for medical and hospital systems has pressured hospitals to become more prospective in interactions with patients concerning reimbursement (Dugan, 1987, p. 131). Hospital emergency room staff may raise the issue of payment with patients and families concurrent with, or even prior to, the initial treatment interaction. Regardless of diagnosis, hospitals are financially rewarded for saving time and minimizing treatment procedures. Such financial pressures initiated public concern that patients who could not pay might not be treated and might be "dumped," or transferred to public hospitals or even discharged without treatment. The 1986 federal Emergency Medical Treatment & Active Labor Act forbids hospitals receiving Medicaid money from turning away women in active labor or any other patient in an unstablized condition (U.S. is Putting Patient Dumping . . . 1991). The law stresses that transfers cannot be based on economic reasons.

Caregivers also may provide different types of care to dying patients based on prejudged moral character and on perceptions of the patient's social value. Thus:

> The moribund patient who appears to be of low social class, is shabbily dressed, unwashed, or smells of alcohol, seems to be less likely to receive vigorous attempts at resuscitation, as will the patient with perceived social deviancy—the addict, the suicide, and the vagrant. On the other hand, the great and powerful—like Generalissimo Franco—may be denied the possibility of an unharassed death and may receive bizarrely prolonged and desperate resuscitation attempts (Simpson, 1979, p. 111).

Lasagna (1970) found that the treatment of patients varies according to the social acceptability of the patient as defined by the staff: wealthier people are treated better than poor people; young people better than old people; nonalcoholics better than alcoholics.

Patients with AIDS

That patient treatment may be influenced by social class and status has particular relevancy for patients with AIDS, who must also cope with the stigma society has placed upon them. Cecchi (1986) notes that for many people with AIDS, every contact with the health care delivery system has a potential for a confrontation: for example, ambulance drivers may refuse to transport patients (p. 47). Although there has been a great deal of media attention on the incidence of AIDS among middle- and upper-middle-class Caucasian homosexual men, it is important to remember that 40 percent of persons with AIDS in the United States are members of minority groups (Fowler & Chaney, 1989, p. 228).

Opportunities to choose and reject treatment need to be available to everyone. The issue has been raised of staff recommending AIDS patients sign a Do Not Resuscitate (DNR) consent form on their first visit to the emergency room. This may convey to AIDS patients a message of treatment futility. Nurses have advocated that DNR orders be discussed with patients as part of their care plan, but not at the initial treatment evaluation when little yet is known about patients and their responses to the disease (Bennett, 1987).

Dying Trajectories

Patients' dying trajectories may influence the care given to them in a hospital. Dying trajectories (as discussed in Chapter 2) are *projected* courses of dying; yet a trajectory will, to a large extent, determine where and how a patient will be treated in a hospital. If the patient is admitted via the emergency room (ER), the dying trajectory will be defined there. Patients who are near death may either be treated in the ER, be sent to surgery, or be admitted to an intensive care unit. If the evaluation is that the person may live, care in these areas is concentrated, quick, and efficient, and staff is geared to providing heroic measures to save lives.

Patients who enter the hospital with chronic illnesses or with problems that are not yet diagnosed have more uncertain dying trajectories. They often are sent to medical units where staff and organization of work allow time for establishing diagnoses and dying trajectories. Although such units are more closely geared to providing longer-term care for the dying than in the emergency and intensive care units, staff may still have difficulty in providing this care.

Terminal care may be seen by some caregivers as monotonous and routine. Staff may feel helpless when there is nothing more they can do in terms of life-saving treatments; they may begin to avoid seeing and being with patients. Physicians may disengage with patients as palliative care becomes essentially a nursing prerogative. Conboy-Hill (1986) proposes that physicians may withdraw socially from dying patients while still providing adequate physical care because of their own fears of death or their perception of patient death as failure. However, Williams (1982) suggests that as the patient shifts from the sick to dying role, the nurse assumes the dominant complementary role as the initial dominant role of the physician diminishes. "Although both professions carry responsibilities in the primary domain of the other, the domain of medicine is therapy and treatment, whereas the domain of nursing is care and support" (p. 9). Often when the treatment emphasis shifts from cure to care, patients are discharged from the hospital.

Alternatives to Hospital Care

If patients' illnesses become stabilized and dying trajectories are established that indicate longer-term care than an acute care setting with prospective payments can provide, discharge planning is initiated. Ideally, this planning involves a collaborative effort between hospital staff, patients, and families. It includes assessment of patient and family needs, strengths, resources, and support systems, and attempts to match these with available community resources if these are needed. Hospice care is one alternative to hospital care and is discussed in Chapter 5. Other alternatives include home care, nursing homes, terminal care facilities, and supportive housing.

Home Care

Many patients want to return home, and express a wish to die there. What is important to determine in this decision is what resources are available to carry out the treatment plan while leaving as much control as possible in the patient's hands. Family, friends, and lovers may be supportive of caring for patients at home, but often because of two-career families, single-parent families, and people living alone, this may be difficult. Medicare provides for limited home care service after hospital discharge based on an evaluation of the patient's skilled nursing and rehabilitation needs. Such services can include skilled nursing visits, a home health aide, and physical and occupational therapy if needed. However, when the patient's needs are no longer assessed as requiring acute care, Medicare coverage may cease. Patients must then pay for home care services on their own or find community resources to assist them.

For-profit home health care agencies have proliferated over the past few years. Individual health insurance policies vary a great deal in terms of home care coverage. Some policies provide no nursing or home health aid coverage at all; others provide for such coverage if the need is justified by a physician.

Reimbursement for equipment, supplies, and medication is also variable. Medicaid coverage of services varies from state to state and by locality within each state. In New York City, Medicaid in the past would provide a home health aide for 24 hours, seven days a week, but at this writing this provision is undergoing careful scrutiny. Depending on the patient's nursing needs, it is possible that nursing home care might be less expensive than 24-hour nursing care at home. Based on cost-effectiveness, Medicaid payment may then be allocated for nursing home care rather for home care.

The resulting home care plans often represent a patchwork of independent systems stitched together to provide a treatment approach. Hospitals and health caregivers are attempting to provide more cohesive and comprehensive home care programs. Some hospitals have developed their own home care programs, with nursing staff assessing patient needs while they are in the hospital, coordinating their care at home after discharge, and assisting the family with bereavement after the patient dies.

However, there can come a time when home care is no longer feasible. The patient's nursing needs may intensify, or 24 hour nursing care may be more expensive than institutional care. The most obvious reason is often the exhaustion of family members who are primary caregivers. Nursing is hard work and it goes on day and night. Months of lifting, turning, bathing, and providing pain medication several times during the course of every night can take their toll. The emotional strain of "always being there" can be as energy depleting to a family caregiver as the intense physical care.

Nursing Homes

"What kind of person puts her mother in a nursing home? How can a family condemn Grandpa to an institution?" (Tisdale, 1988, p. 298). Nursing homes are often thought of as terrible places by many people in the United States, and "placing" a family member in one is frequently accompanied by feelings of guilt and shame. Benoliel (1979) noted that "the nursing home industry expanded rapidly after World War II to meet a growing demand for institutionalized services for the incapacitated elderly: these and other custodial services became places for the prolonged dying of individuals with low social value . . ." (p. 146).

But as the saying goes, "times have changed," and indeed nursing home care may be considered appropriate after all options are considered. While many people may enter the extended care facility of a nursing home only to leave it through death, other patients may use its skilled nursing facilities for a short time and leave. Rapid turnover of patients, unheard of five years ago in nursing homes, is becoming a reality. Nursing homes may also offer respite care for families taking care of patients at home.

One aspect of negative feelings associated with placing a relative in a nursing home concerns the fear that the patients are not well cared for, their needs not met. Assuaging that fear is difficult for family and friends feel no institution can replace their own care even though their options have run out. "Acceptance of what is," may be one coping mechanism to use while simultaneously serving as a motivator for many health caregivers and consumers to participate in changing the health care system to include more comprehensive terminal care through professional, community, and political action.

Terminal Care Facilities

Several charitable organizations established institutions to provide care for the terminally ill in the late 1800s. These include the seven facilities throughout the United States run by the Dominican Sisters of Hawthorne and Youville Hospital in Massachusetts.

St. Rose's Home, one of the Hawthorne facilities which is located in New York City, is an example of how these institutions function. St. Rose's is a 60-bed, skilled nursing facility for terminally ill people who cannot afford to pay for any health care services. Because it is funded entirely by public donations, the home does not have to address the issues of prospective payments and regulated use of hospital beds; patients may stay as long as it is necessary for them to receive comfort care.

Calvary Hospital, located in Bronx, New York, is the only fully accredited acute care specialty hospital for advanced cancer patients in the United States. Its mission is to provide palliative care, addressing the symptoms of the disease, not its cure. Calvary is a voluntary, not-for-profit hospital sponsored by the Archdiocese of New York. Founded in 1899 by several Catholic women, it is a 200-bed hospital with more than 650 employees. Any adult person who is diagnosed as having advanced cancer and needing medical services in an acute care setting is a candidate for admission. The hospital also has outpatient programs and a certified home health agency to provide home care services to support patients and their families at home.

Supportive Housing

The AIDS epidemic is straining an already inadequate health care system. People with AIDS can have frequent hospitalizations, resulting in great financial burdens that can leave them penniless and homeless. Dying trajectories are often indefinite. As treatment for the acute infections of AIDS continues to improve, the disease becomes more of a chronic one, and people with AIDS need supportive environments in which to live. Some communities have begun to address this issue. Bailey House in New York City is a six story group residence for 44 people with AIDS. A project of the AIDS Resource Center in New York City, Bailey House offers shelter, health monitoring, counseling, and social and pastoral support (Lone, 1989, p. 490). People may stay as long as they wish, and many choose to die there rather than return to the hospital. Providing supportive housing for people with AIDS is a major priority in health care.

SUMMARY ❧

The history of treatment for people in hospitals evolved over the centuries within a context of providing care and comfort. Nurses and physicians sustained people through distress, attempting to alleviate pain if possible and to offer hope. The twentieth century introduced highly specialized and technical medical procedures, which resulted in physicians organizing their practice around a cure orientation and hospitals structuring their goals to that of cure also. Nurses have continued to maintain their focus of practice within the caring domain.

The establishment of a prospective payment system, coupled with institutional goals of cure, create a tension between the individualized, personal, and interpersonal needs of dying people and the life-saving ethics and values of control and efficiency of the hospital environment. Other factors contributing to determinants of terminal care include staff and patients' role expectations, caregivers' responses to dying patients, patients' social class and status, and dying trajectories. Provision of terminal care may be viewed as a political act in that complex ongoing decisions must constantly be made as to allocation of scarce resources between living and dying patients.

Alternatives to hospital care for people who are dying include home care, nursing homes, terminal care facilities, and supportive housing. Patients, families, and health care professionals can continue to work together in developing and implementing new models and services for dying people that will provide a balance of technology and individualized care.

LEARNING EXERCISES ❧

1. Role play a patient and a nurse, a doctor, or a social worker interacting in each of Glaser & Strauss's awareness states.
2. Eight deaths:
   a. Mary—age 87—at home, after 15 years of feeling more or less "useless" due to aging condition and disabilities.
   b. George—age 69—suddenly, of a heart attack, still active in his job.
   c. Sam—age 72—in a nursing home, six months after his wife died.
   d. Carl—age 57—after four weeks in the hospital, having experienced a lot of pain, but having taken the opportunity to prepare family and close friends.

e. Henry—age 48—shot in the street by a random bullet coming out of a restaurant.
f. Betty—age 37—in an auto accident, leaving husband and two children.
g. Carrie—age 30—from a drug overdose.
h. Keith—age 23—after a kidney transplant and a long, heroic struggle in the hospital, where everybody on the staff loved him.

Choose the "best" death and the "worst" death from the preceding examples. Discuss the reasons for your choice.

3. Read the obituaries of a large city newspaper for one week. What does each obituary tell you about the potential availability, or ability of family to provide home care for a dying family member? What are the implications of your survey for health care policy changes?
4. Explore your community for alternative resources to hospital care for dying people. Are there facilities that are accessible and available to all people or are there restrictions for admission (finances, diagnosis, dying trajectory?)

AUDIOVISUAL MATERIAL ❧

Dying Wish. 52 min/videocassette. Films for the Humanities & Sciences. Box 2053, Princeton, N. J. 08543.
This video portrays how the advances in technology have redefined death and have presented family and professional staff with a new load of ethical, emotional, intellectual and legal dilemmas.

Terminal Illness: The Patient's Story. 28 min/videocassette. Films for the Humanities & Sciences. Box 2053, Princeton, NJ, 08543.
This is the story of Joan Robinson, who at 41 learned she had ovarian cancer. The film covers the last five years of her life and is an account of sorrow, love, and death.

Who Lives? Who Dies? 55 min/videocassette/1987. Filmakers Library, Inc., 124 E. 40 St., New York, NY, 10022.
This video explores many North American health care practices and values that result in an unequal distribution of health care benefits. Poor and uninsured people are ultimately the populations which pay the price for these inequities with an increase in serious illness. This is a video which serves as a consciousness-raiser.

Walk Me to the Water: Three People in Their Time of Dying. 16 min/black & white/film & videocassette/1985. Walk Me to the Water, P.O. Box 258, New Lebanon, NY 12125.

Through listening to the stories of Joe, Anna, and Marian, three people who are dying, viewers of this program learn how to appreciate the individuality and uniqueness of each person's death. Caregivers must take their cues from each patient as what level of help that patient will require in dying.

REFERENCES ❧

Ashley, J. (1976). *Hospitals, paternalism, and the role of the nurse.* New York: Teachers College Press.

Bennett, J. (1987). Nurses talk about the challenge of AIDS. *American Journal of Nursing. 87* (9), 1150–1155.

Benoliel, J. Q. (1979). Dying in an institution. In H. Wass (Ed.), *Dying; Facing the facts* (pp. 137–157). Washington, DC: Hemisphere Publishing Corporation.

Benoliel, J. Q. (1987–88). Health care providers and dying patients: Critical issues in terminal care. *Omega: Journal of Death and Dying. 18* (4), 341–363.

Burling, T., Lentz, E. M., & Wilson, R. N. (1956). *The give and take in hospitals.* New York: Putnam.

Califano, J. A., Jr. (1986). *America's health care revolution.* New York: Random House.

Cassell, E. J. (1976). Dying in a technological society. In C. Muscatine & M. Griffith (Eds.), *The borzoi college reader* (3rd ed., pp. 454–461). New York: Alfred Knopf.

Cecchi, R. (1986). Living with AIDS: When the system fails. *American Journal of Nursing. 86* (1), 45–47.

Charmaz, K. (1980). *The social reality of death.* Reading, MA: Addison-Wesley.

Commission on Hospital Care. (1957). *Hospital care in the United States.* Cambridge, MA: Harvard University Press.

Conboy-Hill, S. (1986). Psychosocial aspects of terminal care: A preliminary study of nurses' attitudes and behavior in a general hospital. *International Nursing Review. 33* (1), 19–21.

Coser, R. T. (1962). *Life in the ward.* East Lansing, MI: Michigan State University Press.

Coser, R. T. (1963). Alienation and the social structure: case analysis of a hospital. In E. Freidson (Ed.), *The hospital in modern society* (pp. 231–265). New York: The Free Press of Glencoe.

Dolenc, D. A., & Dougherty, C. J. (1985). DRGs: The counterrevolution in financing health care. *Hastings Center Report. 15* (3), 19–29.

Duff, R. S., & Hollingshead, A. B. (1968). *Sickness and Society.* New York: Harper & Row.

Dugan, D. O. (1987). Masculine and feminine voices: Making ethical decisions in the care of the dying. *The Journal of Medical Humanities and Bioethics. 8* (2) Fall/Winter, 129–140.

Foucault, M. (1973). *The birth of the clinic.* New York: Pantheon Books.

Fowler, M. D. M., & Chaney, E. A. (1989). Ethical and legal issues. In J. H. Flaskerud (Ed.), *AIDS/HIV infection: A nursing guide for nursing professionals* (pp. 215–229). Philadelphia: W. B. Saunders.

Glaser, B. G., & Strauss, A. C. (1965). *Awareness of Dying.* Chicago: Aldine.

Goss, M. E. W. (1978). Organizational goals and quality of medical care: Evidence from comparative research on hospitals. In H. D. Schwartz & C. S. Kart (Eds.), *Dominant issues in medical sociology* (pp. 276–289). Reading, MA: Addison-Wesley.

Knight, M., & Field, D. (1981). A silent conspiracy: Coping with dying cancer patients on an acute surgical ward. *Journal of Advanced Nursing. 6,* 221–229.

Lasagna, L. (1970). Physicians' behavior toward the dying patient. In O. Brim, H. Freeman, S. Levine, & N. Scotch (Eds.), *The dying patient* (pp. 83–101). New York: Russell Sage Foundation.

Lone, P. (1989). A place to call home. *American Journal of Nursing. 89* (4), 490–492.

Morison, R. S. (1973). Dying. *Scientific American. 229* September, 55–62.

Mauksch, H. O. (1975). The organizational content of dying. In E. Kübler-Ross (Ed.), *Death: The final stage of growth* (pp. 7–24). Englewood Cliffs, NJ: Prentice-Hall.

Merton, R. (1969). Bureaucratic structure and personality. In A. Etzioni (Ed.), *A sociological reader on complex organizations* (2nd ed., pp. 47–59). New York: Holt, Rinehart, & Winston.

Mumford, E. (1967). *Sociology in hospital care.* New York: Harper & Row.

Mumma, C. M., & Benoliel, J. Q. (1984–85). Care, Cure, and hospital dying trajectories. *Omega: Journal of Death and Dying. 15* (3), 275-288.

Noyes, R., & Clancy, J. (1977). The dying role: Its relevance to improved patient care. *Psychiatry. 40,* 41–47.

Roberts, C. M. (1977). *Doctor and patient in the teaching hospital.* Lexington, MA: Heath.

Simpson, M. A. (1979). Social and psychological aspects of dying. In H. Wass (Ed.), (pp. 108–131). *Dying: Facing the facts.* Washington, DC: Hemisphere Publishing Corporation.

Strauss, A., Fagerhaugh, S., Suczek, B., & Wiener, C. (1985). *Social organization of medical work.* Chicago: University of Chicago Press.

Sudnow, D. (1967). *Passing on: The social organization of dying.* Englewood Cliffs, NJ: Prentice-Hall.

Thompson, L. M. (1984). Cultural and institutional restrictions on dying styles in a technological society. *Death education. 8* (4), 223–229.

Tisdale, S. (1988). Harvest Moon: Portrait of a nursing home. *American Journal of Nursing. 88* (3), 297–300.

U.S. is putting patient dumping law to the test. (1991). *American Journal of Nursing. 91* (5), 11.

Williams, C. A. (1982). Role considerations in care of the dying patient. *Image: Journal of Nursing Scholarship. 14* (1), 8–12.

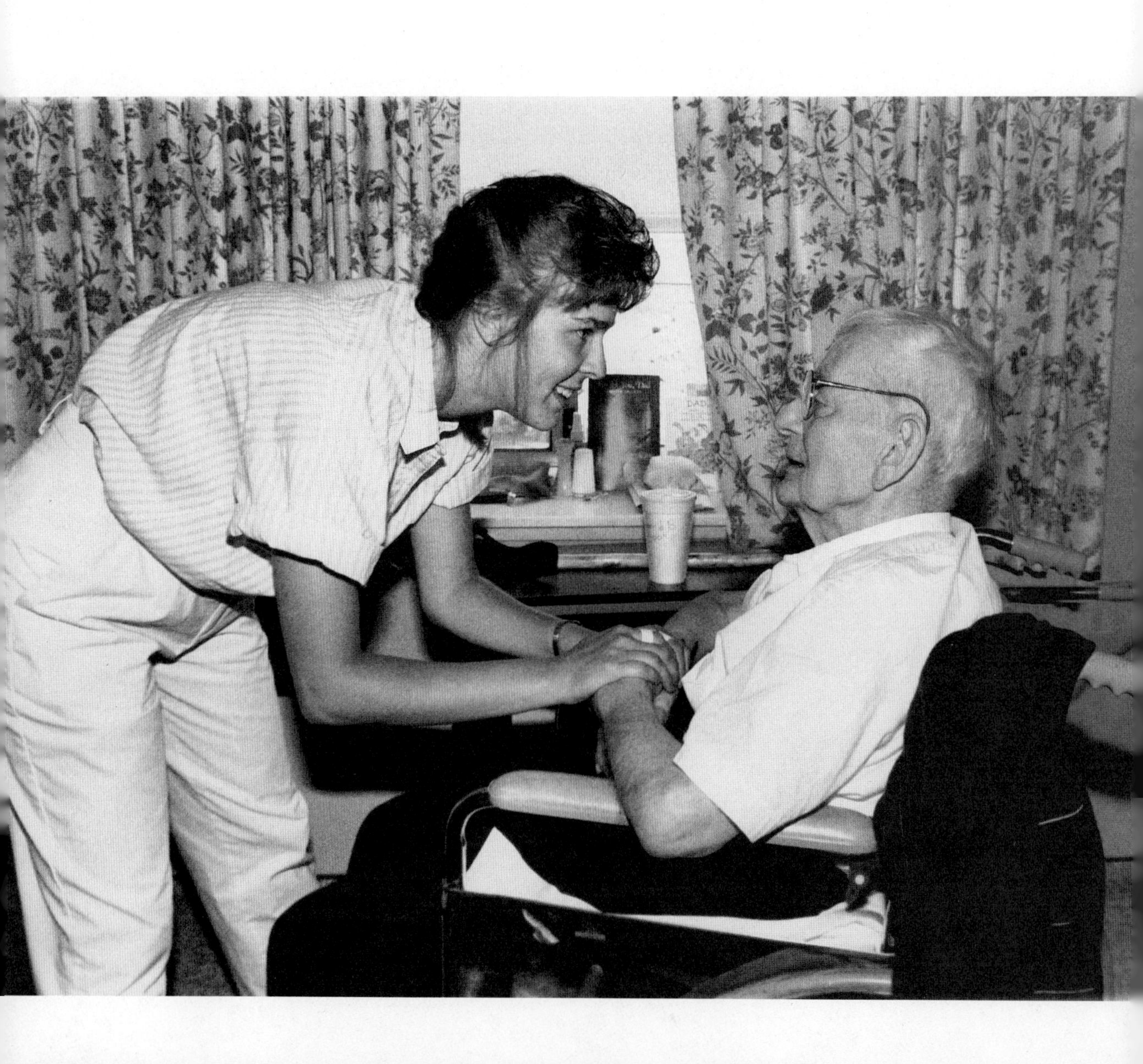

Chapter 5

Hospice Care

In 1974 there was one hospice in the United States; there are now over 1,700 hospices (Dunn, 1991, p.107). Hospice has become an accepted part of the health care system in the United States: it is accredited by the Joint Commission on Accreditation of Healthcare Organizations (JCAHO); and hospice care is reimbursed through Medicare and Medicaid.

This chapter will look at the history of hospice, and hospice today. The issue of pain control will also be discussed since this is such an inherent part of the hospice concept.

Philosophy and Principles

Hospice is a "concept of care, the goal of which is to help a person be alive until he or she dies" (Magno, 1990, p. 111).

The philosophy of hospice as stated by the National Hospice Organization is (cited in Munley, 1983):

> Hospice affirms life. Hospice exists to provide support and care for persons in the last phases of incurable disease so that they might live as fully and comfortably as possible. Hospice recognizes dying as a normal process whether or not resulting from disease. Hospice neither hastens nor postpones death. Hospice exists in the hope and belief that, through appropriate care and the promotion of a caring community sensitive to their needs, patients and families may be free to attain a degree of mental and spiritual preparation for death that is satisfactory to them (p. 320).

Robert Buckingham (1983) enunciates the principles of hospice, which must be followed if hospice is to fulfill its goals of allowing patients to die pain free and with the highest quality of life possible:

Photo courtesy of Marilyn Nolt, Photograper

- The patient should be treated as a person, not as a disease, by professional health caregivers, family, and friends.
- Humanistic care should be integrated with expert medical and nursing care.
- A family facing the impending death of a loved member needs support and advice from health-care professionals.
- The terminal patient must be allowed to give as well as receive.
- We must perpetuate among the dying their continuing self-respect and identity as persons with freedom from being a burden to others.
- The family must feel a sense of participation in caregiving and decision making.
- The primary care person tending to a patient at home needs support and occasional relief from duties to the dying person.
- The patient needs to be as symptom-free as possible so that his energy can be used to live the remaining portion of his life as fully as possible.
- Doctors and nurses must be easily accessible to the patient and to family members.
- Continuity of care should be sustained by the same health team, regardless of whether the patient is in the hospital or at home.
- The patient's and the family's life-style must be maintained and their life philosophies respected by the professional health caregivers.
- Loneliness, isolation, and fears of abandonment are significant sources of anguish to patients who are dying. Professional and lay health caregivers must be prepared to address the problem when it surfaces.
- Twenty-four-hour care must be available to the patient and to family members.
- No one person can fully meet the needs of the dying. A multidisciplinary team must be available for support, counseling, and advice. This team may include doctor, nurse, social worker, clergyman, and lawyer (pp. 16–17).*

History

The hospice concept developed out of the increasing inability of large medical institutions to provide the humanistic and individualized care required by the terminally ill. The pendulum appears to be swinging back

---

*Reprinted with permission of Robert Buckingham.

across centuries, and twentieth-century humanity is echoing the words of the citizenry of sixteenth-century England in petitioning Henry VIII to provide "for the ayde and comforte of the poore, sykke, blynde, aged and impotient persons . . . wherein they may be lodged, cherysshed and refreshed" (Stoddard, 1978, p. 1). Indeed, the concept of hospice care goes back even further to the beginnings of Christianity that had "Hospitia," places run by religious orders which emphasized hospitality for the sick, the poor, and the dying.

During the Crusades, the "hospitium" took on new significance (Amenta & Bohnet, 1986):

> The universal idea that the person who is dying is a metaphorical traveler at a stopping place on a long journey that will be continued after death was highly prominent in the collective consciousness of the Christian Middle Ages. Whether literal travelers to the Holy Land succumbing to fatigue, disease, and wounds or symbolic journeyers on a way station in life, the dying received particular attention. They were honored and treated with great care, and were valued as persons "moving forward more rapidly than others on the metaphysical plane" (p. 51).

Eventually, with the declining influence of the Church and the development of medicine, hospitia became the basis for the modern hospital—a place for curing instead of caring. Yet, some hospice activity continued. In the 1600s, St. Vincent de Paul founded the Sisters of Charity in Paris which opened hospitals to take care of the sick and the dying. Over 100 years later the first Protestant hospice, Kaiserwerth, was opened in Prussia after a Prussian nobleman visited the French institutions.

The first institution to serve as the basis for the modern day hospice was Our Lady's Hospice founded in Dublin by the Irish Sisters of Charity in the late 1800s. It was strictly dedicated to the care of the dying. In 1902, five of these Sisters opened St. Joseph's hospice for the dying poor in England. Two other homes for the dying poor in London were Hostel of God, an Anglican home, and St. Luke's, a Methodist home. Sixty-five years later, Dr. Cicely Saunders opened St. Christopher's Hospice, which became the model for today's hospice care, in London (Hillier, 1983, p. 322).

Cicely Saunders and St. Christopher's Hospice

Cicely Saunders, after leaving nursing because of a health condition, began to study medical social work. While training on a cancer ward, she met David Tasma, a refugee from the Warsaw ghetto. During his terminal illness, he and Cicely Saunders spent hours envisioning the type of institution that could best serve the needs of the terminally ill. Tasma bequeathed 500 pounds to start such a place. More importantly, he served as the inspiration for Cicely Saunders.

After David Tasma's death in 1947, Ms. Saunders began volunteer work at St. Luke's, a home for the dying poor. At St. Luke's, she saw pain being controlled through the use of drugs. Drugs were not given "as needed," but on a regular basis so that pain was prevented as much as possible. She stayed as a volunteer for 18 months, then she decided to return to school to become a physician.

Once she became a physician, she worked at St. Joseph's Hospice where she studied the effects of drugs on controlling pain in the dying. In addition, she helped make St. Joseph's a place where the whole person was treated.

In 1967, she opened St. Christopher's, "a center that would be an ecumenical religious and medical foundation combining the best care for dying patients with opportunities for teaching and research in the fields of medicine, nursing, and allied professions" (Hillier, 1983, p. 322). The aims of St. Christopher's are: (1) to understand, properly diagnose, and treat pain associated with terminal illness and (2) to establish a standard for terminal care. The major focus at St. Christopher's is to assure that each patient is free from pain and the memory of pain.

The floor plan at St. Christopher's encourages patient interaction and prevents the isolation terminally ill patients often experience. The average length of stay is only 10 days (Saunders, 1977, p. 166). This may seem surprisingly low, but it is in large part due to the extensive home care program that is part of the service provided by St. Christopher's. The home care team continues to maintain support in the home as long as it is possible and desired. Frequently, patients enter St. Christopher's for a few days' "rest period" and then return home again.

Each week an interdisciplinary team of physicians, nurses, psychiatrists, pharmacists, clergy, social workers, and volunteers meet to discuss inpatients and outpatients and to evaluate individual care plans. Care of the patient is very family centered. Staff often spend as much time with relatives as with patients, and this contact is maintained after the death of a patient to assist relatives in their bereavement. A sense of community is encouraged, and relatives often return to volunteer or to attend Sunday chapel service. St. Christopher's also has a play group and school club for the children of staff and the nearby community. Children play and mingle with patients on a regular basis. This provides a blending of all ages and encourages the concept that death is a normal, natural life event.

A discussion of St. Christopher's would be incomplete if no mention were made of the sense of spirituality and community among its staff and patients. Although no effort is made to foster faith or philosophy, Saunders (1977) explains: "At any time some may be finding their way through doubt to faith, while others feel they can only go on waiting for the answer, all find the strength of being with others who are also searching" (p. 176).

The care at St. Christopher's is summed up by a story Dr. Saunders tells of a patient (as quoted in Phipps, 1988):

> Mr. P came to us from a teaching hospital with an unsolved problem of pain, unhappy and breathless. He quickly settled to our regime of drugs, and pain was never a problem again. Mr. P used the 10 weeks he was with us to sort out his thoughts on life and faith. . . . He enjoyed meeting students and visitors, and he made good friends in the ward. After Christmas I took him some copies of a photograph I had taken of him at one of our parties. I wanted to give it to him; he wanted to pay for it. We ended by each accepting something from the other. As we were discussing this I held my hand out. At this he held both his, palms upwards, next to mine and said, "That's what life is about, four hands held out together" (p. 67).

Hospice in the United States

The idea of hospice was exported from Great Britain to the United States. Two major reasons for the development of hospice in the United States was the publicity surrounding the British hospice, and the publishing of *On Death and Dying*, by Elisabeth Kübler-Ross. Both Cicely Saunders and Elisabeth Kübler-Ross are charismatic speakers who spoke tirelessly on the need for treating dying patients with dignity and respect and on not using the acute care model for the care of the terminally ill. Hospice was seen to be "a constructive alternative to the patient for when further aggressive therapy could not promise hope of remission or cure" (Lamars, 1986, p. 137). In addition, hospice care was seen as a way to save money. Conventional wisdom was that the cost of hospice care would be less than the cost of caring for the dying in an acute care setting.

In 1974, the first Hospice, then called Hospice Inc., now Connecticut Hospice, began as a demonstration project funded by the National Cancer Institute. The initial program design had the following components: (1) coordinated home care/inpatient beds under a central, autonomous hospice administration; (2) skilled symptom control (physical, sociological, psychological, and spiritual); (3) physician-directed services; (4) provision by an interdisciplinary team; (5) service available 24 hours, seven days a week; an on-call basis with emphasis on the availability of medical and nursing skills; (6) the patient and family regarded as the unit of care; (7) bereavement follow-up; (8) use of volunteers as an integral part of the team; (9) structured staff support and communication systems; and (10) acceptance of patients into the program on the basis of health needs, not ability to pay (Wald et al., 1980, p. 42).

Although the first hospice was to be modeled on St. Christopher's as an inpatient facility, as a result of the funding from the National Cancer

Institute, Connecticut Hospice began as a home care hospice. It was not until 1979 that a 44-bed inpatient facility opened (Paradis & Cummings, 1986, p. 376).

The National Cancer Institute then proceeded to fund other hospice demonstration projects in Arizona, California, and New Jersey. Thus, hospices were launched in the United States.

Today, there are three basic models of hospice:

1. Those affiliated with a hospital.
2. Those affiliated with home health agencies without an inpatient unit.
3. Independent hospices, which may or may not have an inpatient facility.

Vincent Mor (1988) describes a "typical" hospice of each type:

> A *hospital hospice* has eight dedicated beds in a converted wing of a 500-bed general hospital. The staff consist of an administrator, social worker, minister, nursing director, staff nurses (few aides are used), and a medical director. There is a limited home care program consisting of a single coordinator on the staff of the hospital's home care department. There are few volunteers, and although separate from the hospital's regular volunteer program, they are engaged in similar activities. The hospital's medical staff is divided on the value of hospice care; some are strongly committed to it, while others never refer their patients. Hospital hospice patients have a median survival in the hospice of only 30 days; 25 percent survive less than 10 days. Most of the short-stay patients spend their entire hospice stay in the inpatient unit. In general, the preference is to admit terminal patients to the hospice ward rather than treat them at home.
>
> A *hospice home health program* is a special unit of an urban/suburban Visiting Nurse Association. It is staffed almost entirely by nurses, with the addition of a single social worker and an administrative coordinator; a part-time medical director is employed under contract. Aides and homemakers, who provide the bulk of care to patients at home, are assigned from the pool employed by the agency. There is a small volunteer program with a volunteer coordinator. Referrals come largely from the agency's existing network of discharge planners placed in area hospitals. Most patients are internally transferred from the regular home health service or are admitted to hospice care at the time of their discharge from a hospital. Almost all have intact homes with family helpers.
>
> *Independent hospice* programs began as a small group of volunteers, lay and professional, committed to changing the pattern of care for the

> terminally ill. Initially, funding from local foundations, bequests, and other gifts made it possible to hire a coordinator and to formalize a relationship to the local visiting nurse association and hospital. In time, with the potential for Medicare certification and reimbursement, staffs were hired, and both the number of patients served and the amount of service provided increased. Nurses, social workers, supervisory staff, volunteers, a minister, and a clerical staff now comprise the organization. Plans are under way to build an inpatient unit, but currently inpatient services are provided under arrangement with a local hospital. The volunteer program has over a hundred active volunteers involved in direct patient care and administrative functions under the direction of a full-time volunteer coordinator. Patients are frequently referred by family, friends, or initiate contact on their own. Family support is generally very strong (pp. 17–18).

Hence, hospice is not a facility, necessarily, but an organized way of caring for the terminally ill.

Each of these types of hospices should have the following elements, as described by Gonda & Ruark (1984, p. 208):

1. The unit of care is the patient and the family.
2. Home care services in collaboration with inpatient backup facilities are available.
3. Care is provided by a multidisciplinary team with special expertise in symptom control, on which medical, nursing, social chaplaincy, and volunteers services are represented.
4. Skills of the multidisciplinary team are available 24 hours per day, seven days per week.
5. Follow-up care for the bereaved.
6. Ongoing emotional support for hospice personnel is provided.

Today, hospice has become an institutionalized part of health care. It has a national professional organization, the National Hospice Organization (NHO); hospices are accredited by the Joint Commission on Accreditation of Health Organizations (JCAHO); and they are eligible for Medicare reimbursement.

National Hospice Organization (NHO). The National Hospice Organization works "to promote, direct, standardize and monitor hospice activities" (Paradis & Cummings, 1986, p. 376). NHO members lobbied successfully

---

Reprinted with permission of V. Mor, D. Greer, and R. Kastenbaum, eds. *The Hospice Experience*, Johns Hopkins University Press, Baltimore/London, 1988, p. 17–18.

to provide Medicare reimbursement for hospice care and to have hospices accredited by JCAHO. Today they provide education and training for their members and maintain an up-to-date directory of hospices. Their meetings are attended by representatives of almost every hospice in the country (Amenta & Bohnet, 1986).

Joint Commission on the Accreditation of Healthcare Organizations (JCAHO). Working with the NHO, JCAHO began accrediting hospices in 1984. Based on the "Assumptions and Principles Underlying Standards for Terminal Care" formulated by the International Work Group on Death, Dying, and Bereavement and the standards developed by the NHO, (see Table 5.1 and

Table 5.1 Assumptions and Principles Underlying Standards for Terminal Care (Formulated by The International Work Group on Death, Dying, and Bereavement)

GENERAL ASSUMPTIONS AND PRINCIPLES	
Assumptions	**Principles**
1. The care of the dying is a process involving the patient, family, and caregivers.	1. The interaction of these three groups of individuals must constantly be assessed with the aim being the best possible care of the patient. This cannot be accomplished if the needs of family and/or caregiver are negated.
2. The problems of the patient and family facing terminal illness include a wide variety of issues—psychological, legal, social, spiritual, economic, and interpersonal.	2. Care requires collaboration of many disciplines working as an integrated clinical team, meeting for frequent discussions with a common purpose.
3. Dying tends to produce a feeling of isolation.	3. All that counteracts unwanted isolation should be encouraged. Social events and shared work that include all involved should be arranged so that meaningful relations can be sustained and developed.
4. It has been the tradition to train caregivers not to become emotionally involved, but in terminal illness the patient and family need to experience the personal concern of those taking care of them.	4. Profound involvement without loss of objectivity should be allowed and fostered, with the realization that this may present certain risks to the caregiver.

Table 5.1 Continued

Assumptions	Principles
GENERAL ASSUMPTIONS AND PRINCIPLES	
5. Health care services customarily lack coordination.	5. The organizational structure must provide links with health care professionals in the community.
6. A supportive physical environment contributes to the sense of well-being of patients, of families, and of caregivers.	6. The environment should provide adequate space, furnishings that put people at ease, the reassuring presence of personal belongings, and symbols of the life cycle.
PATIENT-ORIENTED ASSUMPTIONS AND PRINCIPLES	
Assumptions	**Principles**
1. There are patients for whom aggressive curative treatment becomes increasingly inappropriate.	1. These patients need highly competent professionals, skilled in terminal care.
2. The symptoms of terminal disease can be controlled.	2. The patient should be kept as symptom free as possible. Pain should be controlled in all its aspects. The patient must remain alert and comfortable.
3. Patients' needs may change over time.	3. Staff must recognize that other services may have to be involved but that continuity of care should be provided.
4. Care is most effective when the patient's life-style is maintained and philosophy of life is respected.	4. The terminally ill patient's own framework of values, preferences, and outlook on life must be taken into account in planning and conducting treatment.
5. Patients are often treated as if incapable of understanding or of making decisions.	5. Patients' wishes for information about their condition should be respected. They should be allowed full participation in their care and a continuing sense of self-determination and self-control.
6. Dying patients often suffer from helplessness, weakness, isolation, and loneliness.	6. The patients should have a sense of security and protection. Involvement of family and friends should be encouraged.

(continued on next page)

Table 5.1 Continued

PATIENT-ORIENTED ASSUMPTIONS AND PRINCIPLES	
Assumptions	**Principles**
7. The varied problems and anxieties associated with terminal illness can occur at any time of day or night.	7. Twenty-four-hour care must be available seven days a week for the patient and family where and when it is needed.
FAMILY-ORIENTED ASSUMPTIONS AND PRINCIPLES	
Assumptions	**Principles**
1. Care is usually directed toward the patient. In terminal illness the family must be the unit of care.	1. Help should be available to all those involved—whether patient, relation, or friend—to sustain communication and involvement.
2. The course of the terminal illness involves a series of clinical and personal decisions.	2. Interchange between the patient and family and the clinical team is essential to enable an informed decision to be made.
3. Many people do not know what the process of dying involves.	3. The family should be given time and opportunity to discuss all aspects of dying and death and related emotional needs with the staff.
4. The patient and family need the opportunity for privacy and being together.	4. The patient and family should have privacy and time alone, both while the patient is living and after death occurs. A special space may have to be provided.
5. Complexity of treatment and time-consuming procedures can cause disruption for the patient and family.	5. Procedures must be arranged so as not to interfere with adequate time for patient, family, and friends to be together.
6. Patients and families facing death frequently experience a search for the meaning of their life, making the provision of spiritual support essential.	6. The religious, philosophical, and emotional components of care are as essential as the medical, nursing, and social components and must be available as part of the team approach.
7. Survivors are at risk emotionally and physically during bereavement.	7. The provision of appropriate care for survivors is the responsibility of the team who gave care and support to the deceased.

Table 5.1 Continued

STAFF-ORIENTED ASSUMPTIONS AND PRINCIPLES	
Assumptions	**Principles**
1. The growing body of knowledge in symptom control, patient-and family centered care, and other aspects of the care of the terminally ill is now readily available.	1. Institutions and organizations providing terminal care must orient and educate new staff and keep all staff informed about developments as they occur.
2. Good terminal care presupposes emotional investment on the part of the staff.	2. Staff needs time and encouragement to develop and maintain relationships with patients and relatives.
3. Emotional commitment to good terminal care will often produce emotional exhaustion.	3. Effective staff support systems must be readily available.

"Standards for Hospice Care: Assumptions and Principles" by Zelda Foster. Copyright 1979 National Association of Social workers, Inc. Reprinted with permission of *Health and Social Work, Vol. 4,* No. 1 (February 1979), pp. 124–127.

Table 5.2), JCAHO developed accreditation standards to monitor the quality of care in hospices. Hospices accredited by JCAHO see their accreditation as "endorsement of their capacity to provide first-rate care" (Amenta & Bohnet, 1986, p. 387). JCAHO is also integrating the principles of hospice care into its standards of accreditation of other health care facilities.

Medicare Certification

The most important influence on the regulation of hospice is the Medicare eligibility. In 1983, hospices became eligible for Medicare reimbursement as part of the Tax Equity and Fiscal Responsibility Act of 1982.

Rhymes (1990) summarizes the Medicare regulations (p. 370):

- Patients must have a terminal illness with a life expectancy of six months or less and be entitled to Medicare part A insurance.
- Election of the hospice benefit requires relinquishing other Medicare benefits (except for reimbursement to the patient's attending physician).
- The benefit is divided into two 90-day periods and one 30-day period, for a total of 210 days.
- Revocation of benefit means losing the remaining days in the benefit period.
- The hospice program must continue to provide care to patients who live beyond 210 days.

Table 5.2 Standards of a Hospice Program of Care

1. The hospice program complies with applicable local, state, and federal laws and regulations governing the organization and delivery of health care to patients and families.
2. The hospice program provides a continuum of inpatient and home care services through an integrated administrative structure.
3. The home care services are available 24 hours a day, seven days a week.
4. The patient and patient's family is the unit of care.
5. The hospice program has admission criteria and procedures that reflect:
   a. The patient or family's desire and need for service.
   b. Physician participation.
   c. Diagnosis and prognosis.
6. The hospice program seeks to identify, teach, coordinate, and supervise persons to give care to patients who do not have a family member available.
7. The hospice program acknowledges that each patient and family has its own beliefs or value system and is respectful of them.
8. Hospice care consists of a blending of professional and nonprofessional services, provided by an interdisciplinary team that includes a medical director.
9. Staff support is an integral part of the hospice program.
10. Inservice training and continuing education are offered on a regular basis.
11. The goal of hospice care is to provide symptom control through appropriate palliative therapies.
12. Symptom control includes assessing and responding to the physical, emotional, social, and spiritual needs of the patient and patient's family.
13. The hospice program provides bereavement services to survivors for a period of at least one year.
14. There will be a quality assurance program that includes:
    a. Evaluation of services.
    b. Regular chart audits.
    c. Organizational review.
15. The hospice program maintains accurate and current integrated records on all patients and their families.
16. The hospice complies with all applicable state and federal regulations.
17. The hospice inpatient unit provides space for:
    a. Patient–family privacy.
    b. Visitation and viewing.
    c. Food preparation by the family.

From *Standards of a Hospice Program of Care.* Reprinted with permission of the National Hospice Organization.

- The hospice is reimbursed at a daily rate that depends on the patient's level of care: routine home care, continuous home care, inpatient respite care, and general inpatient care.
- More than 80 percent of each hospice's care days must be for home care.
- There is an annual payment cap for each hospice based on the number of enrolled patients.
- The hospice must provide medical and nursing care, home health services, inpatient care, social work, counseling (including bereavement counseling), medications, medical supplies, durable medical equipment, and physical, occupational, and speech therapy, as needed, based on a plan of care for each patient.

Many of these regulations are quite controversial, for example, the prognosis of six months or less and the 20 percent payment cap on inpatient days. The emphasis on home care may limit the use of Medicare to those dying patients who have a family caregiver in the home. Claire Tehan (1985) tells of the following case:

> Mary S is a very independent eighty-year-old widow who has lived alone since the death of her husband 15 years ago. She is suffering from chronic obstructive pulmonary disease, a diagnosis for which it is difficult to predict a downhill course with a prognosis of less than six months. Her daughter lives 150 miles away and cares for her own family. Mrs. S does not want anyone living in her apartment with her; neither does she want to move to her daughter's home (p. 12).

The hospice in Mrs. S's area will not accept her: (1) because she does not have a definitive prognosis of six months or less; and (2) more importantly, since she is alone she may need to be institutionalized, and her stay will go beyond the 20 percent cap for institutionalization.

As a result, only half of the eligible hospices have applied for Medicare certification, which "suggests that Medicare reimbursement may have the effect of creating 'haves' and 'have nots' among hospice programs. . . . More important, the 'have nots' among terminally ill patients will be denied the opportunity of choosing hospice care" (Corless, 1988, p. 332).

Effectiveness of Hospice

Does hospice make a difference in the quality of life of the terminally ill? Major research studies do not see hospice care as vastly superior

---

to conventional types of care in the treatment of the terminally ill. Hospice provides quality care for dying patients—but so do conventional care settings.

The National Hospice Study (Mor, Greer, & Kastenbaum, 1988) studied a sample of 1,754 hospice and nonhospice patients nationwide who were identified in 40 hospices and 14 conventional care settings. Of the 1,754 patients, 833 had been in a hospice without beds; 624 had been in a hospice that had beds; and 297 were in a conventional care setting.

The basic finding concerning quality of life was that "the quality of life of terminal care patients served in hospice was not demonstrably different from the quality of life of patients served in conventional settings" (Morris et al., 1988):

- While bedded hospices controlled pain better than home care based hospices and conventional care facilities, there was no difference between the home care based hospices and conventional care facilities in the control of pain.
- There was no discernible difference in the quality of life in either the physical or emotional areas of the patient.
- All three patient groups were rated as having a high quality of social life.
- All three patient groups were generally satisfied with the care they received.

These findings were similar to the findings of Kane et al. (1984) who did a controlled study of hospice care at a V.A. Hospital in Los Angeles. There was no difference found between the hospice patients and the conventional care patients with regard to pain control and quality of life; for example, maintaining the activities of daily living.

Corless (1988) gives some reasons for these findings: 1) being part of a study may lead to changes in behavior on part of the staff; 2) morphine, which eases the pain of dying, is used in conventional care settings; and 3) probably most important, the "traditional programs' incorporation of modalities offered by hospice program." Conventional care settings have begun to use the approach used by hospice toward the dying patient.

Pain Management

One of the major goals of hospice care is that the patient be free of pain and other symptoms that do not allow patients to maintain the quality of their lives. The greatest fear for the dying is caused by terminal pain since "it traps the patient in a situation for which there is no comforting explanation and to which there is no foreseeable end" (Saunders & Baines, 1983, p. 14). Pain is more than simply a bodily response that occurs when tissues are damaged or stressed. According to Chapman (1978), "contemporary theorists stress that pain involves emotional arousal, motivational drive, and cognition in addition to sensory information transmission" (p. 169). McCaffery's (1972) workable definition for nurses presents the idea that pain is whatever the person experiencing it says it is, and it exists when that person says it does. This latter definition supports patients because their reports of pain are never doubted. Both these definitions include the concept that pain can be of functional or organic origin. Management of pain in people who are dying is especially significant, not only in terms of pain relief but also because "one cannot adequately help a man to come to accept his impending death if he remains in severe pain, one cannot give spiritual counsel to a woman who is persistently vomiting, or help a wife and children say their goodbyes to a father who is so drugged that he cannot respond" (Baines, 1980, p. 1).

Pain from a terminal illness such as cancer or AIDS is chronic pain, as opposed to acute pain. Acute pain is pain of a limited duration. It is a reaction to a trauma to a body and will abate as the injured area heals. Chronic pain, however, does not diminish or abate. It is ongoing, and it is experienced from dull and aching to excruciating agony. It may become the "focal point of living" (Amenta & Bohnet, 1986, p. 82). Chronic pain in the dying will also have negative psychological effects since chronic pain from cancer indicates that the disease is escalating and that death is six months to one year away (Kohut & Kohut, 1984, p. 84).

It must be noted that not all cancer or AIDS patients experience pain, and we do not have a very accurate picture of the incidence of pain. Some cancers, such as leukemia, produce little pain, while others, such as bone cancer, produce severe pain. John Bonica (as cited in Free, 1986, p. 17) states that pain is usually not existent in the early stages of cancer. But as the disease progresses, pain begins and gets progressively worse. In the intermediate stages of the disease 40 percent of patients experience moderate to severe pain, and in the later stages, 60-80 percent patients experience severe pain.

Perceptions of Pain

There are three major reasons for pain in cancer patients· (1) the cancer itself (about 70 percent); (2) the therapies used to control the cancer (about 20 percent); and (3) factors unrelated to the cancer (about 10 percent).

The tumor itself does not cause the pain, rather the pain is caused by the tumor's invasion in various areas of the body such as the bones, by compression of the spinal cord, and by causing obstructions in areas such as the gastrointestinal tract.

Pain, however, is not just a physical phenomenon. According to Twycross (1978), "pain is a dual phenomenon, one part being the perception of the sensation and the other the patient's psychological reaction to it" (p. 114). Therefore, a patient's pain threshold may vary according to such nonphysical factors as anxiety, fear, depression, and fatigue. Cultural influences and life experiences may also affect pain thresholds. These nonphysical factors, which are not generally so readily evident as are physiological elements, must be considered as part of the process of pain assessment and management.

A patient's membership in a particular sociocultural group may influence pain sensation and the behavioral response to it. In a well-known study of pain responses of Irish, Jewish, Italian, and "Old American" patients, Zborowski (1952) found that Jewish and Italian male patients were very emotional in their responses to pain, tending to exaggerate the experience and to be very sensitive to it. However, the research material suggests that in the male Jewish patient, "the function of the pain reaction will be the mobilization of the efforts of the family and the doctors toward a complete cure, while in the male Italian patient, the function of the reaction will be focused upon the mobilization of effort toward relieving the pain sensation" (p. 24). A similar overt behavioral response in two different patients may have two very different meanings. Caregivers assessment of pain should include an evaluation of whether patients are more concerned with immediate, palliative pain relief, or with what the pain means to them, or with finding an ultimate cure for the pain.

Age and sex also influence patients' responses to pain. In the United States, women seem to be allowed more freedom for emotional expression of pain than men, although this changes as men grow older and are allowed more freedom in this area. Children's developmental levels need to be considered in assessing pain. Infants and toddlers cannot communicate verbally. Their crying must be interpreted—one must determine whether it is a pain cry or whether it has other meanings such as expressing hunger, wetness, or wanting to be held. Telling a preschool child that a painful treatment "will be all over soon" does not mean anything to the child since temporal relationships are not understood (Gilder & Quirk, 1977). Children at this age still utilize a great deal of concrete thinking; a painful procedure just plain hurts and little relationship is seen between the procedure and getting well. Among school-age children, there is fear of bodily injury although anxieties about this are frequently submerged. However, these children can understand that pain can be limited. Explaining potentially painful treatments and procedures, letting the children know what to expect, and allowing them to ask questions and to express their anxieties are meaningful for children of this age.

The patient's prior experience with pain will also affect the perception of pain. (See Kohut & Kohut, 1984, p. 86; and Amenta & Bohnet, 1986, p. 85.) A patient who has had pain that was not managed well will suffer more than the patient who has had pain relieved in the past.

What pain means to the person is also very important. The pain may serve a purpose for the patient; it may be a way of dealing with an unresolved conflict or with feelings of guilt. Pain may also be seen as a threat to patients' lives; their life-styles or body images might be changed by pain. Pain may be alleviated in many patients if they understand what is causing the pain or understand that staff members are trying to determine the cause, that caring people are available on an ongoing basis to help them, and that they have a part in planning how to cope with the pain. Pain may also be valued since, for some, the experience of pain signifies life.

Assessment of Pain

Patients in pain will often put on a "brave face"; they may not appear outwardly to be in any great distress and may state only that they are having a "little" pain. It is therefore important that caregivers assess patients thoroughly to determine the extent and severity of pain. Assessment includes careful history taking and physical examination. History taking includes not only listening to the patient's description of the pain but also asking the patient such questions as: "When did the pain start?" "What makes it worse?" "What makes it less intense?" "Do any medications help?" "Does it stay in one place or move around?" "Are you in pain all the time, or does it come and go?" It is helpful to have patients describe a normal day's activity pattern and then ask them if pain has interfered in this pattern at all; that is, interrupted sleep, dulled appetite, limited mobility. Interviewing a family member or friend about the patient's pain might also help gain a more accurate picture of what is happening.

Neurophysiological processes may underlie the sensation of pain and should be assessed by physical examination. The results of such an examination may reveal a specific pathology that is causing the sensation of pain and may indicate why the pain is localized in a specific part of the body or why it is perceived as referred pain in another area.

Assessment of the pain may even help alleviate some of the pain. Both a pain assessment survey (Figure 5.1) and a pain assessment flow chart (Figure 5.2) are useful tools. The pain assessment survey provides data on the type of pain the patient is feeling, the location of the pain, and how the patient feels about the pain. The pain flow chart shows when the patient experiences the pain and helps regulate the medication that is being used to control the pain.

Assessment of the pain must be ongoing since new pains may develop as the cancer metastasizes, or management of one pain may lead to the emergence of a different pain. For example, (Twycross, 1986):

> An 85-year-old man with carcinoma of the prostate and pain in the right femur caused by a metastasis was treated with aspirin and morphine. Casual questioning the next day indicated that, although the pain was

Figure 5.1 Pain Assessment Survey

Patient's name ____________ Date ____________ Time ____________ a.m./p.m.
Analgesic(s) ____________ Dosage ____________ Time given ____________ a.m./p.m.
____________ Dosage ____________ Time given ____________ a.m./p.m.

Analgesic time difference (hours): +4 +1 +2 +3

PRI: S ______ (1–10) A ______ (11–15) E ______ (16) M(S) ______ 17–19) M(AE) ______ (20) M(T) ______ (17–20) PRI(T) ______ 1–20)

1. Flickering ____
   Quivering ____
   Pusling ____
   Throbbing ____
   Beating ____
   Pounding ____
2. Jumping ____
   Flashing ____
   Shooting ____
3. Pricking ____
   Boring ____
   Drilling ____
   Stabbing ____
   Lancinating ____
4. Sharp ____
   Cutting ____
   Lacerating ____
5. Pinching ____
   Pressing ____
   Gnawing ____
   Cramping ____
   Crushing ____
6. Tugging ____
   Pulling ____
   Wrenching ____
7. Hot ____
   Burning ____
   Scalding ____
   Searing ____
8. Tingling ____
   Itchy ____
   Smarting ____
   Stinging ____
9. Dull ____
   Sore ____
   Hurting ____
   Aching ____
   Heavy ____
10. Tender ____
    Taut ____
    Rasping ____
    Splitting ____
11. Tiring ____
    Exhausting ____
12. Sickening ____
    Suffocating ____
13. Fearful ____
    Frightful ____
    Terrifying ____
14. Punishing ____
    Grueling ____
    Cruel ____
    Vicious ____
    Killing ____
15. Wretched ____
    Blinding ____
16. Annoying ____
    Troublesome ____
    Miserable ____
    Intense ____
    Unbearable ____
17. Spreading ____
    Radiating ____
    Penetrating ____
    Piercing ____
18. Tight ____
    Numb ____
    Drawing ____
    Dqueezing ____
    Tearing ____
19. Cool ____
    Cold ____
    Freezing ____
20. Nagging ____
    Nauseating ____
    Agonizing ____
    Dreadful ____
    Torturing ____

PPI

0 No pain ____
1 Mild ____
2 Discomforting ____
3 Distressing ____
4 Horrible ____
5 Excrutiating ____

PPI

Comments:

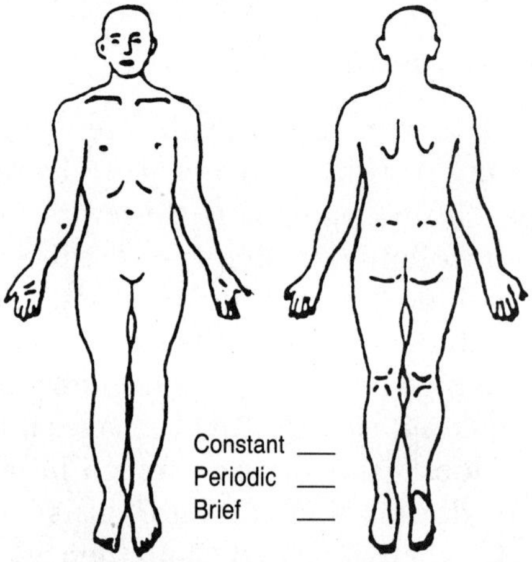

____

Constant ____
Periodic ____
Brief ____

Accompanying Symptoms:

Nausea ____
Headache ____
Dizziness ____
Drowsiness ____
Constipation ____
Diarrhea ____

Comments:

____

Sleep:

Good ____
Fitful ____
Can't sleep ____

Comments:

____

Food intake:

Good ____
Some ____
Little ____
None ____

Comments:

____

Activity:

Good ____
Some ____
Little ____
None ____

Comments:

____

Reprinted by permission of Ronald Melzack.

Figure 5.2 Pain Flow Chart

Date ______________

Patient ______________________________

Rx ______________________________

Purpose: To evaluate the safety and effectiveness of the analgesic(s).

Analgesic order ______________________________

Pain Rating Scale used ______________________________

I. Time	II.* Pain rating	III. Analgesic	IV. R	V. P	VI. BP	VII. Level arousal	VIII.* Other	IX. Plan & comments

**Pain rating*: A number of different scales may be used. Indicate which scale is used and use the same one each time. Two common examples:

- 0 to 10 with 0 being no pain and 10 being as bad as it can be.
- Melzack's scale: 0 = no pain; 1 = mild; 2 = discomforting; 3 = distressing; 4 = horrible; 5 = excruciating.

Possibilities for other columns: respiratory depression, nausea and vomiting, bowel function, other pain relief measures, etc. Identify the side effects of greatest concern to patient, family, physician, nurses.

*Noreen T. Meinhart, Margo McCaffery, *Pain: A Nursing Approach to Assessment and Analysis* (Norwalk, Connecticut: Appleton-Century-Crofts, 1982), p. 361.

less severe, he was still in pain. Further questioning revealed that the site of pain was now retrosternal and epigastric; he had no femoral pain at all. The dose of morphine was, therefore, left unaltered, and the prescription of an antacid resulted in complete relief (p. 110).

Pain Control

Twycross suggests that relief of pain should have realistic objectives. The ultimate aim is always complete relief from pain, but perhaps graded relief is more realistic; that is, (1) a pain-free, sleep-full night; (2) relief at rest in bed or chair during the day; (3) freedom from pain on movement (Twycross, 1978, p. 115). The latter may be the most difficult to achieve, but, if patients can rest comfortably at night and throughout the day, their morale will be better and they may be able to cope more effectively.

Once pain is under control, the continued relief of dying patients is based on preventing any more pain rather than waiting for the pain to reappear and then trying to treat it.

Pain may be controlled by (see Twycross, 1986; and Buchanan, 1986):

1. Modifying the pathological process.
2. Elevating the pain threshold.
3. Interrupting the pain pathways through the use of drugs.
4. Modifying one's life-style.

Modifying the Pathological Process. Chemotherapy, hormone therapy, and radiation may ease the pain affecting the cancer. According to Twycross (1986), pain from bone cancer may be alleviated in 90 percent of patients through the use of radiation (p. 111). The caregiver must make sure, however, that the effect of the treatment is not worse than the pain being caused by the disease.

Elevating the Pain Threshold. Since pain, as noted before, is also a subjective phenomenon, such feelings as worry, anxiety, and depression may intensify the feelings of pain. Allowing the patients to talk about their fears may help relieve the pain.

For patients who want to take control of their situation, biofeedback may be used. Biofeedback involves the use of biophysiological instrumentation to provide patients with information about changes in their bodily functioning of which they are not normally aware. This information may enable patients to control voluntarily some aspect of their physiology that is supposedly casually linked to the pain being experienced (Turk et al., 1979, pp. 1322–1323). Relaxation therapy, which may be as effective and is a great deal less expensive since it requires no equipment, may also help in pain management. Relaxation therapy involves deep breathing, a conscious effort to relax one's muscles, and some visualization of comforting scenes. Therapeutic touch, hypnosis, acupuncture, use of imagery and distraction, behavior therapy, alleviation of anxiety, teaching patients about the nature of pain and its intensity, reduction of stimulus, and the establishment of a trusting relationship between the caregiver and patient are all being used in pain management.

Interrupting Pain Pathways. The most common method of interrupting the pain pathways is through the use of analgesics. This will be discussed in depth in the next section of this chapter.

In cases of intractable pain, chemical nerve blocks may be used. This involves the injection of an agent that damages the nerves involved in pain transmission but minimally affects sensory and motor nerves. Results vary, but certain types of blocks have benefited at least 70 percent of the patients involved for up to three months (Robert, 1986).

Modifying of Life-style or Immobilization. Pain may sometimes be eased by immobilizing a bone or another part of the body or by having a person modify his life-style; for example, using a wheelchair rather than walking. However, since this may involve loss of independence, it should not be done lightly.

The Use of Analgesics

Analgesics are basically either non-narcotic or narcotic. The World Health Organization recommends the use of an "analgesic ladder" beginning with non-narcotics leading to the use of narcotics (as cited in Creagan & Wilkinson, 1989, p. 134).

The non-narcotics include aspirin, acetaminophen, and nonsteroidal, anti-inflammatory drugs such as ibuprofen. The weak opioids, such as codeine, alone will generally work no better than the non-narcotics. However, in combination with the non-narcotic analgesics, the weak opioids will provide an enhanced effect.

For severe pain, the most effective narcotic is morphine. Much has been written on the use of heroin, and the use of "Brompton's Cocktail," a combination of heroin (a narcotic), cocaine (a stimulant), gin, chlorpromazine, and sugar, but recent research has shown that morphine alone is just as effective (Levy, 1988).

The following are guidelines for the use of narcotic analgesics in pain management as delineated by Foley (cited in Creagan & Wilkinson, 1989):

Figure 5.3 World Health Organization Analgesic Ladder

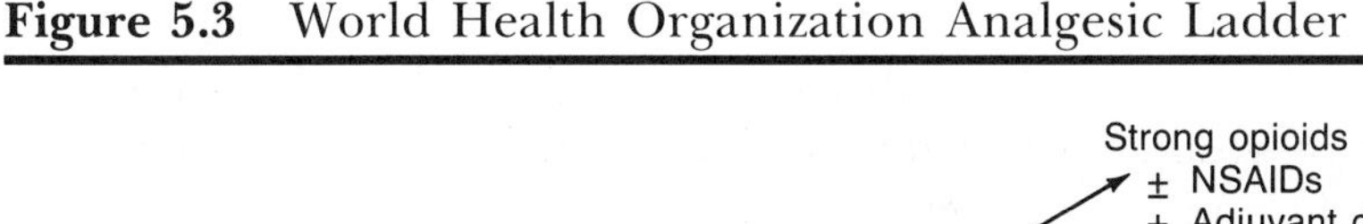
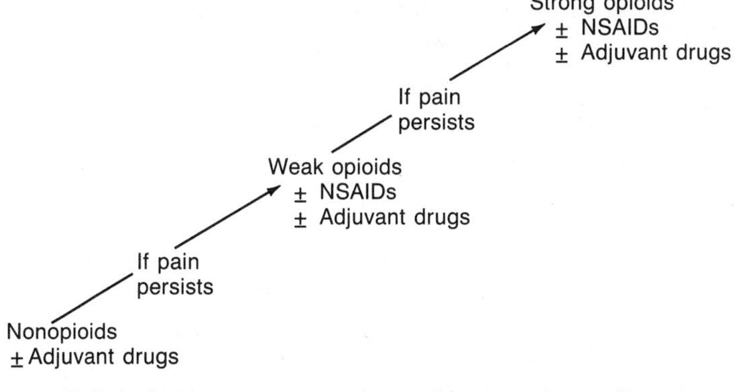

"Pain Relief in Terminally Ill Patients" by E. Reagan and J. Wilkinson. Reprinted with permission of *American Family Physician,* vol. 40. Published by the American Academy of Family Physicians.

1. Start with a specific drug for a specific type of pain
2. Know the pharmacology of the drug prescribed
   a. Duration of the analgesic effect
   b. Pharmacokinetic properties of the drug
   c. Equianalgesic doses for the drug and its route of administration
3. Adjust the route of administration to the patient's needs
4. Administer the analgesic on a regular basis after initial titration of the dose
5. Use drug combinations to provide additive analgesia and reduce side effects (e.g., nonsteroidal anti-inflammatory drugs, antihistamine [Hydroxyzine] and amphetamine [Dexedrine])
6. Avoid drug combinations that increase sedation without enhancing analgesia such as a benzodiazepine (e.g., diazepam [Valium]) and a phenothiazine (e.g., chlorpromazine [Thorazine])
7. Anticipate and treat side effects
   a. Sedation
   b. Respiratory depression
   c. Nausea and vomiting
   d. Constipation
8. Watch for the development of tolerance
   a. Switch to an alternative analgesic
   b. Start with one-half the equianalgesic dose and titrate the dose for pain relief
9. Prevent acute withdrawal
   a. Taper drugs slowly
   b. Use diluted doses of naloxone (0.4 mg in 10 ml of saline) to reverse respiratory depression in the physically dependent patient and administer cautiously
10. Do not use placebo to assess the nature of pain
11. Anticipate and manage complications
   a. Overdose
   b. Multifocal myoclonus
   c. Seizures

An effective new method of pain control is PCA, Patient-Controlled Analagesia. With PCA a patient is hooked to an intravenous line attached

---

"Pain Relief in Terminally Ill Patients" by E. Creagan and J. Wilkinson. Reprinted with permission of *American Family Physician,* vol. 40. Published by the American Academy of Family Physicians.

to a pump and a button. When pain medication is needed, the patient pushes the button and a small dose of morphine is pumped into the vein and goes to work immediately. A computer controls the dosage and the dosing intervals. PCA allows repetitive dosing of pain medication when the patient feels that the pain requires treatment. It does away with the traditional as-needed narcotic dosing. The patient is no longer dependent on the nurse to bring the pain medication. PCA brings a "modicum of control and dignity to patients at a time they badly need both." (Zimmerman, 1990, p. S8) (For excellent discussions of PCA, see Anderson and McCann, 1992; and Camp, 1991.)

Pain Control and Health Care Professionals

Although studies have shown that pain can be controlled in close to 100 percent of patients, lack of education vis-à-vis pain control and attitudes of health professionals toward pain lead to inadequate control of pain in patients.

Caregivers and patients often find themselves in disagreement with one another about the use and administration of narcotics. Patients may feel that they are not obtaining adequate pain relief. Nurses may be reluctant to give regular doses of a narcotic around the clock for fear of accumulation of side effects that could possibly cause death in some patients. Doctors may be concerned about the origin and reality of the patient's pain. Social workers may feel that no one is listening to the patient's reports of pain.

As stated by Amenta & Bohnet (1986):

> Nurses and physicians fall easily into the position of believing that they, and not their patients, are the authorities on patient pain. When this is the case, patients are treated on the basis of what might be beneficial to the health professional according to his or her perception of how much pain should be experienced by the patient in a given situation. We emphasize again, the only authority on pain is the patient (p. 82).

Two major misconceptions health care professionals hold concern patients' tolerance of pain and the fear of addiction. Stoicism and tolerance of pain are generally admired. Along with this is the expectation that patients will respond the same to medications. There is also an expectation that medication will have an instantaneous onset and an extended duration of action. Yet drugs have different periods for onset of relief, and they reach their peak action at different items. Caregivers should be aware of the onset and duration of each drug to help patients plan their activity and rest throughout the day. A person who needs increased mobility at a certain time may well want to plan that mobility around the time of the drug's peak action so that pain will be decreased and function improved.

In addition to caregivers' beliefs about the origin and quality of a patient's pain influencing pain management, their beliefs (as well as the patients') about how, when, and whether to use analgesics will affect pain control (Silman, 1978).

There is also a fear of addiction even though it has been shown that addiction does not occur when narcotics are used to control pain. Actually, "withholding narcotics to prevent addiction may in reality contribute to addiction. The patient in pain who is denied medication or who receives an inadequate dose may become overwhelmingly concerned with the comforting drug and crave the next dose. That this craving disappears with proper administration demonstrates that patients would seem to crave pain relief, not drugs" (Amenta & Bohnet, 1986, p. 83).

The organization of health care itself plays a very significant part in the management of pain, particularly in institutional settings such as hospitals and clinics. Fagerhaugh & Strauss (1977) present three main themes developed from their two-year research study on pain management. The first theme is that pain management occurs within organizational settings that greatly influence the character of the interaction between patients and staff. These interactions, which are extremely important in the management of pain, are affected by the context of the organization itself—its work structure, its goals, its philosophy. An example of this theme may be seen in the difference in pain management in hospices and in acute care centers. In hospices, the philosophy is to help patients on their journey through life. The hospice is considered a place where patients may always come for sustenance. As a result of this philosophy, pain management is collaboratively planned by patients and staff to enhance comfort, alertness, and participation in living. Staff members consistently communicate with one another and with the patient about the effects of pain management—how it is working and what needs to be changed. Pain management in acute care centers may often focus on immediate relief with the intention of ultimately curing the cause of pain; there is often the expectation that the pain should diminish after intensive treatment.

A balancing of decisions is a vital component in the political actions of pain management. "The pain tasks of diagnosing, preventing, minimizing, inflicting, relieving, enduring, and expressing are weighed with the consequences for life and death, carrying-on, interaction, ward work, and personal integrity" (Fagerhaugh & Strauss, 1977, p. 244). For example, a terminally ill patient in an acute care center has morphine ordered for pain relief every four hours p.r.n. (as needed). The patient must decide not only when to ask for the medication and how often but also how requests for medication (a narcotic) will affect her interaction with staff and family, whether or not the medication will affect alertness, and how to deal with personal feelings about continually having to ask for help in pain relief. Components of the staff's decision in administering the medication may include their feelings about drug addiction, the reality of the patient's pain, their knowledge of drug action, and their experience in working with terminally ill patients. Organizational and social contexts that are influential in this decision may include the organization of the unit itself—whether it is primarily set up to care for patients with acute illnesses or for patients with chronic illnesses; how busy the unit is; and the unit's ratio of staff to patients. A balancing of factors such as these contribute to the decision on how, if, and when pain control will be utilized.

Twycross (1983) presents "Ten Commandments" for health care professionals to ensure that patients' pain is managed:

1. Thou shalt not assume that the patient's pain is caused by the malignant process.
2. Thou shalt take into consideration the patient's feelings.
3. Thou shalt not use the abbreviation p.r.n. (i.e., pro re nata, meaning as required.) Continuous pain requires regular preventive pain management.
4. Thou shalt not prescribe inadequate amounts of any analgesic.
5. Thou shalt try non-narcotic analgesics in the first instance.
6. Thou shalt not be afraid of narcotic analgesics.
7. Thou shalt not limit thy approach simply to the use of analgesics.
8. Thou shalt not be afraid to ask a colleague's advice.
9. Thou shalt provide support for the whole family.
10. Thou shalt have an air of quiet confidence and cautious optimism.

By following these commandments, "patients with severe, chronic pain from advanced cancer can be made relatively pain free and permitted to close their life with dignity and purpose" (Levy, 1988, p. 274).

SUMMARY ❧

Hospice is a concept of care in the treatment of the terminally ill. It believes that the dying should be able to experience a pain-free, high quality life. It traces its roots to the beginnings of Christianity, but modern day hospice was modeled after St. Christopher's hospice in London, which was founded by Cicely Saunders.

Today there are over 1,700 hospices in the United States. Hospice has become an institutionalized part of our health care system. Although studies have not shown that the quality of life is different for the terminally ill if they choose hospice or conventional care, hospice has become a viable alternative for dying patients and their families. One reason why there may be little difference is because conventional care is incorporating the ideas of hospice in its treatment of the dying.

A major component of hospice care is the control of pain. Morphine administered by itself has been found to be the most effective means of controlling pain. In order to control pain, health care professionals must remember that their goal is not simply to relieve pain, but to prevent it as well.

LEARNING EXERCISES ❧

1. In Chapter 4 you were asked to role play a nurse, a doctor, or a social worker interacting in each of Glaser and Strauss' awareness states. Now, role play a nurse, a doctor, and a social worker interacting with a patient in a hospice vis-à-vis pain.
2. Discuss whether or not a patient should be given a dose of pain medication that carries a high risk of respiratory arrest. Who should make the decision?
3. Imagine where you would like to go to die. How would the place look? What objects would you have with you? Which people would you have with you?

AUDIOVISUAL MATERIAL ❧

The Heart of New Age Hospice. 28 minutes/videocassette/1989. Carles Medical Communications, 110 West Main Street, Urbana, IL, 61801.
An introduction to the principles and practices of hospice presented through candid interviews, this film uses music and visual scenes to emphasize its points.

Hospice: Medical Care for the Dying. 17 minutes/videocassette/1986. Health Sciences Consortium, 201 Cedar Court, Chapel Hill, NC, 27514.
This videotape shows the roles of physicians in hospice: their responsibilities vis-à-vis pain control, home care, and the team approach.

If I Should Die. 47 minutes/videocassette/1986. Daniel Arthur Simon Productions, P.O. Box 49811, Los Angeles, CA, 90049.
An award-winning film about terminally ill Sandy Simon who helps found the Hospice Program at Cedars Sinai Medical Center in Los Angeles, and then receives her own care there.

The Quality of Mercy: A Case for Better Pain Management. 55 minutes/videocassette/1989. Filmakers Library, 124 East 40th Street, New York, NY, 10016.
The argument for the effective use of narcotics in the treatment of pain is presented.

REFERENCES ❧

Amenta, M., & Bohnet, N. L. (1986). *Nursing care of the terminally ill.* Boston, MA: Little, Brown and Co.

Anderson, J., & McCann, J. (1992). Pain management: Challenging the myths. *Medical World News. 33* (4), 18–23.

Baines, M. (1980). *Principles of symptom control.* Paper presented at St. Christopher's Bar Mitzvah; London, England: June 1–10.

Buchanan, J. (1986). Analgesic drugs. In R. Turnbull (Ed.), *Terminal care.* Washington: Hemisphere Publishing Corp.

Buckingham, R. (1983). *The complete hospice guide.* New York: Harper & Row.

Camp, J. (1991). Patient-controlled analgesia. *American Family Physician, 44* (6), 2145–2150.

Chapman, C. R. (1978). Pain, the perception of noxious events. In R. A. Sternback (Ed.), *The psychology of pain.* New York: Raven Press.

Corless, I. (1988). Settings for terminal care. *Omega, 18,* 319–340.

Creagan, E., & Wilkinson, J. (1989). Pain relief in terminally ill patients. *American Family Physician,* December, *40,* 133–140.

Dunn, D. (1991). Tender care for terminal patients. *Business Week,* March 25, 107.

Fagerhaugh, S. Y., & Strauss, A. (1977). *Politics of pain management: Staff–patient interacters.* Menlo Park, CA: Addison-Wesley.

Foster, Z. (1979). Standards for hospice care: Assumptions and principles. *Health and Social Work,* February, *4,* 124–127.

Free, C. (1986). The nature of malignant pain. In R. Turnbull (Ed.), *Terminal care.* Washington: Hemisphere Publishing Corp.

Gilder, J. H., & Quirk, T. R. (1977). Assessing the pain experience in children. *Nursing clinics of North America,* December, *12,* 631–637.

Gonda, T. A., & Ruark, J. E. (1984). *Dying dignified: The health professional's guide to care.* Menlo Park, CA: Addison-Wesley.

Hillier, E. R. (1983). Terminal care in the United Kingdom. In C. A. Corr & D. M. Corr (Eds.), *Hospice Care.* New York: Springer Publishing.

Kane, R. L., Wales, J., Bernstein, L., Lebowitz, A., & Kaplan, S. (1984). A randomized controlled trial of hospice care. *The Lancet,* 890–894.

Kohut, J. M., & Kohut, S. (1984). *Hospice: Caring for the terminally ill.* Springfield, IL: Charles C Thomas.

Lamars, W. (1986). Hospice care in North America. In S. Day (Ed.), *Cancer, stress and death.* New York: Plenum.

Levy, M. (1988). Pain control in the terminally ill. *Omega, 18,* 265–279.

Magno, J. (1990). The hospice concept of care: Facing the 1990's. *Death Studies, 14,* 109–119.

McCaffery, M. (1972). *Nursing management of the patient with pain.* Philadelphia: Lippincott.

Meinhart, N., & McCaffery, M. (1982). *Pain: A nursing approach to assessment and analysis.* Norwalk, CT: Appleton-Century-Crafts, 361.

Mor, V. (1988). Participating hospices and the patients they served. In V. Mor, D. Greer, & R. Kastenbaum (Eds.), *The hospice experience.* Baltimore, MD: Johns Hopkins University Press.

Mor, V., Greer, D., & Kastenbaum, R. (Eds.). (1988). *The hospice experience.* Baltimore, MD: Johns Hopkins University Press.

Morris, J., Sherwood, S., Wright, S., & Gutkin, C. (1988). The last weeks of life: Does hospice make a difference? In V. Mor, D. Greer, & R. Kastenbaum (Eds.), *The hospice experience.* Baltimore, MD: Johns Hopkins University Press.

Munley, A. (1983). *The hospice alternative.* New York: Basic Books.

Paradis, L., & Cummings, S. (1986). The evolution of hospice in America toward organizational homogeneity. *Journal of Health and Social Behavior*, December, *27*, 370–386.

Phipps, W. (1988). The origin of hospice, hospitals. *Death studies, 12,* 91–97.

Robert, M. (1986). The Anesthetist as a pain therapist. In R. Turnbull (Ed.), *Terminal care.* Washington: Hemisphere Publishing Corp.

Rhymes, J. (1990). Hospice care in America. *JAMA*, July 18, *264*, 369–372.

Saunders, C. (1977). Dying they live: St. Christopher's Hospice. In H. Feifel (Ed.), *New meanings of death.* New York: McGraw-Hill.

Saunders, C., & Baines, M. (1983). *Living with dying, the management of terminal disease.* New York: Oxford University Press.

Silman, J. (1978). Reference guide to analgesics. *American Journal of Nursing*, January, *79,* 74–78.

Stoddard, S. (1978). *The hospice movement: A better way of caring for the dying.* New York: Vintage Books.

Tehan, C. (1985). Has success spoiled hospice? *Hastings Center Report*, October, *15,* 10–13.

Turk, D. C., Merchenbaum, D. H., & Berman, W. H. (1979). Application of biofeedback for the regulation of pain: A critical review. *Psychological Bulletin*, November, *86*, 1322–1338.

Twycross, R. G. (1978). Continuing and terminal care—overview of analgesics (historical and chronological evolution). In I. Goldberg, A. Kutscher, & S. Malitz (Eds.), (1986) *Pain, anxiety and grief, pharmaco-therapeutic care of the dying patient and bereaved.* New York: Columbia University Press.

Twycross, R. G. (1983). Principles and practice of pain relief in terminal cancer. In C. A. Corr, & D. M. Corr (Eds.), *Hospice care, principles and practice.* New York: Springer Publishing.

Twycross, R. G. (1978). The assessment of pain in advanced cancer. *Journal of Medical Ethics*, September, *4*, 112–116.

Wald, F., Foster, Z., & Wald, H. (1980). The hospice movement as a health care reform. *Nursing Outlook*, March, *28*, 173–178.

Zborowski, M. (1952). Cultural components in responses to pain. *Journal of Social Issue, 8*, 16–30.

Zimmerman, D. (1990). Freedom from pain; a revolution in the care of hospital patients. *The New York Times Magazine, 139*, S8.

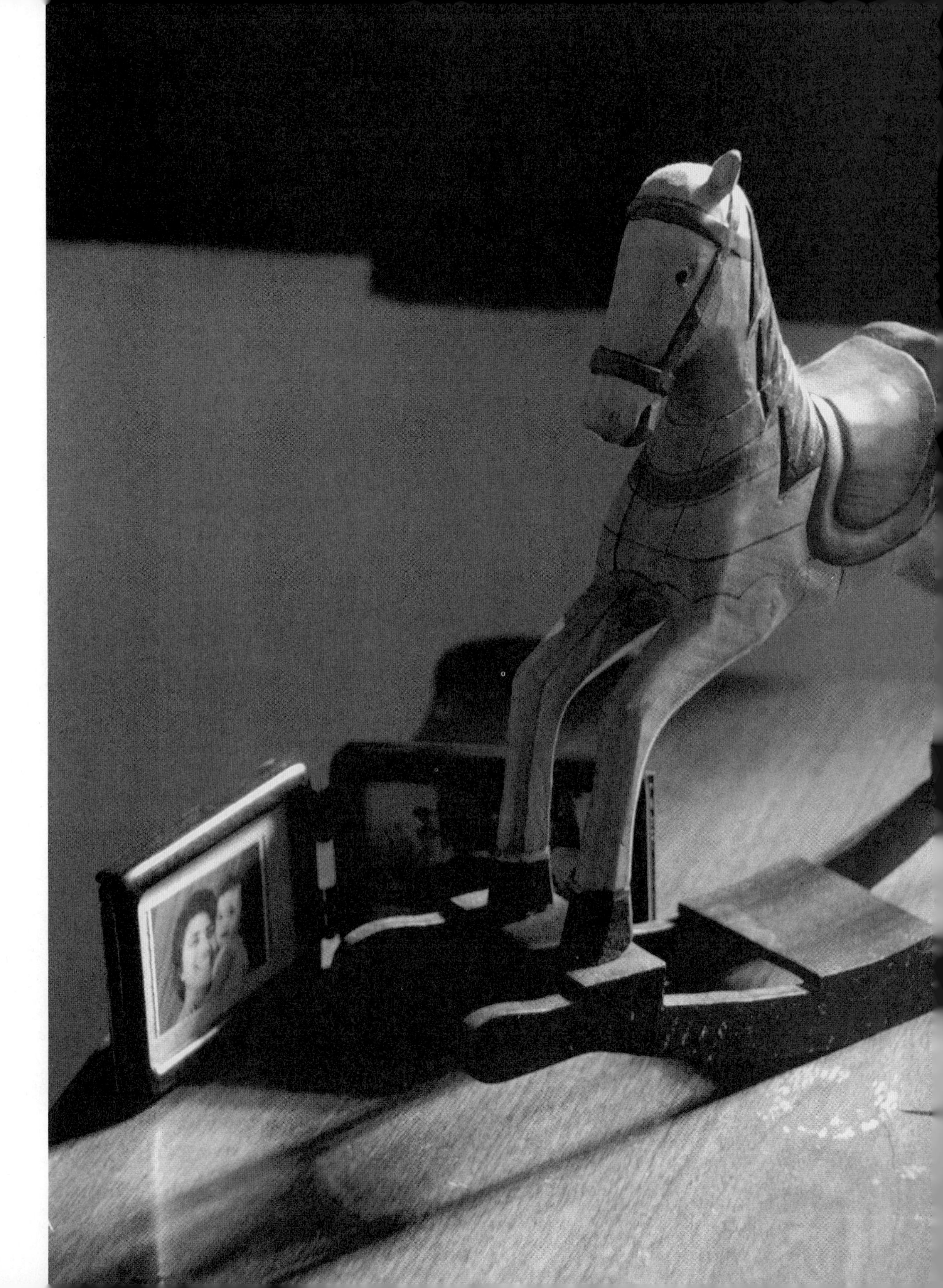

Chapter 6

Children and Death

A child's death evokes fears, questions, and anxieties about death and the emotional responses of grief, pain, and sadness. Questions are asked such as, "Why? Why must a young life be taken? Why this particular child?" The impartiality of death—and hence one's own vulnerability to death—are felt: if a young child can die, then all are indeed mortal. For many adults, the adaptive sense that life will go on growing and getting better is shattered by the death of a child. Relief is felt for the child whose death has brought an end to her pain and suffering. Relief may also be felt for self since it is no longer necessary to have to invest so much feeling and so much energy in the dying process. The hurt is real, as is the grief that this child will never know the joys and sorrows of a human being developing over a life span of years. There is, however, some solace in the knowledge that the child did experience the uniqueness of life, if only for a short time.

The loss of a child has many meanings for parents. Perhaps the first and most obvious loss is the loss of the child itself, with the concomitant loss of love, enjoyment, and the special relationship with that particular child (Purpura, 1986). A child may be seen as an extension of the parents, a part of their immortality; this is lost when the child dies. The child is also a personal creation of the parents, and this is lost. Parents' hopes and aspirations for the child must be relinquished. Another child born into the family never really replaces the child who has died.

Children who are dying also experience loss and significant changes in their life-styles. If they have a terminal illness, they often undergo changes in their actual physical condition and body image. They may feel tired and sick. As a result of different treatments, such as radiation or medication, they may have reactions that include itching, loss of hair, and loss or gain of weight. Family responses and roles may change. Parents and relatives may hesitate to set limits with dying children; siblings who were once fierce

---

Photo courtesy of and © by Dalia Migdal, Photographer

rivals may become very pleasant friends. These changes add to the already bewildering questions the child may be wondering about, including "What is wrong with me, and why do I feel so badly?" Children also react to the deaths of parents or siblings or friends with deep feelings which may go unexpressed unless significant adults in the child's life are alert to the existence of these feelings.

This chapter discusses children's responses to death and dying, family responses to the dying and death of a child, and how caregivers may offer the support and care children and families may need in these experiences.

Children's Concepts of Death

Children's concepts about death develop through a natural maturational sequence and specific life experiences. There have been numerous research studies on the development of the concept of death in childhood. A pioneering study done by Nagy (1959) was one of the first to present an outline of the developmental levels of children, 3 to 10 years old, concerning the meaning of death. The study involved 378 children in Budapest, Hungary. The children were asked to express their feelings about death in words and pictures. Nagy found that the children's replies about the meaning of death could be categorized into three developmental stages.

In Stage I, there is no definitive death. Children who are less than 5 years old usually do not recognize death as an irreversible fact; life and consciousness are attributed to the dead. Death may be seen as a departure, as sleep, or as gradual or temporary. The following conversation with a child is presented by Nagy (1959) as an example of these concepts:

T. P. (4 years 10 months)

> A dead person is just as if he were asleep. Sleeps in the ground, too.
>
> How do you know whether someone is asleep or dead?
>
> I know if they go to bed at night and don't open their eyes. If somebody goes to bed and doesn't get up, he's dead or ill.
>
> Will he ever wake up?
>
> Never. A dead person only knows if somebody goes out to the grave or something. He feels that somebody is there, or is talking (pp. 81–82).

Children in this group seem to accept death to a certain extent. They do not completely deny the finality of death, but they think of death as a gradual occurrence. At this point, they seem to have arrived at a compromise situation.

Stage II indicates children's personification of death. This seemed to be most characteristic between the ages of 5 and 9.

B. T. (9 years 11 months)

> Death is a skeleton. It is so strong it can over turn a ship. Death can't be seen. Death is in a hidden place. It hides in an island (Nagy, 1959, p. 89).

An increased sense of reality is seen in this second stage. Children accept the existence of death, yet the thought of it is still so frightening that they conceive of it as remote and external in the form of a person.

Stage III illustrates an acknowledgment of the cessation of bodily activities. Starting at the age of 9 or 10, children reach the point where they recognize that death is universal and signifies a cessation of bodily life.

F. E. (10 years 0 months)

> It means the passing of the body. Death is a great squaring of accounts in our lives. It is a thing from which our bodies cannot be resurrected. It is like the withering of flowers. (Nagy, 1959, p. 94).

Nagy's study emphasizes the developmental view of children's concepts of death. The fact that this study was conducted with European children who had experienced the effects of World War II could have affected the study's conclusions in terms of cultural influences and life experiences. However, subsequent follow-up studies have supported some of Nagy's findings.

Childers & Wimmer's (1971) study of children's concepts of death concluded that a moderate relationship exists between increasing age and an acceptance of the universality of death. The concept of the universality of death was almost unanimously upheld by the 9 to 10 year olds in this study, but the irrevocability of death was found to be much more tenuous. There was no age group in the study that was clearly sure of death's irrevocability.

In contrast to the above findings, an earlier study by Gartley & Bernosconi (1967) studied the death concepts of 60 Roman Catholic schoolchildren, ages 5½ to 14 years, and found that these children dealt with death in a very matter-of-fact and realistic way. "All believed in the finality of death rather than its reversibility as documented in other studies" (p. 83). The researchers suggested an environmental influence here in that religious training was provided in school, and the children had definite concepts of dying and going to heaven or hell. Anthony & Bhana's (1988–89) study of 40 Muslim girls' understanding of death concepts also indicated that by six years of age, the children were able to describe the universality and finality of death. It seemed to the researchers that Muslim religious education or training may have played a vital role in this understanding: the Muslim religious beliefs regarding death are very explicit.

Nagy's (1959) findings of children's personifying death between the ages of 5 and 9 years were not substantiated in the latter two studies. Kastenbaum (1986), in a review of research on children's concepts of death, has also noted that the tendency to personify death has not appeared in most follow-up studies. He suggests that "perhaps the world of childhood has changed enough from the time of Nagy's research to replace personification with more objective and scientific-sounding responses" (Kastenbaum, 1986, p. 252).

Meleor (1973) studied 41 children in Colorado who were asked about their concepts of death, and found that their concepts could be classified into four categories:

1. There is relative ignorance of the meaning of death. (Ages 3–4)
2. Death is a temporary state and is not seen as irreversible. The dead have feelings and biological functions. (Ages 4–7)
3. Death is final, but the dead can function biologically. (Ages 5–6)
4. Death is final and there is cessation of all biological functioning. (Ages 6 years and older) (Meleor, 1973, pp. 359–360).

This study found a maturational progression similar to Nagy's in children's development of death concepts. The awareness of the death concepts of irreversibility, nonfunctionality, and universality in children 5 to 7 years of age is supported by other studies in the literature (Speece & Brent, 1984; Lansdown & Benjamin, 1985).

Menig-Peterson & McCabe's (1977–78) study of narratives written by 96 children of important experiences in their lives showed that narratives about death were almost nonexistent for 3½ to 5½ year olds, but that over half of the 5½ to 6½ year olds produced 14 narratives about death. The most death narratives, 22, were produced by the 7½ to 8½ year olds (p. 306). The researchers suggested that older groups of children had a greater conceptual capacity to deal with the topic of death and more curiosity about it than younger children. Children less than approximately 9 years of age had very little if any affective responses to death and dying, whether of animals or people (p. 316). This finding could suggest a developmental progression in being able to cope with death emotionally, and it has implications for how, and when, caregivers and parents may want to talk with children about death and dying. The study also indicates that factors other than maturational development contribute to children's understanding of death.

Using questionnaires and survey instruments, Cotton & Range (1990) studied 42 children ages 6 to 12 years old concerning acquisition of death concepts. Results indicated the best predictors of the formation of accurate death concepts were cognitive level *and* past experience with death. Joy, Green, Johnson, Caldwell, & Nitschke (1987) examined differences in the concepts of death between 32 healthy children and 32 children with cancer (aged 3 to 16 years). There was no evidence that children with cancer exhibited more advanced concepts of death than physically well children. However, statistical correlations conducted within the cancer group indicated 3- to 6-year-old children who had personal experiences with death (loss of a loved one) were more likely to exhibit the concepts of universality, personal death (acknowledgment that "I" can die), and irrevocability.

Experiences with death for children currently growing up in the United States can include those involving the immediate family and beyond. Children may be exposed to different types of violence, including witnessing spousal abuse, homicide, rape, and suicidal behavior, as well as being victimized by juvenile gang violence and community violence (Pynoos & Nader, 1990, p. 335). The media, primarily television, brings pictures and sounds of violence and death into most households. Wass, Raup & Sisler (1989), discussing the results of a follow-up study on adolescents' television viewing habits and perceptions, state that the teenagers reported high proportions of violent death on their favorite television programs and on the news.

As the 1991 Persian Gulf War was being fought, children were watching the relentless bombing of Iraq and asking, "Who is being killed? Will it happen here?" A woman, attempting to explain the fighting to her 6-year-old daughter, talked about the war occurring in a distant land: " 'I'm not afraid,' said her daughter at the end, because the fighting is far away, right?' 'Right,' answered the mother, wondering what parents who aren't far away could possibly tell *their* children" (Telling the Kids, 1991, p. 18E).

Schonfeld & Smilansky's (1989) cross-cultural comparison of Israeli and American children's death concepts using the Smilansky Death Concept Questionnaire indicated the Israeli children scored higher than the American children on factors of death irreversibility and finality, and for total death concept score. The authors hypothesize that the difference in the scores may reflect differences in the rate or quality of exposure to experiences that might serve to advance a child's understanding of the concepts and to differences in the nature of explanations that accompany the experiences. The ongoing military activity and political unrest in Israel are a part of everyday life for the children.

However, there are parents and children who aren't living far away, who are living in the United States with violence and death on a daily basis. Kotlowitz (1991), in his book *There are No Children Here,* describes this as "the other America," our embattled inner cities. He talks about two boys, Pharoah and Lafayette Rivers, their mother LaJoe Rivers, and their family growing up in a public housing project in Chicago. The children confront death continuously in relation to gang wars and drug dealings.

> One night in July, amid the *rat-a-tat-tat* of a semi-automatic weapon, LaJoe heard a noise in the hallway. She turned to see what it was. In his sleep, Pharoah was crawling in the hallway to escape gunfire.
>
> A few days later, Pharoah, now eleven, told a friend: "I worry about dying, dying at a young age, while you're little. I'll be thinking about I want to get out of the 'jects. I want to get out. It ain't no joke when you die" (Kotlowitz, 1991, p. 264).

Theoretically, children growing up in inner cities and in areas of political unrest may be exposed to death in a way that can affect their concepts of it. In a study done by McIntyre, Angle, & Struempler, (1972), data indicated that low socioeconomic clinic patients, ages 6 to 10, conceived death to be due to aggressive causes (accidents, violence, war, suicide) whereas nonclinic children, from middle and upper-middle socioeconomic levels, believed death to be caused by disease or old age. The researchers suggested that their results reflect the fact that the lower socioeconomic status (clinic) children had "early and repeated exposure to death, chronic illness, violence, and exploitation, whereas the middle-class (and nonclinic) children were familiar with all the death-delaying tactics of modern medicine" (p. 531).

Studies such as these begin to give some indication of factors other than maturation that influence children's concepts of death. Much more attention needs to be directed to the unique set of variables, including ethnicity, race, class, and gender, that may be associated with a sample of children at any one point in time. Driven by the most visible change in its population in four centuries, the United States is redefining itself in multicultural terms (Roberts, 1991). Research on children's concepts of death incorporating this cultural diversity may yield new results.

To summarize, the pattern of research findings, despite considerable variability, indicates that both maturation and specific life experiences contribute to children's understanding of concepts of death. Children tend to move from conceptualizing death as a temporary and reversible state, such as sleep or a separation, to an internal and universal biological process (Stambrook & Parker, 1987). Children's concepts of death are also influenced by many other factors, including death experiences, socioeconomic class, social and cultural environments, family and religious attitudes and values, and other factors—some of which are probably not yet known and all of which interact with one another to form a concept and awareness of death for each child. Their concept of death and their maturational level will affect how dying children view their own death.

The Dying Child

Using a cognitive developmental framework based in part on Piaget's (1973) approach to cognitive-affective development (Schonfeld & Smilansky,

1989, p. 594), this section will look at how terminally ill children experience their dying.

The infant's world is centered on the meeting of personal needs of hunger, warmth, and security. After about six months of age, infants become more aware of their mothers as individuals separate from themselves. It is at this time that infants may exhibit some separation anxiety. They are aware of their mothers' absence and of the lack of gratification of their needs (Jackson, 1975).

Although infants do not yet conceive of death, feelings of loss and separation are a part of developing death awareness. That very young children experience these feelings is indicated in Bowlby's (1965) studies of infants and young children who have been separated from their mothers. Behavior changes in these children, such as listlessness, quietness, unresponsiveness to a smile or coo, and physical changes, such as weight loss, decrease in activity, and lack of sleep, indicate that feelings of loss and separation are being experienced. Therefore, if terminally ill infants are hospitalized, it is important that parents be allowed to stay with their children. Parents may also need encouragement to plan so they may be able to spend time with the rest of their family as well.

During the preoperational period of cognitive-affective development (18 months to 6 or 7 years), children's thoughts are egocentric and magical. Toddlers are very much concerned with themselves and with their ability to do things. They are developing motor ability, self-awareness, and feelings of power in relation to the environment. However, along with these powerful feelings are feelings of fear related to maintaining body integrity and safety. It is important in caring for toddlers to very simply explain any procedure that may be performed on them. Also, separation continues to be a primary concern, and parents again may need help in planning how to meet other family obligations if they decide to stay with hospitalized children.

The preschool child may have no clear concept of the finality of death. Death is often seen as reversible. Indeed, some of the current life experiences of preschool children seem to confirm this concept. The actor on television is shot dead one day but appears alive and well on another program the next day.

Preschool children are developing language skills and their communications give evidence of their lively and curious interest in the world. They are beginning to collect knowledge related to death and like talking and asking questions about heaven, God, and burials (Codden, 1977). One four-year old boy, attending his grandmother's funeral, asked his father, "Where is grandma?" When told that grandma went to heaven to be with God, the child replied, "Then who is in that box?"

The child's concept of death may involve magical thinking, that thoughts can cause action. Children may feel they have done or thought something "bad" in order to become ill, or if a loved one dies, it was because of some personal thought or wish of the child's (Hymovich, 1986). Parents and caregivers must listen to cues from dying children. The children may feel guilty about something they have done that would bring this illness upon them, and they need reassurance that they have not done anything wrong. Children also need reassurance that they are not alone, as well as simple explanations of what is going to happen to them at the time of each treatment and procedure.

Another important feature death has for children at this developmental stage is immobility. This concept is demonstrated in their play, as they lie motionless depicting death, and then bounce up quickly to show their aliveness. Thus young children who are immobilized in hospitals by casts, traction, and other restraining devices may have some anxiety related to death with these treatments.

During the period of concrete operational thought (7 to 12 years) children are beginning to realize the finality and inevitability of death. They note that when grandparents or friends die, there is no return. They see death as a separation and a loss. Children may cope with this anxiety-producing realization by developing rituals to ward off these frightening thoughts such as "always running fast if you have to pass a cemetery" or the rhyme, "If you step on a crack, you break your mother's back."

Children at this age may use intellectual coping, trying to find out how things work, or thinking through the cause-and-effect nature of an illness. Perhaps by understanding how things happen, one may then prevent one's own death. School-age children who are dying are nonetheless developing their independence and may need time away from their parents and hospital staff to continue to do this. Maintaining normal daily activities such as school, for even a short period of time, is important to enhance children's self-esteem and to indicate that adults have not given up on them because of their illness. Children need to have their questions answered about their illness and to be reassured that someone will be with them when necessary.

The period of formal operations, or logical thinking, begins around 12 or 13 years. Adolescents generally have sufficient ego development to understand the meaning and ramifications of death, but the reality of personal death is difficult to accept. Adolescence is a busy time, and death anxiety may be denied or used in new ways to affirm the ideals of life, such as relating to meaningful values and goals and developing emotional and intellectual capacities. Denial of mortality may be seen in the adolescent's death-denying involvement with speeding vehicles and experimentation with consciousness-altering substances (Hostler, 1978, p. 19). Safe sex practices involved in the prevention of HIV/AIDS and other sexually transmitted diseases may be scoffed at as part of this mortality denial.

Adolescence is also a tumultuous time. Starting with puberty, important physiological changes occur. A group of adolescent girls, responding with true teenage candor to a group of adolescent boys who were teasing them, shouted, "Get your hormones together!" Peer group approval is important, and peer group pressure and judgment are often harsh. There are strong sexual urges to become intimate with another person, yet these urges may be accompanied by ambivalence. Tension within the family originates from the adolescent's need to separate from parents while still wanting to maintain a closeness. Parents are typically criticized by their adolescent children; teenagers may fantasize that these people could not really be their parents, that they indeed must be adopted, that their "real" parents would be more understanding. All these developmental tasks will influence adolescents' responses to the issues of their own death and dying.

Adolescents are concerned with their future, with preparing for a career, with becoming somebody. Terminally ill adolescents experience much frustration in that, developmentally, they have decided upon goals they want to accomplish in life, but they now will not be able to attain them. Adults who are dying have some chance to review what tasks they have completed and what goals they have met, but adolescents have not had the chance to try out their newly formed values, beliefs, and dreams.

> Glen is a 17-year-old boy with a rapidly progressive neuromuscular disease. Discussions by staff concerning possibilities of tracheostomy, assisted ventilation, and deterioration of his blood gases are continually met with disinterest by him. His parents are concerned by what they interpret as increased anxiety at home. Hospital school teachers and therapists talk about the "strangeness" of Glen's behavior. An invitation to talk with his primary physician about his depression reveals he is not concerned directly with dying but with his virginity. Sexual fulfillment, previously a future goal, has become an immediate one, "before I get hooked up on all that machinery" (Hostler, 1978, pp. 22–23).

As illustrated in the above vignette, adolescents who are dying may need encouragement to talk about their anger, sadness, and disappointment about not being able to continue their lives.

Talking with Children about Death and Dying

Chapters 1 and 2 discussed the American culture's denial of death. The family system often incorporates this culture-bound inability to integrate death as a natural part of the process of living (Pattison, 1976). Parents wonder if, how, and when to include children in the family's mourning of a dead uncle, parent, or grandparent. They may develop various stories or be very vague about what has happened to a family member who has died, telling a child that "Grandpa has gone to sleep and you won't see him anymore." Families may avoid discussing the death or showing their feelings in front of children. Children can cope with death, but they have difficulties coping with family avoidance about death.

Talking with Children about the Death of a Loved One

Koocher's (1974) study of well children and their ideas about death lead to some suggestions for discussing death with children who have suffered a loss:

1. Children are interested in the subject of death, seem to want to talk about it, and are capable of discussing it. Silence about death only indicates to them that the subject is taboo and does not help them deal with their loss.
2. Explanations and discussions about death are most helpful if they are simple and direct, especially if children are younger than six or seven years old.
3. It is helpful, when explaining about death to a young child, to ask the child to explain back to you what has been discussed. Young children often use magical thinking and have many fantasies and misperceptions about death. Having the child explain to you what has been discussed may help clear up some of these distortions (p. 410).

Children may ask, "Mom, Dad, are you going to die?" Parents often are at loss at how to respond to this. It is important to find out what the child is actually asking. Readers may recall here the well-known story of a child asking where she came from, the parent giving an involved biological answer, and the child responding, "That's funny, Shauna says she came from New York!" Parents may respond in many ways to the question, depending on the age of the child, but it is helpful to remember that children are concerned about being cared for and about what will happen if a loss occurs. Parents may want to reassure children of their love for them, and what arrangements have been made if anything does happen. Many parents can let children know that they do not expect to die while the children are still young and need their help (Pattison, 1976).

However, some children do have parents who are terminally ill, perhaps with AIDS or cancer, and other children lose a parent through an accident or a sudden fatal illness. Talking with these children about death and their grieving feelings is very important in helping them cope with the emotional and psychological impact of loss in their lives. In addition to recognizing that children's coping will be influenced by their perception of death and the meanings attributed to it at different maturational stages, their responses to death and loss must be viewed within the family context.

Bowlby (1980) noted that family variables that he believed were associated with more favorable outcomes of childhood bereavement included: (a) what children are told about the death and what opportunities are given to them subsequently to inquire about what happened, (b) the patterns of family relationships prior to the loss, and (c) the family relationships after the loss. Within a supportive family context, supplying children with explicit information about the terminal illness of a parent is likely to enhance their ability to cope with anxiety (Rosenheim & Reicher, 1985). Dubik-Unruh & See (1989) suggest that, if at all possible, children "should be allowed to visit the parent during the illness, to permit as much interaction as possible and also to enable the child to become gradually aware that the parent is sick, that the illness is serious, and develop some understanding of death in that context rather than the parent simply disappearing out of his or her life" (p. 13).

Family relationships before the loss of a parent, such as family adaptability and the participation of the children in family rituals associated with death, may affect children's coping (Weber & Fournier, 1985). Research done by Vess, Moreland, & Schwebel (1985–86) suggests that families characterized by open communication and flexible power structures will more effectively reallocate family roles following the death of a spouse or parent than those characterized by more closed communication and rigid power structures.

Children need rituals in order to memorialize loved ones just as adults do, and they can be allowed to participate in funeral or memorial services to the degree to which they feel comfortable (Krupnick, 1984). However, Schaefer (1988) emphasizes the importance of explaining to children what they will see at the funeral home and the funeral service before they go there. They need to know about the casket, the flowers, the people visiting. "I have found that about 85 percent of the children between the ages of four and twelve who come to a funeral home and see a half-closed casket do not realize or believe that the deceased's legs are in the bottom of the casket" (Schaefer, 1988, p. 141). One small girl thought her grandma had been cut up because she only saw half of her. Children may not totally understand what is happening at a funeral, but the importance of the ceremony, of saying goodby and seeing other people who are sad about the death can assist them in integrating this loss.

The death of a parent means something very different in various phases of childhood than any loss in adulthood. To the adult, the loss of any one love object does not represent an almost total loss of object love (Furman, 1974, p. 128). During mourning, adults can usually rely on other relationships for support. The child, however, has invested love in one or two persons, and, when one of these persons dies, it is a special tragedy.

Immediate reactions of children who have lost a loved one will depend upon their stage of emotional and cognitive development, but may include feelings of sadness, anger, and fearfulness. Their behaviors may include appetite and sleep disturbances, withdrawal, concentration difficulties, dependency, regression, restlessness, and learning difficulties. "There are at least three questions, whether articulated or not, that will occur to most children following a loss: (a) 'Did I cause this to happen?' (b) 'Will it happen to me?' (c) 'Who will take care of me now (or if something happens to my surviving caretaker?')" (Krupnick, 1984, p. 119). It is important to listen for these questions and to provide answers.

Children are not as able as adults to seek out reassurance about their grief reactions and to share these with others; they need help in doing this from parents, teachers, and significant others. Their lack of sustained periods of sadness may sometimes belie the nature and intensity of their grief reactions; children strongly defend themselves against intolerable feelings that might overwhelm them. Pynoos & Nader (1990) observed that school-age children in particular monitor their parents' reactions and are afraid of adding to their parents' grief or anxiety (p. 341).

"Children who have lost a parent are at increased risk for physiological and psychological problems if the loss is accompanied by disruption in routine, changes in environment such as moving to a new home, or changes in other caretakers" (Dubik-Unruh & See, 1989). These children may also fear the loss of the remaining parent. The results of a study of acute parental bereavement in preschoolers indicated the surviving parents' ability to cope with their own grief and their capacity to provide for the emotional and other needs of their young children were important mediating factors in the children's responses to the loss (Kranzler, Shaffer, Wasserman, & Davies, 1990).

Additional conditions then that can influence children's coping with a parental loss are the quality of the surviving parent–child relationship, the parenting that children receive following the loss, and the stability of the children's environment. Such conditions, while important to the children's adjustment, may also place stress on the remaining parent who is also trying to cope with her own grief.

Siegel, Mesagno, & Christ (1990) note: "The death of a spouse is generally regarded as the most stressful life event an adult can experience . . . parents cannot be expected to engage effectively in an intervention focusing on their children unless their own needs are acknowledged and they feel supported in expressing their own grief" (p. 169). A psychoeducational program developed by the above-mentioned authors indirectly targets children through intervention with the healthy parent, providing that parent with support in dealing with her own grief and in continuing parental functions (Siegel, Mesagno, & Christ, 1990).

The impact of AIDS on a family can be catastrophic. More than one family member may have HIV/AIDS. A child may not only have to cope with the loss of one or both parents, but possibly also of siblings and of self. Families with AIDS experience fear: fear of losing their most precious possessions, their lives, and the lives of their children (Karthas, 1989, p. 158).

Little psychological support may be provided to the child attempting to make some sense out of these events. The parent or parents with AIDS may not have resolved the fears associated with their own death(s) and may find it difficult to help their child cope with death (Kirkland & Ginther, 1988, p. 307). Parents may develop symptoms that make it difficult or impossible to continue to take care of their children. One mother with AIDS desperately wished that her child with AIDS would die before her so the child would not have to be an orphan.

Parents may need a great deal of help and support in making arrangements for who will take care of their child after they are unable to do so, as well as making funeral arrangements for themselves and possibly for their child. Some families may be able to sufficiently work through the anger, guilt, depression and fear associated with AIDS to remain involved in making decisions for their child even though they may no longer be primary caregivers. However, the family system may become increasingly chaotic as addiction, illness, hospitalization, abandonment or court removal of children, and sibling separation or homelessness contribute to family death (Dubik-Unruh & See, 1989, p. 10). Even though a child may need to be placed in foster care or a residential home, maintenance of bonding between parent and child is encouraged. The child continues to look to the parent as a source of security and love, no matter how society may view the actions of that parent.

Talking about Death with Terminally Ill Children

Children who are dying are no different from well children in their abilities and in their need to discuss death. They are extremely perceptive and can see through the smoke screen of silence about their illness. Children know from their bodies, if from nothing else, that they are not well; their appetites change, they are tired, and they may not be very interested in anything. Bluebond-Langner (1978), in her study of hospitalized leukemic children, found that the children were very much aware of the social system of the hospital unit; that is, who had what authority and what the pecking order was. Although not all the children knew the name of their disease, acute lymphocytic leukemia, this proved no barrier in their learning as much as any lay adult about it and about its treatment, process, and prognosis (p. 157).

Bluebond-Langner (1978) found it quite remarkable that the children were able to find out so much about the hospital, staff, rules, and procedures, as well as about their disease, in a situation in which both parents and staff consciously tried to keep them from learning this information. All the children studied knew their prognosis and that they were dying before their death was imminent. However, they did not all express their awareness in the same ways:

> Some children said directly, "I am going to die," or "I'm going to die soon. . . ." Other children were less direct. They talked about never going back to school, of not being around for someone's birthday, or of burying dolls that they said looked the way they used to look (p. 165).

In a study designed to ascertain dying children's anxiety about and awareness of their prognosis, Waechter (1977) found that children were significantly knowledgeable about what was happening to them. The study indicated that giving children the opportunity to discuss their fears and prognoses does not heighten death anxiety; on the contrary, allowing children to do this may decrease feelings of isolation and alienation. Waechter concludes that asking whether children should be told that their illnesses are fatal is a meaningless question; what is significant is that the questions and concerns that are meaningful to children threatened with death are dealt with in such a way that the children do not feel more alone, different, and alienated from parents and other meaningful adults (p. 27).

Greenham & Lohmann (1982) note that in the late 1960s and 1970s a more open approach to talking to children about their dying began gaining ground after it was discovered that terminally ill children are often aware of their prognoses even if they are not told and that secrecy often sets up a circular process of interaction in which the evasions and deceptions of parents and caregivers erode trust in others and provoke excessive fear, withdrawal, anxiety, and frustration (p. 90).

However, some parents and caregivers may still focus on shielding the children from knowledge of their illness in an attempt to protect them as much as possible from fear of death. Often families (and sometimes staff) overprotect, cover-up, hedge, evade, stifle, or even lie to terminally ill children, to make their lives, short as they are, "easier" (Gyulay, 1989, p. 36). Vianello & Lucamante (1988) interviewed 30 pediatricians and 30 parents regarding children's concepts of death and discussing death with children. Both parents and physicians tended to believe children's understanding of death is less evolved than it really is, and they tended to avoid talking about death with children. Other researchers have noted that "while the open communication approach is gaining favor with medical systems, it is not universally championed, and there are still many medical systems that still adhere to the protective approach" (Chesler, Paris, & Barbarin, 1986, p. 514).

In Bluebond-Langner's (1978) study, only two children were able to bring about open awareness (p. 220). Both children initiated this process by similar overt statements about their dying, and their parents were able to acknowledge and respond to them. However, mutual pretense was the dominant mode of interaction between the terminally ill children and staff and parents. (See Chapter 4 for a discussion of open awareness and mutual pretense.) Bluebond-Langner hypothesized that this mutual pretense interaction provided individuals a way to do what society expected of them: children were allowed to act as children; that is, as if they had a future; parents could to some extent continue their roles of nurturing and protecting their children; and caretakers could continue their treatment roles (p. 229).

In thinking about what to tell children about their dying, it may be helpful to consider the same basic rule of thumb as in deciding what to tell children about sex; tell them only what they want to know, what they are asking about, and on their own terms (Bluebond-Langer, 1978). Most children become aware of their prognosis whether or not adults reveal it to them. Therefore, it is important to listen very carefully to what children are asking and saying, to understand their perceptions of what is happening to them, and to help them articulate their concerns so they can receive help in coping with them (Adams-Greenly, 1984).

Talking with children about their dying does not occur in isolation. Awareness of the family's culture, religion, and previous ways of dealing with crisis is vital. Parents and caregivers need to work together in what is being explained to the child. Parents may need time themselves to react, to respond to their child's diagnosis before they can begin to talk about it. Also, it cannot be assumed that telling is a one-time event. As the illness progresses, new experiences and evidence may alter what parents feel they must tell their child (Chesler, Paris, & Barbarin, 1986).

Children and family needs are thus both considered. The children may need to talk about their questions and concerns about dying but also need their parents to be with them. The parents may need to be with the children too, but may also need to avoid talking about the prognosis. Children may need to talk to caregivers, because they often are inhibited from expressing thoughts that may displease, alienate, or frighten other members of the family system (Lonsdale, Elfer, & Ballard, 1979). It may be possible to help children work out interactions of open awareness with people who can cope with this, while maintaining mutual pretense with people who need this type of interaction. Children are aware that they assume different roles with different people, and they can do this very well. The issue, then, is not so much to tell or not to tell but how to tell so that children's many varied needs, and their needs for different interactions, are respected.

Caregivers and Terminally Ill Children

Caregivers can offer support to children regarding their needs by careful and attentive listening to what the children are trying to express, especially in dealing with fantasies. Children may have many fears based on their perceptions of what they see in hospitals and on what is not explained to them. For example, such statements as "I'm going to give you a shot now" or "I'm going to take some of your blood," without further explanation, could evoke fears of mutilation and death within a child. Depending on children's developmental levels, explanations can be given as to what procedures they are going to experience, what medications they will receive, what the proposed treatment plan is.

The sharing of information and involvement of children in treatment discussion is most important in dispensing with fantasies. With younger children, who often cannot express their own feelings directly, listening to their "play talk" will give indications of what they really are feeling. A child's comment about a beloved teddy bear hurting or crying or being scared can tell staff much about that child's feelings. Also, children's drawings can be helpful in understanding how they are feeling. A group of children, all hospitalized with leukemia, consistently drew pictures of disasters—fires, accidents, bridges breaking. They were drawing their feelings about their lives ending soon.

Caregivers' awareness of their own feelings and reactions to dying children are basic and vital to all these interactions with children. Chapter 3 presents a discussion of health professionals responses to dying patients, but responses to dying children may be somewhat different. The death of a child in American culture, of which caregivers are a part, is still difficult to accept. "The death of a child is out of order chronologically, emotionally, socially, physically, and spiritually. A family should not bury the youngest generation" (Gyulay, 1989, p. 35).

In caring for a child with a terminal illness, staff may feel even more reluctant than when caring for an adult to change from an aggressive treatment program of cure to a palliative one of care and comfort. Anger at not being able to cure the child can be vented upon one another, with physicians and nurses accusing each other of inadequate communication or of not providing a certain type of care.

> It is often striking that, when the staff and/or parents are not yet in touch with the child's sense of dying and have not yet been able to accept the reality, they are not only at odds with the patient but also with one another—frenzied, irritable, and full of mutual dissatisfaction (Furman, 1984, p. 155).

Staff members also respond to a dying child in terms of their own developmental levels. Young nurses and physicians may respond with youthful rage, feeling death must be kept away at all costs and initiating all types of treatment to try and accomplish this (Easson, 1968, p. 206). In addition, violence is a daily phenomenon for many people, and victims of this violence are often cared for in emergency rooms and intensive care units. "Nurses often become angry at the needless suffering and loss of life that this violence entails. This is particularly true, for example, when a child is a victim of abuse or when drugs have compromised the life of a newborn" (Small, Engler, & Rushton, 1991, p. 104). It is possible that when a child dies both professional caregivers and lay helpers, who may have had a long-term relationship with the child and family or a very intense short-term experience, may acutely grieve this loss.

Caregivers need to be committed to providing support to, and openly communicating with, one another as well as with dying children. It is within the context of this sharing of hopes, feelings, and goals that the comforting and sustaining of each other and of patients can occur.

Families and Terminally Ill Children

It is often difficult for parents, siblings, relatives, and friends to know how to respond to dying children, either at home or in the hospital. Children develop self-confidence and trust from those closest to them (Miya, 1972, p. 220). Children need large quantities of love and support, but they also need to know the boundaries and limits in which they may live or die. They turn to adults for these needed limits and love, for, with both of these, children can feel safe and accepted. Adults may have difficulty in providing these needed qualities, finding it too painful to continue to love a dying child. Or, in feeling so much sorrow and pity for the dying child they may forget all limits and submit to the child's every whim and demand. If this happens, children may feel confused, lost, and without hope, for the source of their feelings of safety and comfort has become inconsistent. They do not know what to expect.

It is most helpful if "business as usual" can be carried on as much as possible with dying children. This means the offering of discipline as well as love. "Business as usual" at school as well as at home conveys to dying children that people have not given up on them. It also weakens the idea that these children are different. Special privileges and inflated grades need not be given, and as normal a school day as possible should be encouraged. If parents can live with the child as normally as possible during the illness, can refuse special privileges, not be overprotective, and—most important of all—enjoy the child, the child will get more satisfaction from each day she lives. However, family members themselves often have special needs as they live with their dying child or sibling.

Parents of Dying Children

Caregivers must listen not only to the needs of dying children but also to what their families say and need in this crisis. Today's nuclear or single-parent family often does not have the emotional support of a stable, extended family. Parents therefore may go through the psychic shock and emotional trauma of the death of a child in relative isolation, with little support from extended family or community. They may need some help with the mourning process in terms of knowing what to expect of their own feelings and reactions and how to cope with these both during and after their child dies. Koop (1965) has commented that families of dying children lose their children twice—once when the diagnosis and prognosis are explained and again when the child actually dies. It is during these times and the time in between that caregivers can help families develop the needed supports and coping mechanisms that will enable them to deal with this crisis.

The retrospective study of Binger, Ablin, Feuerstein, Kirscher, Zoger, & Mikkelsen (1969) of families who had lost a child to acute leukemia indicated that parents felt the most difficult time they experienced was when they first learned their child's diagnosis. "During the first few days or weeks after learning the diagnosis, most parents experienced symptoms and feelings of physical distress, depression, inability to function, anger, hostility, and self-blame" (pp. 414–415). These symptoms gradually subsided, to be followed by a more accepting attitude of the diagnosis and a desire to meet the needs of the ill child.

In their study of hospitalized children with leukemia, Friedman, Chodoff, Mason, & Hamburg (1963) found that when the parents initially learned of the children's diagnosis, they had what appeared to be an insatiable need to know everything about the disease. Parents not only sought out extensive information from the hospital staff but also compared notes carefully with the parents of other ill children. Such seeking out of information could be seen as a coping behavior for the parents in terms of gaining some control in a situation where they felt so helpless.

Parental reactions of loss of control and authority over what was happening to their young was also a finding in Bluebond-Langner's (1978) study. Parents felt powerless before the disease, the hospital staff, the treatment plan, and with their children. They felt they could not care for their children even on a daily basis. Mothers felt that nurses were taking over their nurturing functions. One way of coping with this was to assume a "Why bother?" attitude.

Caregivers should be aware of these initial parental responses and lack of affect, for there is a risk of labeling parents as cold or noncaring or intellectual when, in actuality, they are suffering greatly. When first explaining the child's diagnosis to parents, it is important to state it simply and directly. More detailed explanations can be discussed later as the parents gradually accept the painful reality. Caregivers can facilitate the maintenance of parental control by including parents in the care of the child as much as possible and in providing them with alternatives to consider when making decisions about care (Ross-Alaoblmolki, 1985).

Parents may often feel guilty about something they think they may have done to inflict this fatal illness on their child. A mother may review her pregnancy and wonder whether she took too many vitamins or whether she did not take enough; a father may feel he has not been an adequate provider for the child. Of special significance here is the family whose child is dying of hereditary disease or the family whose child is dying of AIDS.

The parents of a child with hereditary disease not only carry the guilt feelings of transmission but are also concerned about future pregnancies and whether siblings will get the disease. A child's diagnosis of AIDS not only confronts parents with the realization of one or more family member's terminal illness: the family is also confronted for the first time with the high-risk behavior involved—often bisexual activity or intravenous drug use (Karthas, 1989, p. 158). In order for families to function in any of these situations, they must move beyond trying to lay blame or guilt and begin the process of learning to live with the dying child.

Parents want to hold and cuddle their children, but often because of the pain from the disease process, the children do not want to be held or hugged. Also, parents are not able to protect their children from painful procedures. These realities further contribute to their guilt in not being good parents.

Anger is not an uncommon reaction to the impending loss of a loved person. The intense feelings of loss and of deprivation of a significant relationship can be difficult for many parents to express and may emotionally surface as anger. The anger in turn may be directed towards those with whom parents feel safe. Within families, parents may turn their anger on each other or may become easily irritated with siblings. Families may vent their anger on physicians, nurses, and the health care system, complaining about the poor care their child is receiving. If caregivers can understand that this anger is often part of the grieving process and not take it personally, they may be able to help the family members identify and channel their feelings appropriately. Discharging tension through physical activities, talking with other parents in support groups, or participating in fund-raising activities for medical research are some ways to vent anger.

Fear may be present in the parents' grieving process and may relate not only to what is happening to their child but also to family expenses and income, whether the disease will occur in other children, what other people and relatives will say, and how the family will manage after the child dies. Again, including the parents in active planning and treatment of the child can be helpful in reducing parental fear and anxiety. Caregivers can also help parents begin to cope with the realization that their child is dying by assessing with them the strengths the family has and how they may use and build upon these in this crisis. Family strengths can include the ability to communicate with one another; a support system of friends, relatives, and church groups in the community; and the willingness to ask for help when needed.

Coping Behaviors of Parents

In most instances, parents facing the death of a child will develop a variety of coping behaviors. It is important that caregivers understand that each family will cope in its own unique way and in terms of its own developmental life cycle; for example, coping behaviors may be different if this is a single-parent family, married couple, an unmarried couple, a family with young children, a family with adolescents, a family experiencing separation or divorce, or a temporary foster family. In addition, the AIDS epidemic has introduced a new constellation of family coping needs in the death of a child—that of aging parents who are facing illness, loneliness, and poverty in their own lives as well as facing the loss of an adult child. One 80-year-old woman tearfully spoke of her 30-year-old son dying of AIDS 3,000 miles away from her, "I so regret that I'm too old to go and take care of him now. I can't bear that he's so far away and with no family."

Parents may develop coping behaviors in response to situational tasks arising as a result of the child's illness. Hymovich (1986) has identified possible parental situational tasks as: (a) learning to understand and manage their child's illness and death, (b) assisting their child(ren) in understanding and coping with the child's illness and death, (c) understanding the impact of their child's illness and death on all family members, (d) meeting the needs of all family members as well as those of the terminally ill child, and (e) developing a feeling of control over their situation (p. 107). Mann (1974) suggests that parents have to master the following contradictory adaptational tasks: (a) making sense out of a disease that seems senseless, (b) experiencing the inclination to both fight and run away, (c) accepting and preparing for their child's death while attempting to maintain or discard hope for the child's life, (d) caring for and nurturing the child while preparing for separation, and (e) grieving for the child without giving in to an extent resulting in neglect of the child or other family members (pp. 83–86).

To accomplish these tasks, parents will need to trust themselves in developing coping skills and be supported in this trust by caregivers. Parents will also need to trust in the availability and capability of caregivers to provide information, guidance, and support throughout the terminal phase of the child's illness. One mother's way of coping with the deteriorating illness of her 11-month-old daughter was to search for information about the cause of the disease and, at the same time, to control the amount and timing of information she received about the child's condition. She elected to call the nursing staff to inquire about her child's condition rather than having the nurses call her on a regular basis. As the child's condition worsened, she began gradually to withdraw and to spend more time with her other child, her home, and her friends. When the baby died, she seemed calm and almost relieved that her daughter's struggle was over (Coddington, 1976, p. 44).

Contact with other parents who are experiencing a similar situation with a dying child can be helpful. The sharing of feelings and experiences in a group discussion gives parents the opportunity to realize that their grief reactions are not abnormal, to learn how others are coping with these reactions, and to mourn with others. In the study previously cited by Friedman, Chodoff, Mason, & Hamburg (1963), the primary source of emotional support for most parents during their child's hospitalization was other parents who were going through the same experience. The parents were role models for one another. When a child died, parents could learn that, although it was a most painful experience, they did not have to fall apart (p. 619). Most parents in this study also expressed the feeling that religion was of comfort to them.

Heller & Schneider (1977–78) attempted to build on the parental support system described in the latter study by forming a group of parents of dying children and using a peer-oriented, self-help approach called *reevaluation counseling*. The authors' basic goal was to establish support through teaching peer counseling—". . . that is, to have the parents learn to alternate between being counselors and clients with each other" (p. 324). This goal was met, and parents were able to provide mutual support for one another in the setting of these meetings.

Many families coping with stress may desire alternatives for help other than the often time-consuming, expensive, and traditional professional therapy modalities. They need people to listen to them, to reinforce their effective coping mechanisms, and to sustain them in their grief. These activities are not the sole prerogative of professionals. Peer counseling is one alternative to helping families in stress. Centers, such as the MacDonald Houses in New York, Philadelphia, and Chicago that serve as a home away from home for families of children being treated in city hospitals, are also places where parents can share their experiences and responses with one another.

The study by Binger, Ablin, Feuerstein, Kirscher, Zoger, & Mikkelsen (1969) found the following to be sources of support to parents: (a) physicians; (b) other parents; (c) clergy (if there had been a meaningful relationship with clergy before the illness; there seemed to be little value in introducing the family to religion at the time of illness if this was not previously present); (d) social workers, who offered practical assistance as well as listening to feelings; (e) parents of other leukemic children; (f) house officers and nursing staffs; and (g) morticians or funeral directors (fifteen families expressed positive feelings toward the mortician or funeral director for helping them with their grieving) (p. 431).

These studies indicate that parents can benefit from the offer of supportive help from peer groups as well as from professionals. To know that their responses are normal, to have someone available to answer their questions, can help parents a great deal with their anticipatory grief work. Anticipatory mourning, beginning to grieve before the child's death occurs, is an important concept to consider in reducing the seriousness and duration of psychological reactions in families after a child's death. (See Chapter 10 for further discussion of anticipatory mourning.)

Hope is an important component of parents' coping throughout the child's terminal illness. At the time of initial diagnosis there is hope that medical technology will find a cure or bring about a remission. "When that hope is taken away, the hope is then centered on palliative care, moving toward the hope that the child will die with dignity, without pain to the child or the significant others surviving with subsequent grief" (Gyulay, 1989, p. 33). Hope is valuable then for parents of dying children—not hope in the sense of denial of the disease but hope that the child will be comfortable, may be well enough to stay up that night and watch a television movie, or may just have one more good day.

Children's Responses to Death of a Sibling

"The well siblings of terminally ill children live in houses of chronic sorrow: the signs of sorrow, illness, and death are everywhere, whether or not they are spoken of" (Bluebond-Langer, 1989, p. 9). Siblings pick up very quickly that something is different about a sick child who is dying other than simply having an illness.

Children may feel jealousy, anger, and fear toward their dying brother or sister. They see their parents leave to visit the child at the hospital with presents; special favors and privileges may be given to the dying child and not to the other children. Friends and relatives visit and inquire about the ill child and not about the other children. Parents look tired and there is little time to share with the well siblings. Family plans must often be changed because illness does not adhere to schedules. All these events may be resented by siblings. Siblings may also fear that they have caused the illness, and, as a result, they feel tremendously guilty. At one time or another, children normally wish their siblings would go away or die. If a sibling does actually die, frightening fantasies may develop in the child who made such a wish (Gyulay, 1977).

Siblings' behavior often reflects these many feelings. School grades may drop and school attendance may be poor. Frequent visits to the school nurse may indicate the sibling's need for adult attention. The inability of many adults to talk directly about death only enhances children's fears and fantasies.

Once the ill child has died, siblings may express their grieving in many ways, including sleep disorders, acting out, acting like the deceased, regressing, losing their appetites or overeating, and feeling depressed (Bluebond-Langer, 1989). Older siblings may also show their distress through physical symptoms as well as seeking affection, and complaints about disorganized family routines. Many siblings are frightened about dying from the same disease that the ill child had. In the situation of a child dying from AIDS, the possibility of siblings having been born with HIV/AIDS is often real.

Parents can be encouraged to talk with their children about their responses. Parents may also need to discuss sibling reactions with caregivers. Perhaps the relaxing of some hospital visiting regulations, such as allowing siblings to visit the ill child, may help to clear up fantasies and misunderstandings. Siblings need to be comfortable with adults, parents, and caregivers with whom they can ask questions, touch, cry, laugh, and act out if necessary. They need to know they are accepted and loved, and they need to be told the truth about what is happening. They need to be included in the family grieving process both before and after the ill sibling dies (Bendor, 1989). Some families may be able to do this alone; others may need help, perhaps in the form of family conferences with caregivers. Kaplan, Grobstein, & Smith (1976) call for early family-centered intervention to facilitate the health and functioning of all family members when a child is dying.

Once the ill child has died, changes occur within the family structure. There is a shift in family dynamics and role relationships. Parents may have lost an idealized son or daughter. Siblings may have lost a big brother, a protector, or a scapegoat. Siblings are also confronted with a new status in the ordinal structure of the family. In a two-child family, the remaining child is the only child, and may not understand the concerted parental attention now being focused on her. A middle child may become the oldest child, with new privileges and responsibilities that may be both pleasurable and frightening. Siblings may become caretakers of younger siblings or parent to the parents. Surviving siblings' interactions can contribute to the coping of each other as well as of their parents (Rubin, 1986, p. 380).

Grandparents

Grandparents are often the forgotten grievers of a dying grandchild. They are grieving not only for their grandchild but also for their own daughter or son and for themselves. They feel helpless and out of control in this situation, feeling that they should be able to offer more help in coping. They may also be feeling guilt and anger that they were not able to prevent this from happening. Frequently, grandparents are separated from their children and grandchildren by long distances, and this, often coupled with less than the best physical and emotional health, makes it difficult for them to be with their families to provide actual physical care or to help with the emotional strain of the child's illness and dying. In families with parents and children dying from AIDS, grandparents may have to assume the role of parents for the remaining children. As with siblings, caregivers can help grandparents to cope by including them in family planning sessions regarding care of the ill child, and, after the child's death, in bereavement counseling sessions if indicated. Grandparents may want to participate, along with the parents, in self-help groups for bereaved parents such as Compassionate Friends, Candlelighters, and Mothers-In-Crisis.

Caregivers can sustain families through the child's dying process by acknowledging that dying children have a right to receive adequate pain control, enjoy unrestricted contact with people of their choosing, retain as much control and autonomy as possible, and receive affirmation that their lives have had meaning (Price, 1989, p. 53). Parents may decide to care for their child at home so that they may be with the child as much as possible in providing this kind of care.

Home Care for Dying Children

Home care for the dying child may be considered as an alternative to hospitalization; it may or may not be connected with hospice care. Home care can greatly enhance and maximize the quality of the family's and child's remaining time together and can make the separation and loss of death easier for all to bear. However, parents and caregivers need to consider both the advantages and drawbacks of home care in making this choice.

An overall beginning consideration for home care needs to center around what resources are available to provide the service. A study designed to examine the prevalence, utilization, and efficacy of home care services for children dying from cancer indicated institutions that provided their own home care services had a larger proportion of families accept this option and had a smaller proportion of children return to the institution to die than institutions that used community agencies (Lauer, Mulhern, Hoffman, & Camitta, 1986, p. 102). Problems identified in use of community agencies included inexperience with pediatric issues and procedures, inadequate pain management, and reluctance of families to work with unfamiliar staff. Institutionally administered programs were more likely to provide regularly scheduled home visits by pediatric oncology nurses and bereavement follow-up.

The study serves as an indicator of some factors to assess in deciding upon home care. Certainly pain control can be a major issue. All the people involved—parents, nurses, and the child—need to understand that pain control is possible and can be effective at home. If this is doubted by any of the people involved, the child may experience unnecessary trips to the hospital for pain relief. With the recent development of the computer-based, patient-controlled analgesia pump (PCA), children can administer small, preprogrammed doses of analgesic through an intravenous line; this eliminates the need for injections and offers the child a significant degree of control in pain management (Price, 1989). However, parents living in high crime areas where drug dealings are rampant may be reluctant to have any kind of medication or needles in the home. It is also important to assess what respite services are available for parents and children should either need some "time off" from home care (Dominica, 1987). Hospice programs may offer such services, as may some community agencies through a Visiting Nurse Service or a municipal Department of Social Services.

Advantages of home care include the child's continuing to remain a part of the family—its happenings, its joys, its arguments. Familiar surroundings, foods, people, toys, and pets enhance feelings of security. Siblings have a chance to participate in the child's care, and some of the mystery of what is happening is removed. The child receives the care, love, and discipline from parents that is consistent with her view of them. This may not occur in hospitals where parents may feel intimidated and delegate such parenting functions to caregivers.

"Home care then, puts the child into a comforting environment and gives the parents an active role in care as well as control over the immediate situation" (Martinson, 1979, p. 471). Parents and siblings are able to spend more time with the child. It is easier for many parents to care for the child at home because of the transportation, distance, expense, and time often involved in commuting from home to the hospital. Parents have talked about the constant conflict they feel about being in one place and feeling they should be in another, and about the strains and tensions that can arise in the family because a parent (either the husband or wife) is always at the hospital. Home care can help reduce these types of tensions and conflicts.

There are some possible drawbacks to home care. Children may sense that family and friends feel uncomfortable about their dying at home. Some children may feel insecure about being away from hospital-level acute care. The commitment of the family to the child's care can cause some physical and emotional strains. Relatives and friends may not approve of the parents' decision for home care and may evoke guilt in the parents for not providing what they consider to be appropriate care for the child.

Martinson, Gees, Anglinn, Peterson, Nesbig, & Keasey (1977) suggest that home care be offered as an alternative to hospitalization when the following conditions are met:

1. Cure-oriented treatment has been discontinued.
2. The child wants to be at home.
3. The parents desire to have the child at home.
4. The parents recognize their ability to care for their ill child.
5. The nurse is willing to be an on-call consultant.
6. The child's physician is willing to be an on-call consultant (p. 817).

Home care for the dying child may involve various methods of implementation. One common method involves the parents as the primary caregivers, with the health professionals providing support, teaching, and care suggestions as needed. Parents assuming responsibility for the care of their child may need support in their decision to try home care as opposed to hospital care. They may also need support in maintaining their relationship with their child while experiencing anticipatory grieving. Parents perhaps may need help in understanding that priorities of children change with a diagnosis of terminal illness. "Not unlike an adult with a terminal condition, a child may find the interests and pursuits of other children trivial to his or her present life experiences" (Cassidy, 1990, p. 36). Nonetheless, children and parents both need encouragement to play and to enjoy each other. Nurses may be involved in teaching the family such procedures as administering oxygen, using suction apparatus, and changing dressings. Suggestions for improving the comfort of the child, including positioning, hygiene, and nutrition, may be needed and helpful.

Home care may be an alternative choice to hospital care for dying children and their families. Key factors in this choice seem to be family acceptance of the impending death and the child's wish to be at home (Martinson, 1978, p. 88). Caregivers may help people to cope with the death and dying of a family member by providing alternative choices to hospitalization when possible.

Death of an Infant

The death of any child is full of grief and initially incomprehensible, yet the death of an infant seems particularly difficult to experience. The birth of a baby is seen as a happy event in the American culture; parents often do not give much thought to the idea that their baby may die. However, the infant mortality rate in the United States is one of the highest among industrialized nations; some 40,000 infants die each year in this country (Children's needs . . . 1991, p. 1).

The grief of parents after their baby has died is as intense and prolonged as that experienced at the death of an older child. The pain, the ache, the sorrow felt over the loss of a longed-for baby is so acute that it can hurt as much as any physical pain. One mother described her feelings about the loss of her 3-day-old son:

> I cannot bear to think that he is gone, that I will never know him as a person, that he will not experience the joys as well as the sorrows of life. I hurt inside—it is like an empty, painful void within me. I long for sleep so I won't feel this loss, and yet it is so difficult to sleep. I wake up and perhaps for a split-second life seems possible but then

once more this overwhelming ache, this pain of his death, engulfs me like a wave and I feel like I cannot go on. I will live, but right now that has little meaning for me.

Lemmer (1988) examined mothers' and fathers' experiences of perinatal bereavement by interviewing 15 women and 13 men (representing 15 couples) who had experienced the death of a baby through third trimester stillbirth or neonatal death. Qualitative data analysis revealed that all parents experienced grieving through a process involving devastating numbness, intense hurtfulness, and empty sadness before being able to put the experience to rest with precious memories (Lemmer, 1988, pp. 4754–4755).

The process of grieving the death of a child is usually facilitated by memories of that person. Families experiencing the death of an infant, particularly a stillbirth infant, have few if any memories of their baby. Grief responses may therefore be inhibited. Caregivers may assist families in developing memories of their baby by providing them with the opportunity to make a decision about whether they would like to see and hold their infant—an opportunity that should be offered daily as long as the baby's body is available (Lake, Knuppel, & Angel, 1987, p. 86). Parents can also be given the choice of receiving a lock of the baby's hair and photographs of the baby. Table 6.1 suggests options that may help create memories for parents.

Parents can feel very isolated in their grieving and may seek social support for this (Feeley & Gottlieb, 1988–89). Friends and relatives may ignore the fact that the couple had a baby who died; the baby and the death are not discussed. While the parents have a great need to talk about their feelings friends and family may continually avoid it. Parents may

Table 6.1 Options for Providing Memories Following Perinatal Death

Offer opportunity to see, hold, and spend time alone with baby
Offer opportunity for photographs
Offer mementos such as identification bracelet, footprints, lock of hair, articles of clothing worn in the nursery
Encourage naming the baby
Offer complimentary birth certificate with confirming data: weight, length, time of birth
Offer opportunity for baptism

M. F. Lake, R. A. Knuppel, & J. L. Angel (1987), The rationale for supportive care after perinatal death. *Journal of Perinatology*, 7 (2), p. 87. Copyright 1987. Reprinted by permission of Appleton & Lange, Inc.

begin to feel that they are behaving inappropriately in grieving their baby's death (Helmrath & Steinitz, 1978, p. 788).

Caregivers can recognize that parents may need support and help in verbalizing their feelings about the death of their baby. Their grieving can be acknowledged as appropriate and important. Parents need to be aware of the whole range of feelings that can accompany a loss—despair, loneliness, anger, guilt, abandonment—and that these feelings may come and go over varying degrees of time (Costello, Gardner, & Merenstein, 1988).

However, caregivers may have their own difficulties in coping with the death of an infant. People selecting obstetrics as a professional specialty expect to bring life into the world; they may not be prepared to cope with death. Obstetricians may view stillbirth as a serious medical crisis rather than a situation involving the death of a son or daughter (Kirkley-Best, Kellner, & Ladue, 1984–85). Constant exposure to perinatal deaths produces a tremendous stress on the staff, and caring for the bereaved parents can be emotionally exhausting. Caregivers themselves may need to explore more about their own responses to perinatal loss, and to share the responsibility of caring for each other as well as for patients.

Sudden Infant Death Syndrome—SIDS

A particularly shocking and devastating experience for parents is the death of an infant from Sudden Infant Death Syndrome—SIDS. This syndrome, commonly referred to as *crib death,* is the leading cause of death in infants between the ages of 1 week and 1 year in the United States; 6,000 to 7,000 babies die of SIDS every year (The Sudden Infant Death, 1989). SIDS is the sudden and unexpected death of an apparently healthy infant; the death remains unexplained after the performance of a complete postmortem investigation, including an autopsy, an examination of the scene of the death, and a review of the child's medical history.

The cause of SIDS is unknown. Current research studies into possible causes of SIDS include those involving the nervous system, the heart, breathing and sleep patterns, body chemical balances, autopsy findings, and environmental factors (The Sudden Infant Death, 1989). Researchers speculate that no one single area of study will provide the final solution, but that each area may contribute to a more comprehensive understanding of the problem. Although a death from SIDS is impossible to predict or prevent, Herbst, Kelly, Naeye, & Valdes-Dapena (1988) have studied a number of factors that may place an infant at a possible risk for SIDS: (a) maternal cigarette smoking or use of methadone HCL during pregnancy, (b) preterm delivery, (c) maternal anemia during pregnancy, (d) teenage mother, (e) male infant, (f) low socioeconomic level, and (g) overcrowded housing (p. 62). However, most babies dying from SIDS have few or none of these risk factors. Studies that indicate the low rate of SIDS in Asian-American groups (Grether, Schulman, & Croen, 1990) and in Latino groups

(Black, David, Brouillette, & Hunt, 1986) suggest that cultural factors may also be a factor in the incidence of SIDS. There is a high incidence of SIDS among Native Americans and Alaska Natives compared with whites, with a significant difference in the higher incidence of SIDS in Northern tribes than in Southwestern tribes (Bulterys, 1990). A prevalence of maternal cigarette smoking during pregnancy among Northern tribes as compared with Southwestern tribes indicates the need for programs to stop smoking targeted toward Native Americans (Bulterys, 1990, p. 185).

Parents' emotional, cognitive, psychological, and behavioral responses to SIDS are usually very intense. The infant's death is sudden, without warning, and totally unexpected. There has been no chance for anticipatory mourning. Denial and anger are common reactions. Guilt feelings may be overwhelming, and parents may feel they are literally going crazy with grief. They may ruminate over and over, "If only I had left the window closed that night . . ." or "I should have looked in on the baby one more time. . . ." Parents may blame themselves for the infant's death, and uninformed friends and relatives may also do so, sometimes even equating the death with child abuse.

Immediately after the child's death, parents need to know two important points about SIDS: (1) "Your baby died of a definite disease entity (SIDS)," and (2) "It could not be predicted or prevented; you are in no way responsible for the death" (Loscari, 1978, p. 1286). Other points helpful for parents to know are that: (a) the cause of death is not suffocation, (b) there is no sound or cry of distress from the infant, (c) there is no suffering, and (d) SIDS is not hereditary or contagious. It often helps to give parents written information about SIDS.

The crisis nature of this death, coupled with the many questions and feelings arising within the family, creates a need for extensive psychosocial support for parents and siblings. Family and friends may be able to provide such support, but families may need to use community resource systems as support networks. Special groups of people who are likely to come in contact with families involved in SIDS and who may provide help include nurses, physicians, social workers, police, funeral directors, emergency room personnel, ambulance drivers, clergy, school teachers and counselors, and SIDS parent groups. Weinfeld (1990) suggests that an organized, comprehensive approach to perinatal bereavement support must be established and describes a medical center program that includes the development of hospital bereavement protocols, provision of educational programs for nurses and physicians, and assistance in the establishment of local support groups in the community.

The American public needs to be educated about this cause of infant mortality and also about what services are, and should be, available to families who have lost a child to SIDS. Organizations that provide information about SIDS include those listed in Table 6.2.

Table 6.2 Resources Providing SIDS Information

International Council for Infant Survival
9178 Nadine River Court
Fountain Valley, CA 92708

National Sudden Infant Death Syndrome Foundation
Two Metro Plaza, Suite 104
8200 Professional Place
Landover, MD 20785

National Center for the Prevention of Sudden Infant Death Syndrome
330 N. Charles Street
Baltimore, MD 21201

National Sudden Infant Death Syndrome Clearinghouse
8201 Greensboro Drive, Suite 600
McLean, VA 22102

The Sudden Infant Death Syndrome Alliance
10500 Little Patuxent Parkway, Suitc 420
Columbia, MD 21044

SUMMARY ❧

Children's concepts of death are influenced by such factors as developmental levels, life experiences, family attitudes and values, cultural and social environments, and socioeconomic status. Dying children need to know that they will be cared for and that they will not be left alone. Their questions about their own deaths should be answered on their own terms with regard to what it is they are really asking and with regard to the total family picture of culture, religion, support systems, and past coping with crises. Children who are dying may be cared for at home or in a hospital. It is helpful for parents and siblings to be involved in planning and providing care for the ill child. Anticipatory mourning may help parents cope with the impending death of their child. Interactions with other parents of dying children may also be an effective coping mechanism.

Children, too, must cope with the death of significant others in their lives, be that person a parent, a sibling, a friend. Children grieve a death, although in different ways than adults, and may need help and support in this based upon their developmental level.

After a family member dies, family members may grieve in different ways, and family roles and relationships may change. Family members need to grieve not only individually but as a family unit, for it is this unit as a whole that is experiencing the changes brought about by the death of one of its members. Parents may need support in their own grieving process so they in turn may help their children cope with grief.

A child's death affects each one of us in a different way; we may feel love, hate, relief, anger, impotence, sadness. We may look at ourselves, at our own lives, differently. We will not be exactly the same people we were before. For better or worse, this child has touched us, and we cannot go back. Hopefully, we move on, with more awareness for others and for each person's uniqueness and place in life.

ANNOTATED BIBLIOGRAPHY OF CHILDREN'S BOOKS ❧

One way adults can encourage children to discuss and express their feelings about death openly is through the reading and discussion of children's stories with them. Parents and teachers may find these stories as comforting and enlightening as the children do. The following annotated bibliography is adapted from *The New York Times Parent's Guide to the Best Books for Children* by Eden Ross Lipson. Copyright 1988 by Eden Ross Lipson. Reprinted by permission of Times Books, a division of Random House, Inc.

Pre-School:

MY GRANDSON LEW

Written by Charlotte Zolotow
Illustrated by William Pène du Bois
Cloth: Harper & Row/HarperCollins
Paper: Harper Trophy
Published: 1974

Lew's grandfather died when he was quite small, but it turns out that Lew remembers him in vivid fragments while he and his mother talk about remembering.

NANA UPSTAIRS & NANA DOWNSTAIRS

Written and illustrated by Tomie dePaola
Cloth: Putman
Paper: Puffin
Published: 1973

As a grown-up, Tommy remembers the rituals of his visits to the house his active grandmother (Nana Downstairs) shared with his bedridden, ninety-four-year-old great-grandmother (Nana Upstairs), both of whom he loved dearly. Death is a fact, presented and accepted. Even now Tommy sees the Nanas' spirits in shooting stars. A very fine book.

SWAN SKY

Written and illustrated by Tejima
Cloth: Philomel
Published: 1988
Prizes: New York Times Best Illustrated Book

A companion of sorts to the beautiful and celebratory *Fox's Dream,* this story by a Japanese master, using astonishingly supple woodcuts, tells of the illness and death of a mother swan as spring arrives and her family must leave and fly to their summer home. Do not grieve. On their arrival she appears as the brilliant white blaze of the summer sky. An enthralling and comforting story from nature.

THE ACCIDENT

Written by Carol Carrick
Illustrated by Donald Carrick
Cloth: Clarion
Paper: Clarion
Published: 1976

This is the pivotal book in a series of three about a boy named Christopher and his dog, Bodger. In *Lost in the Storm,* the boy must wait out a storm before searching for his dog. In *The Accident,* his dog is hit by a truck and killed, and Christopher must grieve. In *The Foundling,* Christopher concludes his mourning. The stories are all sensitively and thoughtfully done, worthwhile if read separately or serially. The illustrations are low-key and unobtrusive.

ANNIE AND THE OLD ONE

Written by Miska Miles
Illustrated by Peter Parnell
Cloth: Joy Street/Little, Brown
Paper: Joy Street/Little, Brown
Published: 1971
Prizes: Newbery Honor

A little Indian girl recognizes that her grandmother is going to die and learns to accept the cycle of life and death. The story is told with delicacy and caring, and the fine illustrations are a perfect complement.

EVERETT ANDERSON'S GOODBYE

Written by Lucille Clifton
Illustrated by Ann Grifalconi
Cloth: Henry Holt
Published: 1983

Everett Anderson, a little black boy, must deal with his father's death. His feelings are eloquently evoked in simple poems and underscored in gentle pencil illustrations. Two other Everett Anderson books have been reissued—*Some of the Days of Everett Anderson* and *Everett Anderson's Nine Month Long.*

I HAD A FRIEND NAMED PETER: TALKING TO CHILDREN ABOUT THE DEATH OF A FRIEND

Written by Janice Cohn
Illustrated by Gail Owens
Cloth: Morrow Junior Books
Published: 1987

This is bibliotherapy, but there is no natural way for the subject to arise, and yet it does. Betsy's friend Peter was killed by an automobile. This is the story of how her parents and nursery school helped Betsy understand what happened. Very young children find death, even the death of a peer, unimaginable and there is no right way to address it. However, this book has an introduction by a social worker who has some thoughtful suggestions.

ROSALIE

Written by Joan Hewett
Illustrated by Donald Carrick
Cloth: Lothrop, Lee & Shepard
Published: 1987

Rosalie is an old dog. She can't run and her hearing isn't so good, but every member of the family loves her and makes adjustments for her infirmities. If your family has an elderly pet, this might be comfortingly familiar.

SAYING GOODBYE TO GRANDMA

Written by Jane Resh Thomas
Illustrated by Marcia Sewall
Cloth: Clarion
Published: 1988

A young girl tells about going with her parents to her grandmother's funeral. Her account captures the stunned uncertainty about what happens very well—family commotion, games with her cousins, a visit to the funeral home, the service itself. The understated illustrations fit perfectly.

THE TENTH GOOD THING ABOUT BARNEY

Written by Judith Viorst
Illustrated by Erik Blegvad
Cloth: Atheneum
Paper: Aladdin
Published: 1971

When Barney the cat dies, his young owner struggles to think of good things about his pet, and to understand both the finality of death and the unity of life. This is a splendid book, deservedly a classic, suitable for readers of all ages. In its simplicity and the genuine comfort it offers, it is one of the best books for children about death.

THE TWO OF THEM

Written and illustrated by Aliki

Cloth: Greenwillow

Paper: Mulberry

Published: 1979

This is a quiet story about a grandfather who loved his granddaughter from the time she was born, and how, when he died, she was able to remember things he had made for her and the time they had spent together, and thus absorb their special relationship.

Middle Readers:

BRIDGE TO TERABITHIA

Written by Katherine Paterson
Illustrated by Donna Diamond

Cloth: T. Y. Crowell/HarperCollins

Paper: Harper Trophy

Published: 1977

This is an astonishingly powerful novel about an improbable friendship between Jess, a poor local boy, and Leslie, the willful, brilliantly imaginative girl who moves into a house nearby. They establish a secret hiding place they call Terabithia and develop a rich friendship that is severed when Leslie is accidentally killed. There are only a few novels for children about death and they are generally unsatisfactory. This one succeeds brilliantly and speaks to the resolution of grief among the living. But because the writing is so fine and persuasive, the impact on readers of all ages is deep. This is a six-Kleenex late-night-talk-time story, and worth the effort.

EIGHTY-EIGHT STEPS TO SEPTEMBER

Written by Jan Marino

Cloth: Little, Brown

Paper: Avon

Published: 1989

The setting is Boston in the summer of 1948, and the subject is death within the immediate family. Amy Martin's thirteen-year-old brother is dying of leukemia. Amy's denial and anger and fear are captured poignantly, and by the end of the book, she is accepting the new condition of her family's life.

HOW IT FEELS WHEN A PARENT DIES

Written and illustrated by Jill Krementz
Paper: Knopf
Published: 1981

Some eighteen children of different ages and backgrounds talk about the death of a parent—how it felt, how it feels. Their health and well-being in the photographs is subtle reinforcement of the implicit message that life goes on.

LEARNING TO SAY GOOD-BYE: WHEN A PARENT DIES

Written by Eda LeShan
Illustrated by Paul Giavanopoulos
Cloth: Macmillan
Published: 1976

This book is written like a conversation with children about some of the feelings they might encounter if they had to deal with the death of a parent. The author has a compassionate but frank tone. Among her other thoughtful books about problems are *What Makes Me Feel This Way: Growing Up with Human Emotions; What's Going to Happen to Me: When Parents Separate or Divorce;* and *When Kids Drive Kids Crazy.*

A TASTE OF BLACKBERRIES

Written by Doris Buchanan Smith
Illustrated by Charles Robinson
Cloth: T. Y. Crowell/HarperCollins
Paper: Harper Trophy
Published: 1973

In this short, thoughtful novel, a young boy describes his friendship with Jamie and Jamie's sudden death. This is not a substitute for parental support in real life; it is a good novel and not bibliotherapy.

THANK YOU, JACKIE ROBINSON

Written by Barbara Cohen
Illustrated by Richard Cuffari
Cloth: Lothrop, Lee & Shepard
Paper: Scholastic
Published: 1974

A poignant story tells about a young, fatherless white boy and an old black man who are passionate fans of the Brooklyn Dodgers and especially Jackie Robinson. Good deeds are done before the old man dies.

Young Adults:

GOING BACKWARDS

Written by Norma Klein
Cloth: Scholastic
Paper: Scholastic
Published: 1986

In this thoughtful domestic-problem novel, Charles's beloved Grandmother Gustel has Alzheimer's disease. The ending is arbitrary; however, the plot development and the descriptions of the disease affects everyone in the family are particularly well done.

MY BROTHER STEALING SECOND

Written by Jim Naughton
Cloth: Harper & Row/HarperCollins
Paper: Harper Trophy
Published: 1989

The title of this affecting novel of emotional recovery refers to Bobby's favorite memory of his older brother, Billy, who died in an accident before the story begins. The author, a sportswriter, uses baseball scenes deftly.

NIGHT KITES

Written by M. E. Kerr
Cloth: Harper & Row/HarperCollins
Paper: Harper Trophy
Published: 1986

Erick Rudd has a difficult, provocative girlfriend, a rather pompous father, and a kind older brother, who, it turns out, has AIDS. The novel deals with the problem of AIDS within a family, and acknowledging the sexual preference of an adult child with skill and tact as the background to Erick's own maturation.

TIGER EYES

Written by Judy Blume
Cloth: Bradbury
Paper: Laurel Leaf
Published: 1981

One of the most serious of the Blume novels, addressed to older readers, is about a girl called Davey. Her father was killed in a holdup of his store, and she must cope with grief and fear and learn to go on. Davey and her mother head west, to visit relatives in New Mexico, where Davey is befriended by a boy called Wolf.

LEARNING EXERCISES ❧

1. Review children's fairy tales such as "Snow White and the Seven Dwarfs" and "The Sleeping Beauty." Discuss how these relate developmentally to young children's concepts of death.
2. Debate the pros and cons of death education in the public school system.
3. What would you say to a 5-year-old child who asks you, "Where do I go when I die?" What factors would you consider before answering the child?
4. You are a member of a community school board that is meeting to establish a policy for children with HIV/AIDS remaining in the school system. What data are necessary to know to establish this policy? What policy would you recommend?
5. Explore the resources in your community that could be made available to parents and families who are grieving the death of a child.

AUDIOVISUAL MATERIAL ❧

Some Babies Die. 54 minutes/videocassette/1986. University of California, Extension Media Center, 216 Shattuck Avenue, Berkeley, CA, 94704.
Elisabeth Kübler-Ross is the narrator of this film. An Australian counseling team consisting of a pediatrician, nurse, and psychologist help grieving families cope with the feelings that accompany stillbirth and neonatal death. The video focuses on the families of two women, one dealing with the loss of her third child, and the other who has experienced three stillbirths.

Bereaved Parents. 28 minutes/videocassette. Films for the Humanities and Sciences, Box 2053, Princeton, NJ, 08543.
This film addresses the issues of loss and guilt and suggests that parents can better cope with the death of a child by sharing their grief with others and by talking about the lost child.

Children And The Grief Process. 21 minutes/videocassette/1983. Coronet, The Multimedia Co., 108 Wilmot Road, Deerfield, IL, 60015.
This film features Rabbi Earl Grollman, D.D., discussing death with a group of young children. It illustrates ways to help children cope with their feelings about death in a positive manner.

Sudden Infant Death Syndrome . . . A Family's Anguish. 15 minutes/videocassette/1986. Colorado SIDS Program, 1330 Leyden Street, # 134, Denver, CO, 80220.

Medical and statistical information is presented on SIDS. Family issues are presented through interviews with parents—including a single parent—who have lost children to SIDS, and with surviving siblings.

The Forgotten Mourner. 28 minutes/videocassette/hosted by Phil Donohue. Films for the Humanities and Sciences, Box 2053, Princeton, NJ, 08543.
This is a discussion of the mourning needs of siblings and grandparents which are frequently overlooked when there is a death in the family.

REFERENCES ❧

Adams-Greenly, M. (1984). Helping children communicate about serious illness and death. *Journal of Psychosocial Oncology, 2* (2), 61–72.

Anthony, Z., & Bhana, K. (1988-89). An exploratory study of Muslim girls' understanding of death. *Omega: Journal of Death and Dying, 19* (3), 215–227.

Bendor, S. J. (1989). Preventing psychosocial impairment in siblings of terminally ill children. *Hospice Journal: Physical, Psychosocial, and Pastoral Care of the Dying, 5,* March 4, 153–163.

Binger, C. M., Ablin, A. R., Feuerstein, R. C., Kirscher, J. H., Zoger, S., & Mikkelsen, C. (1969). Childhood leukemia: Emotional impact on patient and family. *New England Journal of Medicine, 280* (8), February 20, 414–418.

Black, L., David, R. J., Brouillette, R. T., & Hunt, C. E. (1986). Effects of birthweight and ethnicity on incidence of Sudden Infant Death Syndrome. *Journal of Pediatrics, 108* (2), 209–214.

Bluebond-Langner, M. (1978). *The private worlds of dying children.* Princeton, NJ: Princeton University Press.

Bluebond-Langner, M. (1989). Worlds of dying children and their well siblings. *Death Studies, 13* (1), 1–16.

Bowlby, J. (1965). *Child care and the growth of love.* Baltimore, MD: Penguin Books.

Bowlby, J. (1980). *Loss, sadness and depression: Attachment and loss* (Vol. 3). London: Hogarth Press, 276–296.

Bulterys, M. (1990). High incidence of SIDS among Northern Indians and Alaska Natives compared with Southwestern Indians: Possible role of smoking. *Journal of Community Health, 15* (3), 185–194.

Cassidy, M. (1990). Supportive care and the dying child. *Journal of Home Health Care Practice, 3* (1), 34–38.

Chesler, M. A., Paris, J., & Barbarin, O. A., (1986). "Telling" the child with Cancer: Parental choices to share information with ill children. *Journal of Pediatric Psychology, 11* (4), 497–516.

Childers, P., & Wimmer, M. (1971). The concept of death in early childhood. *Child Development, 42* (4), 1299–1301.

Children's needs challenge RNs. (1991). *The American Nurse,* June, 1.

Codden, P. (1977). The meaning of death for parents and the child. *Maternal-Child Nursing Journal, 6* (1), 9–16.

Coddington, M. (1976). A mother struggles to cope with her child's deteriorating illness. *Maternal-Child Nursing Journal, 5* (1), 39–44.

Costello, A., Gardner, S. L., Merenstein, G. B. (1988). Perinatal grief and loss. *Journal of Perinatology, 8* (4), 361–370.

Cotton, C. R., & Range, L. M. (1990). Children's death concepts: Relationship to cognitive functioning, age, experience with death, fear of death and hopefulness. *Journal of Clinical Child Psychology, 19* (2), 123–127.

Dominica, F. (1987). The role of the hospice for the dying child. *British Journal of Hospital Medicine, 38* (4), 334–336.

Dubik-Unruh, S., & See, V. (1989). Children of chaos: Planning for the emotional survival of dying children of dying families. *Journal of Palliative Care, 5* (2), 10–15.

Easson, W. (1968). Care of the young patient who is dying. *Journal of the American Medical Association, 205* (4), July 22, 203–207.

Feeley, N., & Gottlieb, L. N. (1988–89). Parents' coping and communicating following their infant's death. *Omega: Journal of Death and Dying, 19* (1), 51–67.

Friedman, S., Chodoff, P., Mason, J., & Hamburg, D. (1963). Behavioral observations on parents anticipating the death of a child. *Pediatrics, 32,* October, 610–625.

Furman, E. (1974). *A child's parent dies.* New Haven, CT: Yale University Press.

Furman, E. (1984). Helping children cope with dying. *Journal of Child Psychotherapy, 10* (2), 151–157.

Gartley, W., & Bernosconi, M. (1967). The concept of death in children. *Journal of Genetic Psychology, 110* (first half), 71–85.

Greenham, D. E., & Lohmann, R. A. (1982). Children facing death: Recurring patterns of adaptation. *Health and Social Work, 7* (2), 89–94.

Grether, J. K., Schulman, J., & Croen, L. A. (1990). Sudden Infant Death Syndrome among Asians in California. *Journal of Pediatrics, 116* (4), 525–528.

Gyulay, J. E. (1977). The forgotten grievers. In L. Wilkenfeld (Ed.), *When children die.* Dubuque, IA: Kendall/Hunt.

Gyulay, J. E. (1989). Home care for the dying child. *Issues in Comprehensive Pediatric Nursing, 42* (1), 33–69.

Heller, D. B., & Schneider, C. (1977–78). Interpersonal methods for coping with stress: Helping families of dying children. *Omega: Journal of Death and Dying, 8* (4), 319–331.

Helmrath, T., & Steinitz, E. (1978). Death of an infant: Parental grieving and the failure of social support. *Journal of Family Practice, 6* (4), 785–790.

Herbst, J. J., Kelly, D., Naeye, R. L., & Valdes-Dapena, M. (1988). New findings shed light on SIDS. *Patient Care, 22* (9), 61–63, 67, 71.

Hostler, S. L. (1978). The development of the child's concept of death. In O. J. Sahler (Ed.), *The child and death.* St. Louis, MO: Mosby.

Hymovich, D. P. (1986). Child and family teachings: Special needs and approaches. *Hospice Journal: Physical, Psychosocial, and Pastoral Care of the Dying, 2* (1), 103–120.

Jackson, P. (1975). The child's developing concept of death: Implications for nursing care of the terminally ill child. *Nursing Forum, 14* (2), 204–215.

Joy, S. M., Green, V., Johnson, S., Caldwell, S., & Nitschke, R. (1987). Differences in death concepts between children with cancer and physically healthy children. *Journal of Clinical Child Psychology, 16* (4), 301–306.

Kaplan, D. M., Grobstein, R., & Smith, A. (1976). Predicting the impact of severe illness in families. *Health and Social Work, 1* (3), 71–82.

Karthas, N. (1989). Identifying special needs: Children with HIV infection. In J. B. Meisenhelder & C. L. LaCharite (Eds.), *Comfort in caring: Nursing the person with HIV infection* (pp. 152–166). Glenview, IL: Scott, Foresman/Little, Brown.

Kastenbaum, R. (1986). *Death, society, and human experience* (3rd Ed.). Columbus, OH: Merrill.

Kirkland, M., & Ginther, D. (1988). Acquired Immune Deficiency Syndrome in children: Medical, legal, and school related issues. *School Psychology Review, 17* (2), 304–310.

Kirkley-Best, E., Kellner, K. R., & Ladue, T. (1984–85). Attitudes toward stillbirth and death threat level in a sample of obstetricians. *Omega: Journal of Death and Dying, 15* (4), 317–327.

Koocher, G. (1974). Talking with children about death. *American Journal of Orthopsychiatry, 44* (3), 404–411.

Koop, C. E. (1965). The seriously ill or dying child: Supporting the patient and the family. *Pediatric Clinics of North America, 16* (3), 555–564.

Kotlowitz, A. (1991). *There are no children here.* NY: Doubleday.

Kranzler, E. M., Shaffer, D., Wasserman, G., & Davies, M. (1990). Early childhood bereavement. *Journal of the American Academy of Child and Adolescent Psychiatry, 29* (4), 513–520.

Krupnick, J. L. (1984). Bereavement during childhood and adolescence. In M. Osterweis, F. Solomon, & M. Green (Eds.), *Bereavement: Reactions, consequences and care* (pp. 99–141). Washington, DC: National Academy Press.

Lake, M. F., Knuppel, R. A., & Angel, J. L. (1987). The rationale for supportive care after perinatal death. *Journal of Perinatology, 7* (2), 85–89.

Lansdown, R., & Benjamin, G. (1985). The development of the concept of death in children aged 5–9 years. *Child Care, Health & Development, 11* (1), 13–20.

Lauer, M. E., Mulhern, R. K., Hoffman, R. B., & Camitta, B. M. (1986). Utilization of hospice/home care in pediatric oncology. *Cancer Nursing, 9* (3), 102–107.

Lemmer, C.M. (1988). Mothers' and fathers' experiences of perinatal bereavement. *Dissertation Abstracts International, 49,* 4754B–4755B.

Lonsdale, G., Elfer, P., & Ballard, R. (1979). *Children, grief and social work.* Oxford: Basil Blackwell.

Loscari, A. (1978). The dying child and the family. *Journal of Family Practice, 6* (6), 1279–1286.

Mann, S. A. (1974). Coping with a child's fatal illness: A parent's dilemma. *Nursing Clinics of North America, 9* (1), 81–87.

Martinson, I. M., (1978). Alternate environments for care of the dying child: Hospice, hospital, or home. In O. J. Sahler (Ed.), *The child and death* (pp. 83–91). St. Louis, MO: Mosby.

Martinson, I. M., (1979). Caring for the dying child. *Nursing Clinics of North America, 14* (3), 467–474.

Martinson, I. M., Gees, D., Anglinn, M. A., Peterson, E., Nesbig, M., & Keasey, J. (1977). Home care for the child. *American Journal of Nursing, 77* (11), 815–817.

McIntyre, M. S., Angle, C. R., & Struempher, L. J. (1972). The concept of death in midwestern children and youth. *American Journal of Diseases of Children, 123,* 527–532.

Meleor, J. D. (1973). Children's conceptions of death. *Journal of Genetic Psychology, 123* (2), 359–360.

Menig-Peterson, C., & McCabe, A. (1977–78). Children talk about death. *Omega: Journal of Death and Dying, 8* (4), 305–318.

Miya, T. M. (1972). The child's perception of death. *Nursing Forum, 11* (2), 214–220.

Nagy, M. (1959). The child's view of death. In H. Feifel (Ed.), *The meaning of death* (pp. 79–98). NY: McGraw-Hill. (Reprinted, with some editorial changes, with permission from the *Journal of Genetic Psychology* (1948). *73,* 3–27).

Pattison, E. M. (1976). The fatal myth of death in the family. *American Journal of Psychiatry, 133* (6), 674–678.

Piaget, J. (1973). *The child and reality—problems of genetic psychology.* New York: Grossman.

Price, K. (1989). Quality of life for terminally ill children. *Social Work, 34* (1), 53–54.

Purpura, P. A. (1986). The death of a child: The death of an illusion. *Issues in Ego Psychology, 9* (2), 20–24.

Pynoos, R. S., & Nader, K. (1990). Children's exposure to violence and traumatic death. *Psychiatric Annals, 20* (6), 334–344.

Roberts, S. (1991, July 28). Reshaping of New York City hits Black-Hispanic alliance. *New York Times,* pp. 1, L27.

Rosenheim, E., & Reicher, R. (1985). Informing children about a terminal illness. *Journal of Child Psychology and Psychiatry and Allied Disciplines, 26* (6), 995–998.

Ross-Alaobmolki, K. (1985). Supportive care for the families of dying children. *Nursing Clinics of North America, 20* (2), 457–466.

Rubin, S. (1986). Child death and the family: Parents and children confronting loss. *International Journal of Family Psychiatry,* 7 (4), 377–388.

Schaefer, D. J. (1988). Communication among children, parents, and funeral directors. *Loss, Grief and Care, 2* (3–4), 131–142.

Schonfeld, D. J., & Smilansky, S. (1989). A cross-cultural comparison of Israeli and American children's death concepts. *Death Studies, 13* (6), 593–604.

Siegel, K., Mesagno, F. P., & Christ, G. (1990). A prevention program for bereaved children. *American Journal of Orthopsychiatry, 60* (2), 168–175.

Small, M., Engler, A. J., & Rushton, C. H. (1991). Saying goodbye in the intensive care unit: Helping caregivers grieve. *Pediatric Nursing, 17* (1), 103–105.

Speece, M. W., & Brent, S. B. (1984). Children's understanding of death: A review of three components of a death concept. *Child Development, 55* (5), 1671–1686.

Stambrook, M., & Parker, K. (1987). The development of the concept of death in childhood: A review of the literature. *Merrill-Palmer Quarterly: Journal of Developmental Psychology, 33* (2), 133–157.

Telling the kids. (1991, January 20). *New York Times.* p. 18E.

The Sudden Infant Death Syndrome Alliance. (1989). *Facts About SIDS.* Author. (Brochure available from The SIDS Alliance, 10500 Little Patuxent Parkway, Suite 420, Columbia, MD, 21044.)

Vess, J., Moreland, J., & Schwebel, A. I. (1985–86). Understanding family role reallocations following a death: A theoretical framework. *Omega: Journal Death and Dying, 16* (2), 115–128.

Vianello, R., & Lucamante, M. (1988). Children's understanding of death according to parents and pediatricians. *The Journal of Genetic Psychology, 149* (3), 305–316.

Waechter, E. (1977). Children's awareness of fatal illness.In L. Wilkenfeld (Ed.), *When children die* (pp. 222–29). Dubuque, IA: Kendall/Hunt.

Wass, H., Raup, J. L., & Sisler, H. H. (1989). Adolescents and death on television: A follow-up study. *Death Studies, 13* (2), 161–173.

Weber, J., & Fournier, D. G. (1985). Family support and a child's adjustment to death. *Family Relations: Journal of Applied Family and Child Studies, 34* (1), 43–49.

Weinfeld, I. J. (1990). An expanded perinatal bereavement support committee: A community wide resource. *Death Studies, 14* (3), 241–252.

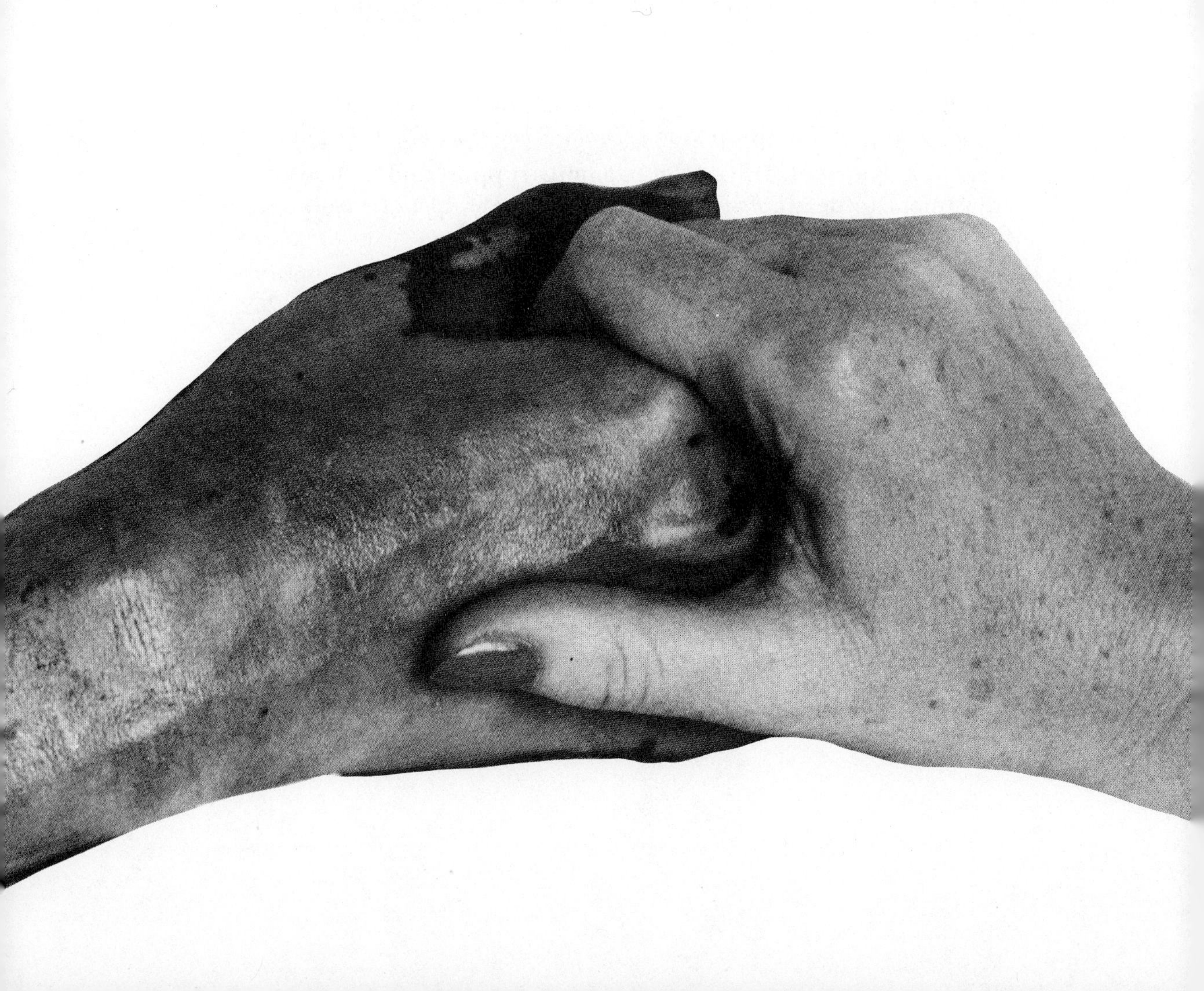

Chapter 7

Living with AIDS

*Kathleen M. Nokes**

In December, 1991, the Centers for Disease Control (CDC) reported that 206,392 persons had been diagnosed with AIDS and 133,232 (64 percent) of these persons were dead. The first 100,000 cases of AIDS were reported in eight years, whereas the second 100,000 cases of AIDS were reported in a two year period (CDC, 1992). Of the 73,160 persons living with AIDS, some are coping with the terminal phase of the illness while others are actively dying. The greatest number of cases of persons with AIDS are found in New York, California, and Florida (42,061, 37,717, and 19,096 respectively) but absolute numbers do not tell the whole story. When the incidence is broken down according to the total population within a specific area, the greatest number of cases per 100,000 persons in that area are found in San Francisco, New York and Washington D.C.

This chapter will explain HIV disease, the concerns facing persons with AIDS and their significant others, and the ethical issues surrounding HIV/AIDS.

Understanding HIV Disease

AIDS is the last stage of a long disease process that depletes the ability of the person's immune system to repond to any infection. Human Immunodeficiency Virus-1 (HIV-1) (otherwise referred to as HIV) has been implicated as the causative organism, but the pathology known as AIDS can only occur when the person's immune system is depressed to a critical

*Special thanks to Ray Woolacott for sharing his experiences.

level. When this critical level of immune depression is reached, the HIV-infected person no longer responds adequately to infections from organisms which would not cause disease in otherwise healthy persons. The course of HIV disease is highly variable in each individual. It seems to be influenced by a variety of factors, including the virulence of the infecting strain of HIV, the mental and physical resistance of the person, the adequacy of support systems, and the presence of other infectious diseases such as hepatitis B and tuberculosis.

The two major routes of HIV transmission are participating in unsafe sex with an infected man or woman and sharing drug-use equipment containing infected blood. Between 5 and 15 years can pass between the time that a person becomes infected with HIV and the appearance of symptoms. Approximately 25–50 percent of persons report flu-like symptoms in the weeks immediately following infection, but most people do not remember experiencing any specific problems.

The window period refers to the time between becoming infected with HIV and the development of antibodies to HIV. This period usually ranges between 6 weeks and 6 months. The blood tests for HIV that are widely used, specifically the ELISA and the Western blot, only test for antibodies to HIV. They do not test directly for the virus. Therefore, a person can be infected with HIV and remain negative on the antibody blood test during the window period.

White blood cells normally provide the first line of defense against any infection. HIV has an affinity for some types of white blood cells, specifically lymphocytes and monocytes. Both of these white blood cells are characterized by having CD4 receptors on their cell membranes. HIV gets into these white blood cells by interacting with the CD4 receptor on the cell. HIV is transported within the infected person's bloodstream by activated monocytes. HIV lives and replicates within a specific type of lymphocyte, the T4 lymphocyte. When HIV infects a T4 lymphocyte, it becomes part of the genetic stucture of the T4 cell. HIV can remain dormant within the infected T4 cell for long periods of time. Through mechanisms that are not entirely clear, HIV gradually depletes the person's supply of T4 lymphocytes.

By examining the blood levels of T cells, some estimate the duration of HIV infection can be derived. Persons with HIV become very familiar with their T cell counts, and it is essential that health care providers are as knowledgeable about these results and their interpretation. Two types of T cells are particularly important: T4 and T8 cells. T4 cells are also known as CD4 cells or as T helper cells. T8 cells are also known as CD8 cells or as T suppressor cells. The normal ranges for T4 and T8 cells vary greatly between laboratories and differ between infants and adults, but the normal ratio of T helper to T suppressor cells is 2:1. An uninfected person has twice as many T4 as T8 cells and this ratio of helper to suppressor cells allows the person to resist infection. The ratio of T helper and T suppressor cells in the HIV-infected person reverses and, over time, there can be many more T suppressor than T helper cells. The health care provider needs to know not only the number of T4 cells but also the ratio of T4 to T8 cells of each patient.

Treatment decisions related to management of HIV infection are linked to T cell counts. Clients are started on antiviral drugs to fight HIV, such as zidovudine (AZT), dideoxynosine (DDI) or deoxycytidine (DDC), when T4 cells drop below 500. They are placed on medication regimens to prevent pneumocystitis carinii pneumonia, such as bactrim or aerosol pentamidine, when T4 cells drop below 200. A health care provider who does not have access to recent blood work can judge the extent of HIV disease by assessing the kind of treatment that a person is receiving. To illustrate, the media announcement that Magic Johnson was started on AZT shortly after it was learned that he was HIV positive, indicates that his T4 cell count was below 500. It is believed that certain opportunistic infections cannot occur unless the T4 cell depression reaches a certain critical level. To illustrate, pneumocystitis carinii pneumonia is not perceived as a potental problem until the T4 cell count drops below 200; cytomegalovirus retinitis (CMV retinitis), an eye disorder that can result in blindness, becomes much more of a problem if the client's T4 cells are below 50.

Defining AIDS

In1985, the Centers for Disease Control (CDC) developed a series of definitions for AIDS; they were revised in 1987 and they have been revised again. The new CDC definition of AIDS created a new category: T4(CD4) cell count below 200. Since many HIV-infected persons have T4 cell counts below 200 but do not meet the 1987 CDC definition of AIDS, the new category has greatly increased the numbers of persons diagnosed with AIDS. While this new category has the benefit of being objective and not based on the skill of a diagnostician, it will confound the issue of when the HIV-infected person becomes terminally ill. One client with 19 T4 cells told this author that he would begin to worry about developing AIDS when his T4 cells dropped to 5—at that point he said he would enter an alcohol detoxification program and continue his three year wait for better housing. Another client, recently discharged from prison, had six T4 cells and 803 T8 cells with a ratio of 0.02 and no AIDS-defining problems according to the 1987 criteria. His major concerns were finding a better place to live and staying drug free. Neither of these clients perceived themselves as terminally ill nor did they appear particularly sick.

The 1987 Centers for Disease Control definition of AIDS was complex but became familiar to many. There were essentially four categories of AIDS-defining problems: opportunistic infections such as pneumocystitis carinii pneumonia; unusual cancers such as Kaposi's sarcoma and non-Hodgkins lymphoma; dementia; and constitutional disease that consisted of loss of ten percent of the body's weight and persistent diarrhea. Documented evidence of one or more of these problems should signal to the health care provider that the client is entering the terminal phase of HIV disease. Multiple recurrent opportunistic infections, recurrent refractory HIV-related lymphoma or refractory wasting have been associated with a poor prognosis (von Gunten, Martinez, Weitzman, & Von Roenn, 1991). Additional indicators that the person with AIDS is terminally ill may be severe wasting syndrome, progressive decline of the person's mental status, generalized deterioration of all body systems, and unresponsiveness to treatment (Martin, 1991). Persons with AIDS lived an average length of 47 days on a hospice program while persons with cancer lived an average of 59 days (von Gunten, Martinez, Weitzman, & Von Roenn, 1991).

The Faces of Persons with AIDS

Although the demographic variables of persons becoming infected with HIV infection are changing, the vast majority of persons with AIDS in the United States in the early part of the 1990s are men who have sex with men or persons of color (CDC, 1991a). While these groups may seem to have little in common with each other, both are stigmatized by the predominant majority. AIDS is used as an additional reason to discriminate against persons in either of these groups. Violence against gay people and racism increased during the 1980s, as evidenced by the rise in bias-related crimes. Learning that one is suffering from a terminal illness is devastating. This devastation increases drastically when that illness is socially unacceptable and associated with behaviors which the ill person preferred to conceal from all but a significant few.

The stereotypic picture of an injecting drug user or gay man is often far from reality. People sometimes create a life story, that is less than complete. They may neglect to mention their bisexuality or "weekend" drug use or occasional sexual experiences with prostitutes for a variety of reasons. Particular cultural practices can also impact on whether these people share information about behaviors; for example, sexual practices tolerated in men of some cultures are abhorred in the women of that culture. Religious teachings that specific behaviors are sinful can reinforce secrecy and guilt. The issues generated when a person is in a stigmatized group cannot be minimized. For example, the major concern of an incredibly caring and loving wife of one man was that the neighbors in the building in which they lived would somehow find out from the hospice nurse that her husband was dying from AIDS.

Women with AIDS present unique problems. The presence of HIV infection is underdiagnosed in women, especially if the woman does not share that she has engaged in risk behaviors such as using drugs or unprotected sex with an injecting drug user. The woman may not know that she has placed herself at risk for becoming infected because her sexual partner is less than candid about his drug use and sexual activities with other female and male partners. Women with HIV infection complain of severe and persistent vaginal infections, especially with the Candida organism, but this infection is not considered by the Centers for Disease Control to be an indicator disease for AIDS. Women with HIV infection may be severely ill, but they do not meet the criteria for an AIDS diagnosis. Since entitlements, such as increased Medicaid allotments and nutritional supplements, have been tied to an AIDS diagnosis, women who are severely ill from HIV disease often do not receive the same benefits as men with AIDS. The new CDC criteria of creating a category of under 200 T4 cells as an AIDS diagnosis is an attempt to address this issue. The Social Security Administration is responding to this potential change in the criteria by moving away from coupling entitlements to an AIDS diagnosis.

Women are also affected by AIDS because they are often the primary caregiver for an adult child who is dying from AIDS. A not uncommon picture is of a family in which the husband is dying from AIDS and the wife is coping with being HIV-infected while she cares for her husband and young children who are dying. Grandparents, often grandmothers, serve as the primary caregiver for their dying adult children and grandchildren of varying ages. The financial and emotional strain that this situation imposes on the grandparents cannot be underestimated.

Concerns of Persons with AIDS

The person with AIDS experiences many milestones during the course of illness, which include starting AZT, taking medications to prevent pneumocystitis carinii pneumonia, and, finally, being diagnosed not with HIV infection but AIDS. Persons with AIDS experience ambiguity because there is uncertainty about death along with an unclear prognosis. Since HIV is a relatively new infectious disease, there is always a hope that the cure will be discovered just in time or that a new drug will be available which will stop the deterioration and prolong life. Each media report of a new treatment or vaccine is received with renewed hope. The uneven course of AIDS, reports of long-term survivors, the lack of standardized medical treatments, and a chaotic health care system all add to the ambiguity. Some clients embrace alternative or complementary therapies such as megadoses of vitamins and homeopathy. Their significant others may be concerned that they may be harming themselves by going on a "health binge," especially if the client refuses to integrate more standardized interventions. The dying trajectory, as described in Chapter 2, is different for each person. Within the dying trajectory, certain junctures are passed, and these parameters are not clearly established for persons with AIDS.

In a study comparing the amount of psychosocial support required by patients with AIDS with non-AIDS hospice patients of the same average age, it was found that AIDS patients required significantly more psychosocial support than non-AIDS patients (Baker & Seager, 1991). Persons with AIDS have multiple concerns, including access to appropriate health care, dealing with multiple losses, trying to plan an uncertain future, pain, and physical deterioration.

Technology sorely limits access to health care for persons with AIDS. The deterioration of the immune system is irreversible and will ultimately result in death. The benefit of technology, such as parenteral nutrition and hyperalimentation to control the weight loss, is often outweighed by the risks of causing an overwhelming systemic infection from the intravenous equipment. Many of the drugs used to treat the opportunistic infections, such as Foscarnet for CMV retinitis, require extensive hydration, intravenous access, and careful monitoring that are not available to all clients.

Financial Concerns

Access to appropriate health care is dependent upon financial status, availability of expert services, and technology. Persons with AIDS are often too weak to continue to work and therefore often lose the health insurance that was one of their employment benefits. Medicare benefits for persons with an AIDS-related disability only go into effect two years after the disability is determined—two years is longer than many persons with AIDS will live.

Medicaid eligibility differs from state to state and requires patience and skill to access. The individual's financial resources will need to be depleted before Medicaid is approved. This process is known as "spending down." The person must first spend any savings and liquidate any property to meet the rather stringent Medicaid criteria. In some states, a person can collect on a pre-existing life insurance policy in order to delay complete exhaustion of resources. The process of applying for entitlements can be particularly difficult for a person who has always been financially self-sufficient. The long waiting periods in crowded offices can be stressful for a person who feels physically ill and may be experiencing frequent bouts of diarrhea. The person with AIDS, recently discharged from a prison where he was receiving health care, is also frustrated by the gap in continuity of treatment necessitated by waiting until Medicaid is reactivated.

Even when persons with AIDS have financial resources, they may not be able to access expert health care providers. Because the treatment of HIV disease changes almost daily, health care providers must continually update themselves about how to tailor the client's treatment. Clients being treated by an HIV-specific interdisciplinary health care team within an inner-city clinic may receive more up-to-date treatment than clients paying out-of-pocket for private medical care from providers who have few

HIV-infected clients in their caseload. The client needs reassurance that different plans of care result from advances in understanding about how to treat HIV disease and not necessarily from confusion. The prescribed treatment plan for pneumocystitis carinii pneumonia is a good illustration of this point. Initially, regular dose bactrim was prescribed but almost half of the clients developed a troublesome skin rash; aerosol pentamidine was then prescribed as the preferred treatment but it was found that this intervention did not work as well as bactrim so bactrim again became the preferred treatment but at lower doses. When the interdisciplinary team treats one to two AIDS clients a week, it is difficult to stay abreast on the latest shifts in treatment.

Limited resources are also a factor in determining whether a person is HIV infected. Unless a client is involved in a research study or can pay out of pocket for special blood tests for HIV, only antibody testing for the virus is available. This lack of access to direct viral testing is a particular problem for HIV-positive mothers. Virtually all babies born of HIV-infected mothers will be positive on the HIV antibody test. These positive HIV antibody test results are very difficult to interpret. It is not known whether those antibodies that are causing the baby to be positive on the blood test come from the mother or are being produced by the baby who is actually infected with HIV. Although technology exists to directly test the person's blood for the virus, it is not readily available. A mother with AIDS may die without learning if her 8-month-old son is HIV positive on the ELISA HIV antibody blood test because he has his mother's antibodies or because he is actually infected with HIV.

Psychological Concerns

Persons with AIDS are coping with multiple losses. Friends; other family members, including children; and a sexual partner may have already died from AIDS. The person with AIDS is losing dreams about living a long life, seeing children grow up, finishing school, becoming a famous lawyer, staying off drugs (Nokes & Carver, 1991). The mother with AIDS loses her infant child, and the infected gay man loses the love of his life at a time when his heart is breaking. The health care provider cannot shield the person with AIDS from knowing about the last stages of the illness. Sometimes, the client knows more about the prognosis of AIDS than the health care provider and will react negatively if the provider tries to create an unrealistically optimistic picture.

Persons with AIDS are concerned about planning for an uncertain future. Because many of the significant relationships in the person's life are not legally recognized, there are concerns about how different people will react after death. Helping persons with AIDS to complete tasks such as making out a will, contacting estranged family, establishing advance directives such as a health care proxy or living will, planning guardianship of minor children, and perhaps prearranging the funeral may help the person with AIDS feel calmer about the future (Moynihan, Christ, & Silver, 1988). As one surviving partner of a person who died from AIDS said: "It really must be impressed upon people to make a will. Even when all is 'cut and dried,' the sudden interest from previously disinterested family members was rather upsetting.

There are many causes of pain from AIDS-related problems and uncontrolled pain is frightening for anyone. Persons with a history of illegal drug use may have the additional fear that the health care provider may not provide adequate analgesic levels because of the provider's value judgements about giving narcotic analgesics to chronic drug users. Because of his former history of illegal drug use, one client with acute pain was denied any analgesic other than tylenol (acetominophen) for a herpes zoster infection which eventually caused blindness of his eye. The health care providers, who could be trusted to know the latest trend in treatment of HIV disease, often lack basic principles of pain management. These providers may prefer to refer the person with AIDS to a hospice for pain management, but this referral may be hindered by hospice policies related to financial constraints, do not resuscitate orders, and the need for a primary care giver (Wallace, 1990).

The chronic intractable diarrhea, blindness, and neurological deficits associated with terminal AIDS cause intense body image changes and physical deterioration. Chronic intractable diarrhea in persons with AIDS is often resistant to most standardized treatments and requires unique approaches. Kaposi's sarcoma, which is a form of cancer, can be incredibly disfiguring. Persons with Kaposi's sarcoma develop multiple skin lesions that vary according to the person's skin color but are often bluish-brown. The picture at the beginning of this chapter shows Kaposi lesions on the hand of a person who died the following day from AIDS. Countless case studies of handsome young men who died shrunken and aged from AIDS fill the literature. At this stage of illness, hospice seems the most appropriate resource, but everyone involved in this decision may be ambivalent. The client, often exhausted by fighting endless battles against innumerable infections, may still be reluctant to admit defeat. The referring health care providers may be having trouble coping with yet another treatment failure of "such a nice person." The hospice personnel may be debating as to whether the HIV-related treatment such as zidovudine, an antiviral drug, has a curative or palliative intent, and if it should be continued after the client is in the hospice program.

Concerns of Family, Lovers, and Friends

The gay man with AIDS often has both a family of origin with biological roots and a family of choice, which often consists of other gays and lesbians. Persons with a history of injecting drug use also have families of origin and those of choice—biological relations and drug-sharing friends. Sexual partners of bisexual men and injecting drug users often identify with more of a nuclear family pattern. These people, usually women, may have been faithful to their steady sexual partner and produced children from the union. The diagnosis of AIDS in a family member produces a crisis in any of the above-mentioned family system patterns. Pre-existing stresses in relationships are often exacerbated as roles change and the person with AIDS grows increasingly dependent on whomever will provide care.

As functional dependency increases and the person with AIDS (PWA) becomes weaker, the primary caregiver takes more control over the situation and may not include significant others. Ray and Jim lived together in a rural setting in Wales for 16 years. Jim's parents lived close by and were disapproving of the gay relationship and made their feelings very clear at every opportunity. When Jim, who was an airline steward, was confined to bed and suffering from growing blindness and increasing cognitive impairment, Ray took over his care. As Jim's dependency grew, Ray grew clearer in his ability to make decisions despite the disruptive influence of Jim's parents. After Jim's death, the strain between Ray and Jim's parents worsened and the grieving process was delayed by a failure to resolve important issues. Involvement in a bereavement group may help to resolve some of those feelings (Oerlemans-Bunn, 1988).

Sowell, Bramlett, Gueldner, Gritzmacher, & Martin (1991) asked eight surviving partners of gay men with AIDS the question, "Please describe your experience of losing a lover to AIDS." Three categories emerged from the interviews: 1) isolation/disconnectedness; 2) emotional confusion; and 3) acceptance/denial. The first category included themes of isolation from their family and their lover's family, friends, and self. Themes of guilt, loneliness, anger, and ambivalence emerged from the category of emotional confusion. Six of the eight men were HIV positive and were coping with their own vulnerability and HIV illness. The survivors were coping with their ambivalence about surviving and forming new relationships. Social support was a significant factor as all respondents described feelings of isolation and loneliness following the loss of their lover and very limited social support.

When the injecting drug user family member finally becomes too weak to go outside, it may be a relief for the family members. They know that their son, daughter, husband, or wife can no longer access drugs because they are too weak. The family members don't have to fear having their property sold for drugs, answering the phone to learn that the person has been arrested again, or being physically abused by the person "crazy on crack." Often cultural and religious beliefs support the family as they take the person back into their home for the last time.

The sexual partner of the person with AIDS fears that she or he will become HIV infected despite the use of safer sex practices. Sexual behaviors change as a result, and both partners may start to distance from one another because of an inability to communicate their perspectives about this fear.

Health care providers are often also ambivalent about assisting couples to deal with their sexuality, especially when there are no guarantees that safer sex practices such as consistent condom use are 100 percent effective. When one client was reminded to use condoms, he remarked that something funny had happened the last time he and his wife had made love. This remark was shortly followed by a statement that the nurse would probably not think that the event was so funny. The client was correct in his assessment of the nurse's reaction. She did not think that his failure to hold the condom in place during withdrawal, which resulted in the semen-filled condom remaining in his uninfected wife's vagina, was funny. For some partners, the person's increasing weakness and the subsequent disinterest in sex is a relief.

Despite counseling of family members that HIV is not spread by casual contact, some people persist in isolating laundry, dishes, and small children from the client. A few days before a client's death, his father helped the client's lover carry him upstairs to bed wearing bright red rubber kitchen gloves although latex gloves were available in the home. Eight months after the client's death, the lover says "I felt incensed—how did Sam really feel about that?" When family members understand that HIV is spread by blood and sexual contact; when they are instructed to use chlorax bleach to kill any HIV that may be in the blood on the person's clothes; when they are provided with the needed equipment such as gloves to use when touching the person's bodily fluids, and they still persist in isolating the client, a deeper fear than that of contagion may be present. The health care provider then needs to balance the benefits that the family member is providing the client such as shelter, food, and medications against the isolation and shame that the client may be experiencing. Options in these situations are very limited and the health care provider can serve as a role model by touching the client without using barriers when giving a back rub or simply shaking hands, active listening, reinforcing what precautions are necessary, and not overemphasizing the negative.

Despite the fact that the first case of AIDS was identified in 1981, the embarrassment of having a family member diagnosed with AIDS persists. People make up stories about why their son or daughter is sick or dying. This inability to share the details about the illness of a significant family member with long-standing support systems impedes the resolution of grief (Worden, 1991). In a study of families of AIDS patients (n = 26) and other hospice patients with terminal illness (n = 26), families of AIDS patients had significantly more stress, more rules prohibiting emotional expression, lower trust levels, and more illness anxiety than the other families (Atkins & Amenta, 1991). Support groups in neutral settings—often far from the community where the person lives—can be safe havens (Bowes & Dickson, 1991). Family members can express anger, fear, frustration, helplessness, revulsion, rejection, and guilt in support groups.

Sharing these feelings with group members who have also experienced them, facilitates their resolution.

Even after death, the family may face discrimination from a funeral director who wants to charge more to arrange the funeral of the person who died from AIDS or who insists on a closed casket. State laws vary about acceptable practices, but health care providers should instruct family members about their rights. Community resources are also very helpful in ensuring that discriminatory practices are not allowed. Sometimes a simple phone call can result in a total change in attitude. Health care providers need to act as advocates for family members who are trying to cope with yet another embarrassing situation.

Because of limited finances, burial arrangements may be problematic. Veterans of the United States military can be buried through the services provided by the government. Medicaid provides a small amount of money for burial. Some AIDS community organizations, recognizing this problem, have asked people to donate extra burial plots. It is not unusual for a family to have one or two extra plots that will go unused; these plots can be donated to persons who have died from AIDS who are alone or whose families do not have the financial resources to pay for the desired burial.

Concerns of Health Care Providers

Perhaps the major barrier to caring for persons with AIDS is fear of being infected with HIV. While the risk of becoming infected through an occupational exposure is very slight (less than one half of one percent) the possibility still generates fear even for those who accept the low risk and choose to work with persons with AIDS. Knowledge about occupational exposure can help to control the fear, but it will not completely erase the fear. It is helpful for any health care provider who is administering direct care to understand that the major risk behavior occurs during contact with the infected client's blood.

Three factors need to be considered in judging an occupational exposure situation. These are the route of exposure, the amount of infected bodily fluids, and the extent of HIV within the infected person's blood. Piercing of the skin through a needle stick or sharp object is more risky than contact with infected blood on an intact skin surface, but either exposure should be taken seriously. Barrier equipment such as gloves will not stop needle sticks, but they will be an effective barrier from skin contact with infected blood. The amount of infected bodily fluids may be a significant factor both in determining whether the health care provider becomes infected and how quickly their disease progresses. The registered professional nurse who died from AIDS in 1991 as a result of occupational exposure had injected herself with about 3 to 5 cc of the AIDS client's blood. She was resting against the client's bed to stabilize her hands while she drew his blood. The bed moved, she felt herself falling, and she inadvertently injected her thigh with the syringe filled with his blood. Another registered nurse in Iowa, who has HIV infection through occupational exposure, used her ungloved fingers and a gauze pad to stop the bleeding at an intravenous puncture site.

The amount of HIV within the client's blood is also perceived as a factor in determing whether the health care provider will become infected with HIV. As HIV continues to infect T4 cells, the probability increases that more blood will actually contain virus. Clients with AIDS have large numbers of infected T4 cells. Exposure to their blood may be more risky than exposure to the blood of an HIV-positive person who has relatively large numbers of T4 cells.

Because of the legal need to determine whether an occupational exposure resulted in HIV infection, health care providers who have been exposed to HIV will be asked to establish that they are HIV negative at the time of the occupational exposure. In many health care facilities, the policies developed to address occupational exposure to HIV require that the health care provider consent to HIV testing in the 24-hour period after exposure in order to establish a negative baseline. HIV testing is then repeated every six weeks, three months, six months and, sometimes one year later. A health care provider who is negative at baseline and HIV positive 6 months later is assumed to have become positive through that occupational exposure. In a Centers for Disease Control Study of occupational exposure, the HIV seroconversion rate of health care providers (N = 1372 between August 15, 1983, to June 30, 1990) after an occupational exposure to HIV was approximately .3 percent (CDC, 1991b). Workers' Compensation and other disability benefits are then available to that health care provider. The use of AZT after occupational exposure is extremely controversial. When a health care facility offers AZT to the health care provider who has experienced significant occupational exposure to HIV, the drug should be started as soon as possible, preferably within the first hour after exposure.

The issue of HIV-infected health care providers providing health care to uninfected health care consumers remains controversial. During the summer of 1991, the Senate of the United States passed the Helms amendment which would have required any HIV-infected health care worker to notify any potential client that he was infected. Failure to notify the potential client would result in criminal penalties of 10 years in jail and a $10,000 fine. This amendment died in Congress, but it should not be forgotten because it illustrates the attitude of a significant number of persons within the United States on the issue of HIV-infected health care providers.

Risks to Health Care Providers

While the risk of becoming infected with HIV through occupational exposure is very low, the risk of becoming infected with other infectious diseases experienced by persons with AIDS should not be minimized. Many persons with AIDS also have hepatitis B, and the risk of infection with hepatitis B after exposure ranges between 6 and 30 percent (Stehlin, 1990). There is now a vaccine available against hepatitis B. In addition, the health care provider who did not have chickenpox may become infected if they are exposed to a client with herpes zoster.

Pulmonary tuberculosis is an infectious disease that results from a defect in the cellular immune system. One standard skin test for exposure to TB is the PPD. When HIV-infected clients lose a significant amount of immune system functioning, perhaps when their T4 cell levels drop below 400, they often cannot have a normal PPD skin response. Their PPD skin test is interpreted as normal or negative because there is no skin reaction. This interpretation is wrong because the absence of the skin reaction is due to depression of the immune system and the resulting inability to produce a accurate response. Even the chest X ray of the HIV-infected client may not show changes from tuberculosis althogh the infection is present.

Health care providers are at risk for contracting tuberculosis, especially from undiagnosed patients (Allen & Ownby, 1991). Tuberculosis epidemics in hospitals, hospices, shelters, and prisons are predicted, and at least four New York and Miami hospitals are presently coping with outbreaks of drug-resistant tuberculosis among persons with AIDS (Headlines, 1992). Within the New York State correctional facilities, outbreaks of drug-resistant tuberculosis were reported in 1991. Adequate ventilation, ultraviolet lights, and environmental modifications are essential to protect the health care providers from tuberculosis infection. Health care providers, working with immune-depressed, HIV-infected clients, must assess their PPD status frequently—every 6 months is probably a good idea. Children in the household who are PPD negative should be temporarily relocated until the patient's tuberculosis infection is controlled by medication (Allen & Ownby, 1991).

The Rewards of Working With Persons With AIDS

AIDS is perceived by some to be the health care challenge of the latter part of the twentieth century. Health care providers who want to make a difference accept the challenge of working with persons with HIV infection. The risks are outweighed by the benefits of believing that the work is truly meaningful. Persons with AIDS are young, often well educated, interesting to speak with, demand equality in decision making, and are very appreciative that someone cares about them. The health care provider is excited by being on the frontlines fighting an infectious disease that will probably be cured, or at least prevented, at some point in the future. The work is stressful but rewarding.

A survey of hospice staff showed they felt that working with persons with AIDS was both more time consuming and more stressful than working with terminally ill patients with other diagnoses (Baker & Seager, 1991). The health care provider may need to deal with the anger, guilt, or shame generated by identifying with the person with AIDS (Miller, 1991). Health care providers need to come to terms about existential issues such as their own mortality and recognize the limits of their interventions. It helps to focus on the joys of the present moment. Although the cure is on the horizon, it will take many years of sustained work before this epidemic is controlled. The health care provider needs to pace for the long run.

Ethical Issues

The HIV epidemic highlights the conflicts between the individualistic and public health ethics (Nokes, 1991). Health care providers are most comfortable with the individualistic approach that emphasizes the rights of specific persons. The public health ethic forces a broader perspective since the rights of the individual are weighed against the rights of others. Contact notification of persons who have a need to know that they should take precautions against becoming infected with HIV is a good illustration of how these two ethical theories conflict. The case of the person dying from AIDS who wants to be discharged to his parent's home, but refuses to tell his parents his diagnosis is not that atypical. In this case, the health care providers need to weigh the rights of the client to confidentiality against the rights of the parents to protect themselves against exposure to bloody fluids.

The economic impact of the AIDS epidemic is expected to be great. One study forecasts that the cumulative lifetime health care costs of treating all people diagnosed with AIDS during a given year to be about $3.3 billion in 1989, $4.3 billion in 1990, $5.3 billion in 1991, $6.5 billion in 1992, and $7.8 billion in 1993 (Hellinger, 1990). Financial constraints generate issues of distributive justice—who gets treated and for what. As the picture of this epidemic continues to evolve, the economic toll that AIDS is making on every person within the United States will start to be recognized.

Perhaps there is no ethical issue that generates more discussion than when the HIV-infected woman becomes pregnant. The risk of actually producing an HIV-infected child is between 25 to 30 percent, which means that between 75 and 70 percent of the offspring will not be infected with HIV (Pizzo & Butler, 1991). Pregnancy does not seem to accelerate the infected woman's HIV disease. Giving birth to one HIV-infected child does not seem to be a good predictor about whether the next offspring will also be HIV infected. Religion, economics, equality, culture, and a need to continue the lineage all impact on whether a HIV-positive woman becomes pregnant, and if she then chooses to continue the pregnancy.

Society, through insurance programs such as Medicaid, pays for the medical care of HIV-infected children—many of whom require extensive technology over long periods of time. Health care providers need to examine their feelings about women with AIDS who choose to continue pregnancies. These feelings need examining because they will impact on the formation of a trusting client–provider relationship. The issue of women with AIDS who choose to continue pregnancies needs to be examined in the context of how women with other life-threatening problems that affect the offspring are regarded by society. The contributions of the male partner to the pregnancy cannot be ignored, and the ethics of this situation needs to be examined through the perspective of the dyad.

There seem to be two groups of children with AIDS, those that die within the first 3 years of life and those who live an average of 7 years. The first group of children is characterized by repeated infections, failure to thrive, regression of developmental milestones, and often mental retardation. The second group experiences more frequent bacterial infections, but they seem to be essentially well. Medical treatment of the HIV-infected child continues to develop, and many of the drugs that are used to treat adults are now being used successfully with children. In addition, intravenous immunoglobulin seems to control many of the bacterial infections. Although the research is scanty, there does seem to be a trend for mothers who have children to live longer than those whose children have died. The needs of the orphans left from these families in which so many people have died from AIDS can be overwhelming, and services for these physically healthy children are not covered by most forms of health insurance. Special programs are now recognizing these needs, but much more attention must be paid to these children who have experienced tremendous loss and grief at relatively young ages.

Community Resources

Although community resources to assist persons with AIDS exist in most geographic areas throughout the United States, they are most extensive in the areas hardest impacted by the epidemic. The list of community resources for persons with HIV infection in the New York City area covers many pages. Because of budget cuts and uncertain funding, some of these agencies have been forced to close or decrease services. The largest community agencies, such as the Gay Men's Health Crisis in New York, have "hot line" phone numbers listed in the telephone directory. Volunteers answering these phones can give information about resources available in different communities. It is best to be as clear as possible about the services needed, and one should expect to make a number of phone calls before the available provider is identified. If a health care provider or friend is calling for a person with AIDS, it is essential to first clarify with the PWA that confidential information will have to be shared with the community resource. Written permission to release confidential information about HIV may be mandated by state law.

SUMMARY ❧

The issues generated by the AIDS epidemic are taxing our society. Young people are dying while leaders in the government and health care industry debate philosophical dilemmas. Persons with AIDS feel tremendous urgency since their time is limited. Many others would still like to ignore the problem. On one level there is turmoil, agitation, and chaos, while on a different level there is an attempt to act as if nothing is happening. According to the Federal government, by the end of 1991 over 200,000 persons within the United States have AIDS. Countless persons throughout the world have died from AIDS. This epidemic will continue to challenge everyone into the 21st century.

LEARNING EXERCISES ❧

1. If you had AIDS, who would you tell? How do you think they would react?
2. Your son comes home to visit from San Francisco. He looks thin and when you ask him what is wrong, he says that he has AIDS. What do you say that night? two weeks later? two months later?
3. Imagine that you have AIDS. Think about what changes you will need to make in your activities of daily living, and plans for your financial future.
4. Imagine that you have AIDS and you have been dating someone and s/he is interested in having sexual intercourse. Do you tell the person that you have AIDS? How do you negotiate safer sex?
5. You are a health care provider who just experienced an occupational exposure to HIV infected blood. How do you feel? What do you do?

AUDIOVISUAL MATERIAL ❧

The Last Laugh. 57 minutes/videocassette. Fanlight Productions, 47 Halifax Street, Boston, MA 02130
Celebrating the healing power of laughter, hope, and positive thinking, *The Last Laugh* documents a three-day comedy workshop for People with AIDS.

Not Ready to Die Alone. 52 minutes/videocassette. Films for the Humanities and Sciences, PO Box 2053, Princeton, NJ 08543
This documentary examines how one man lives with AIDS. It follows him in his fight to be accepted by his family, to protect his right to continue working, and to come to grip with his illness.

Roger's Story: For Cori. 28 minutes/videocassette/1989. Fanlight Productions, 47 Halifax Street, Boston, MA 02130
This documentary about Roger, a 44-year-old recovering heroin addict, and his struggles to continue in his recovery and to cope with his diagnosis of AIDS.

A Gift Of Time. (Pediatric AIDS) 15 minutes/videocassette. The Multimedia Company, 108 Wilmot Road, Deerfield, Deerfield, IL 60015
The video speaks to parents, teachers, and medical professionals about the frequently minimized crisis of pediatric AIDS.

REFERENCES ❧

Allen, M., & Ownby, K. (1991). Tuberculosis: The other epidemic. *Journal of the Association of Nurses in AIDS Care, 2,* 9–24.

Atkins, R., & Amenta, M. (1991). Family adaptation to AIDS: A comparative study. *The Hospice Journal, 7,* 71–83.

Baker, N., & Seager, R. (1991). A comparison of the psychosocial needs of hospice patients with AIDS and those with other diagnoses. *The Hospice Journal, 7,* 61–69.

Bowes, J., & Dickson, J. (1991). Support group for those affected by AIDS in the family. *The American Journal of Hospice and Palliative Care, 8,* 39–45.

Centers for Disease Control (1991a). *HIV/AIDS Surveillance.* December.

Centers for Disease Control (1991b). Hospital infections program: Health-care worker surveillance project. Slides #L-227.

Centers for Disease Control (1992). The second 100,000 cases of AIDS—United States. *Mortality and Morbidity Reports, 41,* 28–29.

Headlines (1992). Devastating TB epidemics. *American Journal of Nursing, 92,* 9.

Hellinger, F. (1990). Updated forecasts of the costs of medical care for persons with AIDS, 1989–93. *Public Health Reports, 105,* 1–12.

Martin, J. (1991). Issues in the current treatment of hospice patients with HIV disease. *The Hospice Journal, 7,* 31–40.

Miller, R. (1991). Some notes on the impact of treating AIDS patients in hospices. *The Hospice Journal, 7,* 1–12.

Moynihan, R., Christ, G., & Silver, L. (1988). AIDS and terminal illness. *Social Casework: The Journal of Contemporary Social Work, 69,* 380–387.

Nokes, K. (1991). Examining ethical and legal issues generated by the HIV epidemic. *Journal of Association of Nurses in AIDS Care, 2,* 25–30.

Nokes, K., & Carver, K., (1991). What is the meaning of living with AIDS—an examination through Man-Living-Health theory. *Nursing Science Quarterly, 4,* 175–179.

Oberlemans-Bunn, M. (1988). On being gay, single, and bereaved. *American Journal of Nursing, 88,* 472–476.

Pizzo, P., & Butler, K. (1991). In the vertical transmission of HIV, timing may be everything. *The New England Journal of Medicine, 325,* 652–653.

Sowell, R., Bramlett, M., Gueldner, S., Gritzmacher, D., & Martin, G. (1991). The lived experience of survival and bereavement following the death of a lover from AIDS. *Image: Journal of Nursing Scholarship, 23,* 89–94.

Stehlin, D. (1990). Hepatitis B: Available vaccine safe but underused. *FDA Consumer, 24,* 14–17.

von Gunten, C., Martinez, J., Weitzman, S., & Von Roenn, J. (1991). AIDS and hospice. *The American Journal of Hospice and Palliative Care, 8,* 17–19.

Wallace, W. (1990). Hospice and AIDS: Clinical issues which affect care. *The American Journal of Hospice and Palliative Care, 7,* 13–16.

Worden, J. W. (1991). Grieving a loss from AIDS. *The Hospice Journal, 7,* 143–150.

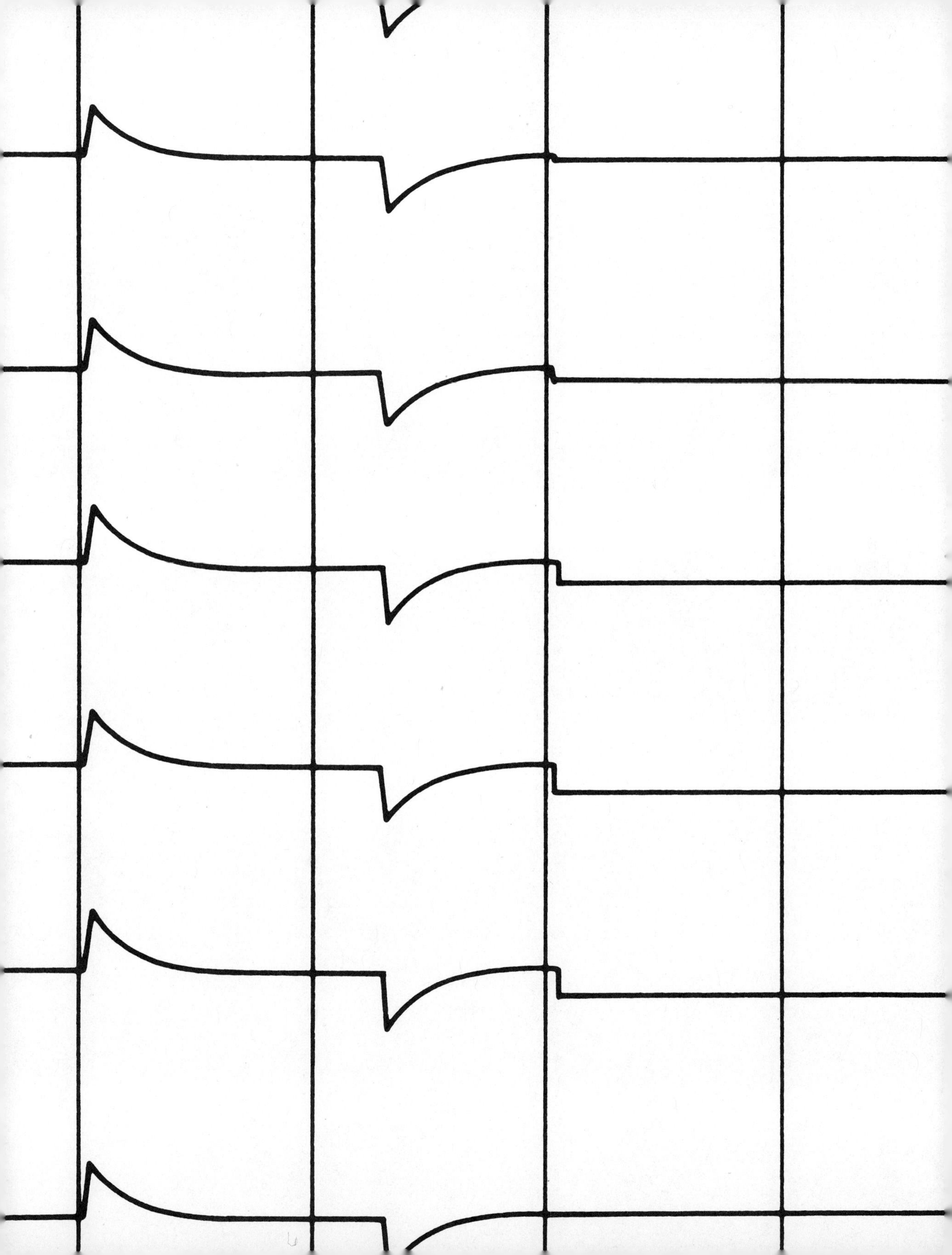

Chapter 8

Ethical Issues

The ethical issues surrounding death have been discussed throughout history, but, because of our advanced medical technology, ethical issues today have become more complex. New machinery, like the heart–lung machine, lead us to question the criteria determining death; new treatments often have painful side effects, and improved forms of treatment maintain the lives of many who would have died in the past. This chapter looks at three major ethical issues surrounding death: the definition of death, the right to refuse treatment, and euthanasia.

The Definition of Death

Within the past twenty years, the controversy surrounding the definition of death has changed. In the 1970s, the definition of death was changed from the irreversible cessation of the heart and respiration to death of the brain; today forty-six states and the District of Columbia authorize the use of brain death as the legal definition of death (Veatch, 1989, p. 45). The present concern is whether death should be defined in terms of the whole brain or the higher brain.

The History of Defining Death

Alexander (1980) argues that defining death was not as simple in the past as we tend to believe. In 1740 "The Uncertainty of the Signs of Death and the Danger of Precipitate Interments and Dissections" set off debate on the criteria of death. Putrefaction was considered the only sure sign of death, and even this criterion was attacked because putrefaction was found in cases of gangrene. The fear of premature burial and premature cessation of medical care motivated the development of safeguards, which took such forms as the creation of mortuaries and legislation delaying burial for at least one day. These developments enabled people to watch the dead to make sure they actually were dead. The following (Alexander, 1980) is a description of a model mortuary:

> The model mortuary contained twenty-three cells for women and the same number for men. Each set of cells was clustered around an observation corridor. The corpse was placed near the cell window through which it could be observed by a guard. The hands of the corpses wore gloves which were attached by strings to an alarm. The slightest movement of a finger caused a large hammer to strike the alarm. The signal was truly frightening, appropriate for the danger it announced. The mortuary also contained a revival room and a pharmacy. On constant duty, guards punched a time-clock every half-hour. A physician directed the mortuary, and physicians made rounds, intervening if necessary (p. 29).

As the medical profession advanced in terms of developing greater scientific standards, a consensus developed that medical knowledge could lead to the best protection against premature burial. In 1875, an article appeared in the *Dictionnaire Dechambre,* an encyclopedia of medicine, that discussed 27 major signs of death. There began to be agreement among physicians that the major signs of death were the irrevocable cessation of heartbeat, respiration, and consciousness.

In the late 1950s and early 1960s there was a push to redefine death in terms of the brain rather than the heart–lung definition. The explicit idea of brain death developed from the work of two French neurologists. In 1959, Mallaret & Goulon presented an article concerning grades of coma; the deepest coma was a state without movement, spontaneous breathing, reflex activity, or temperature regulation. "Essentially this was a state approaching conventional death except for the presence of a beating heart kept alive by artificially controlled lungs" (Black, 1978, p. 213).

Simultaneously, transplant operations of organs were being conducted. In December 1954, Dr. Joseph Murray and his colleagues performed the first successful kidney transplant operation. Then, in December 1967, Dr. Christian Barnard performed a heart transplant operation. Today, up to 25 different organs have been transplanted with different degrees of success, including corneas, teeth, spleen, and pancreas. As a result of this technology, organs became needed for transplantation. If a heart is to be used for transplantation, the donor must be maintained on a heart–lung machine. Other organs would also be of better quality if they were being supplied with oxygen up until removal from the donor. Yet, could a patient be defined as dead if the heart was beating, albeit artificially?

As Glaser (1970) points out, it became imperative to define death in such a way as to protect the "dying patient" *and* to protect the surgeon from violating the law—and so as not to preclude a potentially life-saving operation for the patient who needed a new organ.

But this was not the only reason to redefine death. As pointed out by the President's Commission (1981):

> Of 36 comatose patients who were declared dead on the basis of irreversible loss of brain functions, only six were organ donors . . . thus, medical concern over the determination of death rests much less with any wish to facilitate organ transplantation than with the need both to render appropriate care to patients and to replace artificial support with more fitting and respectful behavior when a patient has become a dead body" (pp. 23–24).

A Framework for Analyzing the Definition of Death

Veatch (1976, pp. 25–54; 1989, pp. 32–34) proposes a framework that would enable us to analyze the various definitions of death. He states that four separate levels must be distinguished:

1. There should be a formal definition of death such as the following: "Death means a complete change in the status of a living entity characterized by the irreversible loss of those characteristics that are essentially significant to it. It would be the point at which the individual is no longer treated as a human being" (p. 25).
2. We must then decide on the concept of death. That is: What is significant about life that when we lose it, there is death? Is life found in the flow of vital fluids, the breath or blood; or in our soul; or in our capacity for bodily integration; or in our capacity for social interaction?
3. Once we have defined our concept of death, we must determine the locus of death. Where should we look to see if death has occurred? If our concept of death concerns the loss of vital fluids, then one must look at the heart and lungs; if one is concerned with bodily integration, then one focuses on the total brain; if the concept is based on social interaction, then death would probably be found in the neocortex. For the soul, one might look for the pineal body, as suggested by Descartes.
4. Then the criteria of death should be decided: What specific tests, for example, the EEG, must be applied at the locus of death to see if death has occurred?

Table 8.1 summarizes the framework presented by Veatch and how it would be applied, depending upon our various concepts of death.

Table 8.1 Levels of the Definition of Death

Formal Definition: Death means a complete change in the status of a living entity characterized by the irreversible loss of those characteristics that are essentially significant to it.

CONCEPT OF DEATH	LOCUS OF DEATH	CRITERIA OF DEATH
Philosophical or theological judgment of the essentially significant change at death.	Place to look to determine if a person has died.	Measurements physicians or other officials use to determine whether a person is dead—to be determined by scientific empirical study.
1. The irreversible stopping of the flow of "vital" body fluids, i.e., the blood and breath	Heart and lungs	1. Visual observation of respiration, perhaps with the use of a mirror. 2. Feeling the pulse, possibly supported by electrocardiogram
2. The irreversible loss of the soul from the body	The pineal body? (according to Descartes) The repiratory tract?	Observation of breath?
3. The irreversible loss of the capacity for bodily integration and social interaction	The brain	1. Unreceptivity and unresponsivity 2. No movements or breathing 3. No reflexes (except spinal reflexes) 4. Flat electroencephalogram (to be used as confirmatory evidence)—All tests to be repeated 24 hours later (excluded conditions: hypothermia and central nervous system drug depression)
4. Irreversible loss of consciousness or the capacity for social interaction	Probably the neocortex	Electroencephalogram

Note: The possible concepts, loci, and criteria of death are much more complex than the ones given here. These are meant to be simplified models of types of positions being taken in the current debate. It is obvious that those who believe that death means the loss of the capacity for bodily integration (3) or the irreversible loss of consciousness (4) have no reservations about pronouncing death when the heart and lungs have ceased to function. This is because they are willing to use loss of heart and lung activity as shortcut criteria for death, believing that once heart and lungs have stopped, the brain or neocortex will necessarily stop as well (p. 53).

The point in distinguishing the levels of death is that the criteria we use to measure death should come from our concept of death. They should not come from our needs for organs for transplantations nor from economic considerations.

Legislation and the Definition of Death

Today, legislation accepts either the brain or the heart and lungs as the locus of death. The first state to legislate a definition of death was Kansas. The statute reads as follows (Veatch, 1976):

> A person will be considered medically and legally dead, if in the opinion of a physician, based on ordinary standards of medical practice, there is the absence of spontaneous respiratory and cardiac function, and because of the disease or condition which caused, directly or indirectly, these functions to cease, or because of the passage of time since these functions ceased, attempts at resuscitation are considered hopeless; and, in this event death will have occurred at the time these functions ceased; or
>
> A person will be considered medically and legally dead if, in the opinion of a physician, based on ordinary standards of medical practice, there is the absence of spontaneous brain function, and if, based on ordinary standards of medical practice, during reasonable attempts to either maintain or restore spontaneous circulatory or respiratory function in the absence of aforesaid brain function, it appears that further attempts at resuscitation or supportive maintenance will not succeed, death will have occurred at the time when these conditions first coincide. Death is to be pronounced before artificial means of supporting respiratory and circulatory function are terminated and before any vital organ is removed for the purpose of transplantation.
>
> These alternative definitions of death are to be utilized for all purposes in this state, including trials of civil and criminal cases, any laws to the contrary notwithstanding. (Kansas Session, Laws of 1970, Ch.378)

By 1980, twenty-five states had a statutory "definition of death." (President's Commission, 1981.) In order to unify the various state legislation, the President's Commission for the Study of Ethical Problems in Medical and Biomedical and Behavioral Research proposed a Uniform Declaration of Death Act (1981):

> An individual who has sustained either (1) irreversible cessation of circulatory and respiratory functions, or (2) irreversible cessation of

all functions of the entire brain, including the brain stem, is dead. A determination of death must be made in accordance with accepted medical standards (p. 2).

Another Definition of Death?

With the definition of death accepted as "the irreversible loss of the capacity for bodily integration and social interaction," and, therefore, located in the whole brain (Veatch, 1989, p. 33) the question now arises if death should be defined as "the irreversible loss of consciousness or the capacity for social interaction" and located only in the higher brain. The higher brain is concerned with consciousness, speech, and feeling. The lower brain, the brain stem, is responsible for "respiration, and spontaneous vegetative functions. . . . It also contributes to the maintenance of blood pressure (Lamb, 1985, p. 42). Although the lower brain can continue to function without the higher brain, the opposite cannot occur.

Changing the definition of death to include only loss of higher brain functions would pertain to two groups: those individuals who are in a persistent vegetative state, and babies who are born anencephalic, or born with only brain stems. Persons in a persistent vegetative state have a higher brain that no longer functions, yet they continue to breathe because of their brain stem. Such was the case of Karen Ann Quinlan. After the courts resolved that she could be removed from a respirator, she continued to breathe on her own. (Karen Ann is discussed further on in this chapter.) If the definition of death had been changed, she would have been considered dead. The fear in changing the definition of death is that persons in a persistent vegetative state may be misdiagnosed, and may be defined dead when there is a chance for recovery. There is also the argument of the "slippery slope." If the definition of death was changed, it "could ultimately lead to declaring people dead who merely lacked certain mental abilities." (Capron cited in Kolata, 1992, p. C13).

Anencephalic babies have only a brain stem; they will continue to breathe after birth. The question of whether they should be considered dead is especially important because of the viability of the babies' organs for transplant. Two cases illustrate the difficulties involved in declaring anencephalic babies as dead. The parents of Baby Gabrielle knew that their baby would be born anencephalic; they decided that they "wanted their infant's organs used for transplantation to touch others and contribute to life in some way." (Blakeslee, 1987, p. A1). The baby was kept on life supports and died naturally two days after birth. Her heart was then transplanted in Baby Paul. In 1992, parents of Baby Theresa Ann made a similar decision. They, however, asked the Florida courts to declare Theresa Ann dead although her heart was beating. The judges refused to do so, basing their decision on the fact that Baby Theresa Ann had brain stem activity and, therefore, did not meet the requirements for the legal definition of death which "requires irreversible cessation of all functions of the entire brain, including the brain stem." (Chartrand, 1992, p. 10). The baby continued to breathe, but her organs deteriorated, and they were unable to be transplanted.

Many ethicists believe that an exception to the brain death definition should be made in cases of anencephaly since the higher brain is absent. The argument that a margin of safety must exist before a person is declared dead, as with someone in a persistent vegetative state, does not seem to hold here. As ethicist Robert Levine states, "with anencephalics you don't have to be extra safe. They never had sentient lives and never will." (as cited in Chartrand, 1992, p. 10).

Yet, if the definition of death were to be changed to include only the higher brain, whether for those in a persistent vegetative state or for babies who are anencephalic, we would need to be able to declare as dead those persons who are still breathing.

The Right to Refuse Treatment

The principle that adults have a right to refuse treatment was stated in 1914 by Judge Cardozo:

> Every human being of adult years and sound mind has a right to determine what shall be done with his own body; and a surgeon who performs an operation without his patient's consent commits an assault, for which he is liable in damages. (As quoted in Grisez & Boyle, 1979, p. 88.)

This right was reconfirmed by the United States Supreme Court in 1990 in the Nancy Cruzan case: "The principle that a competent person has a constitutionally protected liberty interest in refusing unwanted medical treatment may be inferred from our prior decisions," wrote Chief Justice Rehnquist in his opinion. The decision was based on the 14th Amendment of the Constitution, tracing its roots to English common law where "even the touching of one person by another without consent and without legal justification was a battery." This led to the patients' right to informed consent (*New York Times,* 1990, pp. A1, A19).

Informed consent means that the patient must be told of the risks involved in any treatment and that she must consent to the treatment for it to be implemented. Implicit in the principle of informed consent is the principle of informed refusal.

The loophole in the right to refuse treatment is that the adult must be "competent." As discussed by Weir (1989, p. 69) three different groups have suggested that capacity or capability to make a decision, rather than competency, should be the issue. The President's Commission used the terms "decision-making capacity and incapacity"; the office of Technology Assessment used the terms "decisionally capable and decisionally incapable"; and the Hastings Center used the terms of capacity. The Hastings Center's Guidelines on the Termination of Life Sustaining Treatment and the Care of the Dying (1987) define decision-making capacity as:

a. the ability to comprehend information relevant to the decision;
b. the ability to deliberate about the choices in accordance with personal values and goals; and
c. the ability to communicate (verbally or nonverbally) with caregivers (p. 131).

If a person is capable of making a health care decision, then he should have the right to refuse treatment. But, what if a person is not able to make such a decision? As discussed by Weir (1989), the following trends have emerged from court cases:

> An adult patient's right to accept or refuse medical treatment continues even though he or she loses the capacity to make such a decision personally; a patient's incapacity to make a specific decision about medical treatment can differ from a judicial determination of a person's general incompetence; a nonautonomous patient's surrogate has the legal authority to accept or refuse medical treatment on behalf of the patient (p. 145).

This was evidenced in the case of Joseph Saikewicz. Joseph Saikewicz (as discussed by Grisez & Boyle, 1979, pp. 275–277) developed acute myeloblastic monocytic leukemia, which is considered incurable. However, chemotherapy is generally administered with the hope that the therapy will be successful and the patient will go into remission. The treatment is painful, has serious side effects, and requires the patient's cooperation. Without the treatment, the patient will definitely die in a short time, but will die painlessly. The difficulty with this case was that Mr. Saikewicz was a severely retarded, institutionalized 67 year old. A guardian was appointed for Mr. Saikewicz. After investigating the situation, the guardian recommended that Mr. Saikewicz not be given chemotherapy. The recommendation was accepted by the probate court, but the judge also referred the case for review. The Supreme Court of Massachusetts approved the lower court's decision on July 9, 1976. A full opinion was issued on November 28, 1977. Meanwhile, Mr. Saikewicz died on September 4, 1976. The decision to withhold treatment was not based on Mr. Saikewicz's incompetency. Rather, the court reaffirmed "that the noncompetent person has the same rights with respect to care as the competent person" (p. 275).

The reason that treatment was withheld was that it would have led to a great deal of pain and disorientation for Mr. Saikewicz.

Persons may also make out documents when they are capable of making decisions to prepare for when and if they are not capable of making decisions.

Advance Directives

There are two types of advance directives: a treatment directive or a "living will" and a proxy directive allowing a surrogate to make treatment decisions.

Living Wills

The Living Will is a document that allows a person to specify what treatment, if any, she would want given certain conditions. The following is the Living Will distributed by Concern for Dying:

Form 8.1 Living Will

Death is a part of life. It is a reality like birth, growth and aging. I am using this advance directive to convey my wishes about medical care to my doctors and other people looking after me at the end of my life. It is called an advance directive because it gives instructions in advance about what I want to happen to me in the future. It expresses my wishes about medical treatment that might keep me alive. I want this to be legally binding.

If I cannot make or communicate decisions about my medical care, those around me should rely on this document for instructions about measures that could keep me alive.

I do not want medical treatment (including feeding and water by tube that will keep me alive if:

- I am unconscious and there is no reasonable prospect that I will ever be conscious again (even if I am not going to die soon in my medical condition), *or*
- I am near death from an illness or injury with no reasonable prospect of recovery.

I do want medicine and other care to make me more comfortable and to take care of pain and suffering. I want this even if the pain medicine makes me die sooner.

I want to give some extra instructions: *[Here list any special instructions, e.g., some people fear being kept alive after a debilitating stroke. If you have wishes about this, or any other conditions, please write them here.]* ______________________

____

____

Although they are now enforceable in most states, only a small proportion of patients have made out Living Wills (Brock, 1989, p. 337). Another problem with Living Wills is that they are generally couched in general terms, so that a surrogate is needed to interpret the patient's meanings behind the words of the advance directive.

Proxy Directives

A proxy directive is an advance directive whereby an individual appoints someone to make health care decisions if the individual becomes incapable of doing so. It could take the form of a durable power of attorney. The health care proxy suggested by the New York State Department of Health is presented on the next page.

Children and Refusal of Treatment

When a patient is a minor, the parents must authorize the treatment. If the physician (or others) disagrees with the parents' decision, the decision becomes subject to review. Veatch (1976, pp. 125–128) discusses situations in which the courts have been clear about upholding or not upholding the parents' choice. Where the child is not in danger of dying, the courts have made decisions based on the reasonableness of the parents' decision. Generally, if the omission of treatment would lead to the child being damaged, the court will override the parents' decision. There are, however, three acceptable reasons for refusing treatment: where the treatment carries substantial risk; where there is no clear need for treatment; and where the treatment can be delayed until the child can be consulted.

If a child is dying and can be restored to health through medical treatment, the courts will intervene. For example, blood transfusions have been ordered for children of Jehovah's Witnesses. Courts have decided that there is "no parental right to make martyrs of one's children" (Veatch, 1976, p. 125).

Chad Green

The case of Chad Green is one in which a court overturned parents' decision to withhold treatment. His story was presented by Marion Steinman (1978). In August 1977, Chad Green, a 20-month-old boy, contracted acute lymphocytic leukemia, the most common form of childhood leukemia—and the most curable. Chad Green was given intensive chemotherapy in Nebraska, where the family was living at the time, for a four-week period. The therapy was effective and Chad went into remission. However, the next stage of treatment involves injecting drugs into the spinal fluid and/or

Form 8.2 Health Care Proxy

(1) I, ______________________________

hereby appoint ______________________________
(name, home address and telephone number)

____

as my health care agent to make any and all health care decisions for me except to the extent that I state otherwise. This proxy shall take effect when and if I become unable to make my own health care decisions.

(2) Optional instructions: I direct my agent to make health care decisions in accord with my wishes and limitations as stated below, or as he or she otherwise knows. (Attach additional pages if necessary.)

____

____

____

Unless your agent knows your wishes about artificial nutrition and hydration (feeding tubes), your agent will not be allowed to make decisions about artificial nutrition and hydration.)

(3) Name of substitute or fill-in-agent if the person I appoint above is unable, unwilling or unavailable to act as my health care agent.

____
(name, home address and telephone number)

____

(4) Unless I revoke it, this proxy shall remain in effect indefinitely, or until the date or conditions stated below. This proxy shall expire (specific date or conditions, if desired):

____

(5) Signature ______________________________

Address ______________________________

Date ______________________________

Statement by Witnesses (must be 18 or older)

I declare that the person who signed this document is personally known to me and appears to be of sound mind and acting of his or her own free will. He or she signed (or asked to sign for him or her) this document in my presence.

Witness 1 ______________________________

Address ______________________________

Witness 2 ______________________________

Address ______________________________

irradiating the brain. This protects against leukemic meningitis, since leukemic cells will invade the central nervous system where drugs cannot reach them. The Greens decided to go to Massachusetts since Chad's grandparents lived there and because Massachusetts General Hospital did not do cranial radiation. (The Greens were also opposed to radiation of the brain.) In October 1977, Chad had his first injection into the spinal fluid. The Greens also put Chad on a nutritional program. They believed that the chemicals Chad was taking were poisoning his body, and that the nutritional program would counteract the chemicals. After the third injection, Chad needed another drug, which was to be given 10 times daily in injections for two consecutive weeks. The Greens refused to give Chad this treatment. At the same time, Diana Green, without telling the physicians, stopped giving Chad the pills he had been taking. Therefore, all Chad was getting were the spinal injections. By December, Chad was totally off chemotherapy.

In February 1978, Chad again began showing symptoms of a relapse. The Greens, however, refused a bone marrow test and told the physicians that Chad was no longer on chemotherapy. On February 22, 1978, Dr. Truman, the physician in the case, petitioned Plymouth County Probate Court for the appointment of a temporary guardian who could consent to chemotherapy for Chad. The court allowed the petition, and two court-appointed guardians took Chad back for treatment. The same process began again: Chad had the bone marrow test, which showed acute lymphocytic leukemia. He went through the four-week intensive therapy; he went into remission; the spinal injections began. The Greens, however, were still against the chemotherapy, and, on March 29th, the District Court in Higham ruled in favor of the Greens. This decision was overruled by the Superior Court, with whom the Massachusetts Supreme Court ultimately agreed. Meanwhile, in January 1979, the Greens went into exile in Tijuana, Mexico, after a warrant was issued for their arrest on a civil contempt charge. They treated Chad with laetrile and their nutritional program. On October 3, 1979, Chad Green, a 3-year-old leukemia victim, died in Mexico.

The Issue of Defective Infants

In 1984, Congress amended the Child Abuse and Neglect Prevention and Treatment Act to define withholding of treatment from an infant as a form of child abuse except in three cases: "For infants who are irreversibly comatose; for infants for whom such treatment would prolong dying; or for infants for whom such treatment would be "virtually futile" and its provision would be inhumane." Hence, babies born with defects, who are not terminally ill, would be treated (Hastings Center, 1987b, p. 9). These amendments came about as a result of two cases:

Baby Doe of Indiana (1982): Baby Doe was born with Down's Syndrome, and a gastrointestinal malformation. The parents decided against surgery.

The hospital contested the parents' decision, arguing that the malformation was surgically correctable. The Indiana Supreme Court upheld the parents' decision. Baby Doe died six days later (Hastings Center, 1987, p. 9).

Baby Jane Doe of New York (1983): On October 11, 1983, Baby Jane Doe was born with spina bifida, hydrocephalus (water on the brain), and other disorders. The parents refused surgery, which might have extended the child's life from two to twenty years, for the infant. When taken to court, New York's highest court upheld the parents' decision: it was "well within medical standards and there was no medical reason to disturb the parents' decision." Certainly, the child was in no immediate danger (Veatch, 1989, pp. 134–136).

Under the new regulations, Baby Doe of Indiana would have probably had the surgery; it is not clear what would have happened to Baby Jane Doe.

One result of the regulations is that hospitals are now taking a "treat, wait, and see" approach to the care of newborns. Assessments concerning care are then made, and the issue revolves around withdrawing treatment rather than withholding treatment (Hastings Center, 1987, p. 5).

Euthanasia

"Euthanasia," which comes from Greek terms meaning "the good death," has come to encompass four different policies: (1) making the terminal stages as painless as possible but not hastening death; (2) making the terminal stage as painless as possible, but condoning jeopardizing the patient's life in the process; (3) ceasing or not starting treatment; or (4) actively participating in ending the patient's life (Reiser, 1975, p. 31). Euthanasia may be applied to persons with terminal diseases; to persons in irreversible comas; or to patients, although not terminally ill, whose quality of life is unacceptable.

In discussions of euthanasia, major distinctions must be made between active and passive euthanasia; direct and indirect euthanasia; and voluntary and involuntary euthanasia.

Active and Passive Euthanasia

The major difference between active and passive euthanasia is that active euthanasia involves committing an act that would result in a person's death, whereas passive euthanasia involves omission of an act. Other terms for active and passive euthanasia are *positive euthanasia* and *negative euthanasia,* respectively. The ethicists, Joseph Fletcher (1979) and James Rachels (1975, 1986) argue that since the end result is the same—the death of the person—there is no difference between active and passive euthanasia. Despite that the outcomes, and the motives for passive and active euthanasia may be the same, Veatch (1989), and Moreland & Geisler (1990) discuss the differences:

1. The cause of death is different. In omission, the cause of death is the disease, not the action of another;
2. The long-range effects on society may be different. There is a possibility that if we allow active killing of the dying, we may consequently allow active killing of others. This argument, the *wedge argument*, was applied to Nazi Germany. As Leo Alexander (as quoted in Veatch, 1989), a physician who helped draft the Nuremberg Code, stated:

   > The German mass murders started with the acceptance of that attitude basic in the euthanasia movement, that there is such a thing as life not worthy to be lived. This attitude in its early stages concerned itself merely with the severely and chronically sick. Gradually, the sphere of those to be included was enlarged to include the socially unproductive, the racially unwanted, and finally all non-Germans. But it is important to realize that the infinitely small wedged-in lever from which the entire trend of mind received its impetus was the attitude toward the non-rehabilitable sick (p. 66);

3. Letting die may be fulfilling the "principle of respecting autonomy" while killing is always a violation of the "duty to avoid killing."

The law makes distinctions between active and passive euthanasia. Legally, active euthanasia is absolutely prohibited since motive is no defense for killing. Those doctors and laymen who have committed "mercy killings" have been acquitted on the basis of temporary insanity.

Assisted Suicide

Today, as the *New York Times* headline says, "At Crossroads, U.S. Ponders Ethics of Helping Others Die" (1991a), a form of active euthanasia, assisted suicide, has become an important issue: (1) The book, *Final Exit* by Derek Humphrey (1990), is a best-selling suicide manual. It provides the terminally ill information on methods of committing suicide. (2) Jack Kevorkian, a retired physician, developed a "suicide machine" that allows a patient to give himself an intravenous injection of poison. It has been used by non-terminally ill patients such as Janet Adkins, who suffered from Alzheimer's disease (*Time,* 1990). (3) In the state of Washington, there was a referendum to legalize assisted suicide; on November 6, 1991, it was voted down by 54 percent of the voters. The initiative would have allowed doctors to assist in suicide in cases where: (a) the patient was conscious and competent; (b) the patient made a written request to die witnessed by two people; and (c) two physicians certified the patient had less than six months to live.

Although the measure failed to pass, it will probably appear on the ballot in other states (*New York Times,* 1991b, p. B16).

Opponents and supporters of assisted suicide are both concerned about the process of dying, yet they draw very different conclusions (*New York Times,* 1991):

> Both sides worry about introducing euthanasia into a medical system increasingly driven by economic pressures and incentives. Both insist that dying, pain-ridden or anguished patients must be given compassionate care rather than simple prolongation of their lives through technology.
>
> But for some, giving doctors the power of releasing people from life altogether is a necessary form of compassionate care, an essential check on high-tech medicine. For others, it is the ultimate surrender to technology, a dangerous substitute for compassion.
>
> "I think it is the issue of the next 20 years," said Dr. Cassell, "and it won't be resolved on a ballot" (p. B7).

Direct and Indirect Euthanasia

Direct and indirect forms of euthanasia are similar to passive and active forms. The distinction between direct and indirect killing lies in whether or not death is the primary intention of the act. The major indirect form of euthanasia is the use of painkilling drugs. In order to lessen the suffering of the patient, greater and greater dosages of a painkiller may be administered. However, in doing so, death may be hastened. Since the primary intention in giving the medication was to lessen pain, the death would be indirect.

Voluntary and Involuntary Euthanasia

Voluntary euthanasia refers to euthanasia with the patient's consent, while involuntary euthanasia does not involve the patient's consent. The arguments against voluntary euthanasia are that the patient may not be making a decision based on personal wishes, but may be consenting to relieve another's suffering; that people may be under a temporary depression when deciding; and that medication may induce confusion so that the person is unable to make a decision. The problem with voluntary euthanasia is that it is irrevocable (Kamisar, 1958); once the decision is made and the treatment stopped, one cannot change one's mind.

However, proponents of voluntary euthanasia believe that a person has the right to decide whether or not to live, and that safeguards, such as requiring a period of time between the request for euthanasia and the act itself, should be included.

Changing Status of Euthanasia and the Right to Refuse Treatment

Over the past twenty years the legal issues surrounding euthanasia have changed dramatically. There are basically six different positions held on euthanasia (Weir, 1989, pp. 227–268):

1. Life-sustaining treatment should never be withheld or stopped.
2. Treatment with nondying patients should never be withheld or stopped.
3. Life-sustaining nutrition and hydration should never be withheld or stopped.
4. All life-sustaining medical treatment should be withheld or stopped when warranted.
5. Intentional killing is acceptable as an exceptional moral alternative.
6. Intentional killing is acceptable as a moral and a legal alternative.

Although ethicists take these six different positions, only positions 1 through 4 are legal in the United States today. In the years 1976, 1985, and 1990, major changes occurred in the legal status of euthanasia which now allow all "life sustaining medical treatment to be withheld or terminated." (For a discussion of the years 1976 and 1985, see Weir, 1989, pp. 23–26.)

In 1976, there was the Karen Ann Quinlan case; the publication by the Massachusetts General Hospital and Beth Israel Hospital (in Boston) of Do Not Resuscitate (DNR) guidelines; and the passage of the California Natural Death Act.

Karen Ann Quinlan. On April 15, 1975, Karen Ann Quinlan, a 21-year-old woman, went into a coma. She was admitted to St. Clare's Hospital in Denville, New Jersey, and was placed on a respirator. In July, her father, Joseph Quinlan, signed a release to permit the physicians to turn off the respirator, which the physicians refused to do. They felt that to turn off the respirator would be an act of homicide. Joseph Quinlan then went to court to be appointed Karen Ann's guardian "with the express power of authorizing discontinuance of all extraordinary means of sustaining vital processes." Karen's parents argued that she would have wanted to be removed from the machine; they reported that Karen Ann had discussed the fact that she would not want to be kept alive at all costs. The judge of the Superior Court, Judge Muir, decided in favor of the hospital. The judge argued that Karen Ann Quinlan was still alive; she did not meet the Harvard criteria for brain death, and "there is a duty to continue the life assisting apparatus, if within the treating physician's opinion it should be done. . . . There is no constitutional right to die that can be asserted by a parent for his incompetent adult child." He considered that to turn off the respirator would be an act of homicide. The Quinlans then appealed to the New Jersey Supreme Court, which overturned Judge Muir's ruling. One of the major concerns was the violation of Karen's right to privacy:

> We think that the State's interest contra weakens and the individual's right to privacy grows as the degree of bodily invasion increases and prognosis dims. . . . It is for this reason that we determine that Karen's right of privacy may be asserted in her behalf, in this respect, by her guardian and family under the particular circumstances presented by this record (Matter of Quinlan, 1976).

Judge Hughes of the Supreme Court decided that if there were no reasonable possibility of Karen ever becoming conscious, the life-support systems could be removed without any civil or criminal liability. Karen Ann Quinlan was then weaned from the respirator (*Newsweek,* 1975, p. 68).

Massachusetts General Hospital's DNR Regulations. Although hospital authorities already were making decisions about when not to resuscitate patients, in 1976, Massachusetts General specified a formal policy about letting people die ("Helping the Dying Die," 1976):

- Class A: "Maximal therapeutic effort without reservation."
- Class B: Same as A but "with daily evaluation because probability of survival is questionable."
- Class C: "Selective limitation of therapeutic measures." In these cases, there might be orders not to resuscitate, a decision not to give antibiotics to cure pneumonia, and so on.
- Class D: "All therapy can be discontinued."
- Class D is generally only for patients with brain death or those who have no chance of regaining "cognitive and sapient life." (p. 1105).

Patients may be moved into different classes as their situations change.

The California Natural Death Act. California was the first state to recognize the legality of a document, a "Living Will," that allowed a person to specify what treatment, if any, a person would want given a terminal condition.

These three events recognized that it was acceptable to withhold or cease life-sustaining treatment when an individual's wishes were known.

In 1985, another two developments occurred: the Claire Conroy case and an increase in Natural Death Acts.

Claire Conroy. In 1985, the New Jersey Supreme Court handed down the decision that a nasogastric tube, which provided artificial nutrition and hydration, could be removed from incompetent 83-year-old Claire Conroy at the behest of her legal guardian. The decision was based on an individual's "right to reject *any* medical treatment under the doctrine of informed consent" (Annas, 1985 p. 24). The court concluded: "We have no doubt that Ms. Conroy, if competent to make the decision and if resolute in her determination, would have chosen to have her nasogastric tube withdrawn" (Annas, 1985 p. 24).

Increase in Natural Death Acts. Thirteen states passed Natural Death Acts in 1985, containing language on nutrition and hydration. This brought the total of Natural Death Acts to 36 (35 states and the District of Columbia) (Weir, 1989, p. 25).

Hence, in 1985, artificial hydration and nutrition was treated as any other form of medical treatment, and refusal of such could be included in one's "Living Will." This view of artificial hydration and nutrition was affirmed in 1990 with the Nancy Cruzan case.

Nancy Cruzan. In 1983, Nancy Cruzan was in a car accident that left her in a persistent vegetative state; she could breathe, but she had no consciousness. She was maintained through artificial hydration and nutrition. She left no written instructions concerning her wishes if she were in a comatose state. The Missouri Supreme Court upheld the Missouri law requiring "clear and convincing evidence" that a person would want treatment to be discontinued, and denied the parents' request to remove the nasogastric tube. On June 25, 1990, the United States Supreme Court, while upholding Missouri's right (and all states' rights) to require evidence that competent patients would choose to have treatment stopped if they were competent ("The . . . challenging task of crafting appropriate procedures for safeguarding incompetents' 'liberty interests'," Justice Sandra Day O'Connor wrote in her concurring opinion, "is entrusted to the 'laboratory of the states'" [*New York Times*, 6/26/90, pp. A1, A19]), the court ended the distinction between artificial feeding and other medical treatments (Colby, 1990, p. 5). The Supreme Court also acknowledged that competent persons have a constitutional right to refuse medical treatment.

Religion And Euthanasia

Catholicism, Orthodox Judaism, and Fundamental Protestantism are opposed to any form of active euthanasia, but they allow forms of passive euthanasia.

Catholicism

The Catholic view of euthanasia was recently reaffirmed by the National Conference of Catholic Bishops (1984). It was first stated by Pope Pius XII in 1957 in his *allocutio* to Italian anesthetists. Direct euthanasia is strictly forbidden. If self-administered, it is suicide, and, if death is administered by another, it is homicide. Passive euthanasia is limited by the distinction between ordinary and extraordinary procedures. Ordinary measures are always required to be applied to a patient; otherwise, it is morally the same as killing the patient. However, the exclusion of extraordinary treatments where there is no reasonable hope of recovery is acceptable. The difficulty with the distinction between ordinary treatment and extraordinary treatment is that these are relative terms. For example, mouth-to-mouth resuscitation was once considered an extraordinary procedure (Hendin, 1974, p. 18).

There are differences attached to the meanings of "extraordinary" and "ordinary." Paul Ramsey (1970) discusses three differences between the ways in which doctors and moralists would use these terms:

1. The physician is likely to make the distinction between customary versus unusual procedures without taking into account the medical history of the patient, as the moralist would.
2. To the moralist, the decision to stop extraordinary means is basically the same as starting them. For the physician, it is more difficult to stop a procedure once it is begun.
3. Moralists would view the patient as a person and take that into account, while the physician would take a more narrow view.

Gerald Kelly (1958), a Catholic theologian, sees the differences between physicians' and moralists' definitions of "extraordinary" and "ordinary" in the following manner: Physicians would define "ordinary" measures as "standard, recognized, orthodox, or established medicines or procedures of that period, at that level of medical practice, and within the limits of availability. Extraordinary measures are fanciful, bizarre, experimental, incompletely established, unorthodox, or not recognized." Moralists define ordinary measures as "all medicines, treatments and operations which offer a reasonable hope of benefit without excessive pain, or other inconveniences, and extraordinary means offer no reasonable hope of benefit and are excessively expensive, painful and inconvenient" (p. 129).

The differences that Ramsey and Kelly discussed were evident in the case of Brother Joseph Charles Fox, a member of the Order of the Society of Mary. At the age of 83, Brother Fox suffered a heart attack during surgery for a hernia. He went into a coma and was placed on a respirator. His friend, Father Philip Eichner, asked the hospital authorities to take Brother Fox off the respirator, but they refused. Father Eichner took the hospital to court and used, as the basis of his testimony, the fact that when he and Brother Fox had discussed Pope Pius XII's *allocutio,* Brother Fox had stated that he did not want "extraordinary" means used. Father Eichner was defining the word as Kelly and Ramsey said the moralists would. The hospital authorities, however, did not see these measures as extraordinary; furthermore, they did not wish to stop a procedure once it had been started. (The Court granted the petition of Father Eichner on December 6, 1979; the District Attorney immediately appealed but lost his appeal on March 27, 1980; meanwhile, Brother Fox had died in January [Annas, 1980].)

Judaism

Judaism, too, does not sanction positive euthanasia. The biblical basis for this is found in the words of King David. A young survivor of a battle against the Philistines saw King Saul, who was in terrible pain from a wound. The King begged to be killed, and the survivor obeyed him. When David heard of this, he had the man executed, saying, "You have been convicted by the testimony of your own lips of having taken the life of God's anointed" (Silver, 1974, p. 121). However, during the Middle Ages, two types of euthanasia were practiced: it was believed that you could enable a dying person to die more quickly if you removed the pillow or if you placed the synagogue keys under the dying person's pillow. The former was prohibited by law in the fourteenth century; the latter was condemned as being magical (Wilson, 1975, p. 25).

In terms of passive euthanasia, the degree of acceptance is related to the orthodoxy of the theologian. The Orthodox tradition is best reflected by Rabbi Immanuel Jakobovits (1961) writing in the *Hebrew Medical Journal:* "Jewish law sanctions the withdrawal of any factor—whether extraneous to the patient himself or not—which may artificially delay his demise in the final phase" (p. 251). The final phase, however, refers to an individual being expected to live only three days or less. Conservative and Reform Jews would define passive euthanasia with fewer limitations on the prognosis of the dying individual (Hendin, 1974, p. 81).

Protestantism

Protestant theologians provide very different views on euthanasia. Karl Barth (as discussed in Wilson, 1975) believes that human life belongs solely to God, and that we cannot be certain that we are helping a patient when we allow her to die. Allowing a patient to die is as wrong as killing the patient. At the other end of the debate on euthanasia is Joseph Fletcher. Fletcher (1968) defines euthanasia as merciful release from incurable suffering. He feels that the decision for or against euthanasia must depend on the situation. It is not a question of passive versus active euthanasia, nor of using ordinary versus extraordinary measures. For Fletcher, the situation in which the dying person exists is the determining factor. Basically, he sees three positions that can be taken:

1. The absolutist view, which sees life as the highest good and death as the worst evil, and so would be against any form of euthanasia.

2. Stoic-indifference, which sees life as meaningless and assigns no value to life.
3. Pragmatic-situation ethic, in which life and death may both be considered good depending upon the specific circumstances. "In this view life, no more than any other thing or value, is good in itself but only by reason of the situation; and death, no more than any other evil, is evil in itself, but only by reason of the situation" (p. 365).

Different denominations reflect the different views. Southern Baptists are opposed to all forms of euthanasia; while the United Church of Christ passed a resolution affirming "individual freedom and responsibility" in making choices around euthanasia and suicide (*New York Times,* 10/28/91, p. B7).

SUMMARY ❧

This chapter has looked at three ethical issues surrounding death: the definition of death, the right to refuse treatment and euthanasia. Whole brain death has become the standard definition of death. The question concerning the definition of death is whether the definition should be changed to the higher portion of the brain.

With regard to refusing treatment, competent adults have a legal right to do so, including artificial hydration and nutrition. Adults may prepare for a time when they are not competent by writing advance directions, which may involve "Living Wills" or durable powers of attorney. Parents may refuse treatment for children who are terminally ill.

Euthanasia may be active or passive, direct or indirect, and voluntary or involuntary. Legislation, medicine, and religion make a large distinction between active and passive euthanasia. Passive euthanasia, in the form of withholding or withdrawing medical treatment is legal, while active euthanasia is not.

Most religions are against active euthanasia, while acceptance of passive euthanasia differs depending on the orthodoxy of the religious group.

LEARNING EXERCISES ❧

1. Write your own advance directive.
2. If you had cancer, and your life could be extended by six months by undergoing chemotherapy, what would you do? Discuss your decision.
3. Speak to your physician about the ethical issues discussed here. Do you and your physician agree on these issues? How do you feel this discussion will affect your relationship?

4. A baby was born with only a brain stem, no higher brain. The parents wanted to donate the baby's organs, but the courts would not declare the baby dead since he was still breathing. Do you agree with the courts' decision? Why or why not?

AUDIOVISUAL MATERIAL ❧

A Time to Die: Who Decides? 34 minutes/videocassette/1988. Churchill Films, 662 North Robertson Blvd., Los Angeles, CA, 90069.
Three families must make decisions concerning euthanasia: parents for an infant; a sister for her young adult sibling; and a husband for his elderly wife.

Is This Life Worth Living? 57 minutes/videocassette/1988. Filmakers Library, 124 East 40th Street, New York, NY, 10016.
This video focuses on case histories of families who have members who are brain damaged or comatose. It raises questions of when medical care should cease, and who should decide.

The Right to Die: Frontline. 120 minutes/videocassette/1990. PBS Video, 1320 Braddock Place, Alexandria, VA, 22314.
Focusing on the Nancy Cruzan case, this video discusses the various arguments around right-to-die issues.

REFERENCES ❧

Alexander, M. (1980). The rigid embrace of the Narrow House: Premature burial and the signs of death. *Hastings Center Report,* June, *10,* 25–31.

Annas, G. (1980). Quinlan, Saikewicz and Brother Fox. *Hastings Center Report,* June, *10,* 20–21.

Annas, G. (1985). From Quinlan to Conroy. *Hastings Center Report, 15,* 24–26.

Black, P. (1978). Definitions of brain death. In T. Beauchamp & S. Perlin (Eds.), *Ethical issues in death and dying.* Englewood Cliffs, NJ: Prentice-Hall.

Blakeslee, S. (1987). Baby without brain kept alive to give heart. *New York Times.* October 19, A1.

Brock, D. (1989). Death and dying. In R. Veatch (Ed.), *Medical ethics.* Boston: Jones & Bartlett Publishers.

Chartrand, S. (1992). Baby missing part of brain challenges legal definition of death. *New York Times.* March 29, 12.

Colby, W. (1990). Clear and convincing: Missouri stands alone. *Hastings Center Report,* September/October, *20,* 5–6.

Fletcher, J. (1968). Elective death. In E. F. Torey (Ed.), *Ethical issues in medicine.* Boston: Little, Brown.

Fletcher, J. (1979). *Morals and medicine.* Princeton, NJ: Princeton University Press.

Glaser, R. (1970). Innovations and heroic acts in prolonging life. In O. Brim, H. Freeman, S. Levine, & N. Scotch (Eds.), *The dying patient.* New York: Russell Sage Foundation.

Grisez, G., & Boyle, J. (1979). *Life and death with liberty and justice.* Notre Dame, IN: University of Notre Dame Press.

Hastings Center. (1987a). *Guidelines on the termination of life-sustaining treatment and the care of the dying.* Bloomington, IN: Indiana University Press.

Hastings Center. (1987b). Imperiled newborns. *Hastings Center Report, 17,* 5–32.

Helping the dying die: Two Harvard hospitals go public with policies. (1976). *Science,* September 17, *193,* 1105–1106.

Hendin, D. (1974). *Death as a fact of life.* New York: Warner Paperback.

Humphrey, D. (1990). *Final exit.* New York: Hemlock Society and Carol Publishing.

Jakobovits, I. (1961). The dying and the treatment under Jewish law. *Hebrew Medical Journal, 2,* 126–152.

Kamisar, Y. (1958). Some non-religious views against proposed mercy-killing legislation. *Minnesota Law Review,* May, *42,* 969–1042.

Kelly, G. (1958). *Medico-moral problems.* St. Louis, MO: Catholic Hospital Association.

Kolata, G. (1992). Ethicists debating a new definition of death. *New York Times.* April 29, C13.

Lamb, D. (1985). *Death, brain-death and ethics.* Albany, NY: State University of New York Press.

Moreland, J. P., & Geisler, N. (1990). *The life and death debate; Moral issues of our times.* New York: Greenwood Press.

National Conference of Catholic Bishops. (1984). *Guidelines for legislation on life sustaining treatment.*

Newsweek, November 3, 1975, *86,* 68.

New York State Department of Health. (1991). *The health care proxy law: A guidebook for Professionals,* January.

New York Times, June 26, 1990, A1 and A19.

New York Times, October 28, 1991a, A1 and B7.

New York Times, November 8, 1991b, B16.

President's Commission for the Study of Ethical Problems in Medical and Biomedical and Behavioral Research. (1981). *Defining death.* Washington, DC: U.S. Government Printing Office.

Rachels, J. (1975). Active and passive euthanasia. *New England Journal of Medicine,* January 9, *292,* 78–80.

Rachels, J. (1986). *The end of life.* Oxford: Oxford University Press.

Ramsey, P. (1970). *The patient as a person.* New Haven, CT: Yale University Press.

Reiser, S. (1975). The dilemma of euthanasia in modern medical history: The English and American experience. In J. Behake & S. Bok (Eds.), *The dilemmas of euthanasia.* Garden City, NY: Anchor Press.

Silver, D. (1974). The right to die? In J. Reimer (Ed.), *Jewish reflections on death.* New York: Schocken Books.

Steinman, M. (1978). A child's fight for life: Parents vs. doctor. *New York Times Magazine,* December 10, 160.

Time, June 18, 1990, 69–70.

Veatch, R. (1976). *Death, dying and the biological revolution.* New Haven, CT: Yale University Press.

Veatch, R. (1989). *Death, dying and the biological revolution, revised edition.* New Haven, CT: Yale University Press.

Weir, R. (1989). *Abating treatment with critically ill patients.* New York: Oxford University Press.

Wilson, J. (1975). *Death by decision.* Philadelphia: Westminster Press.

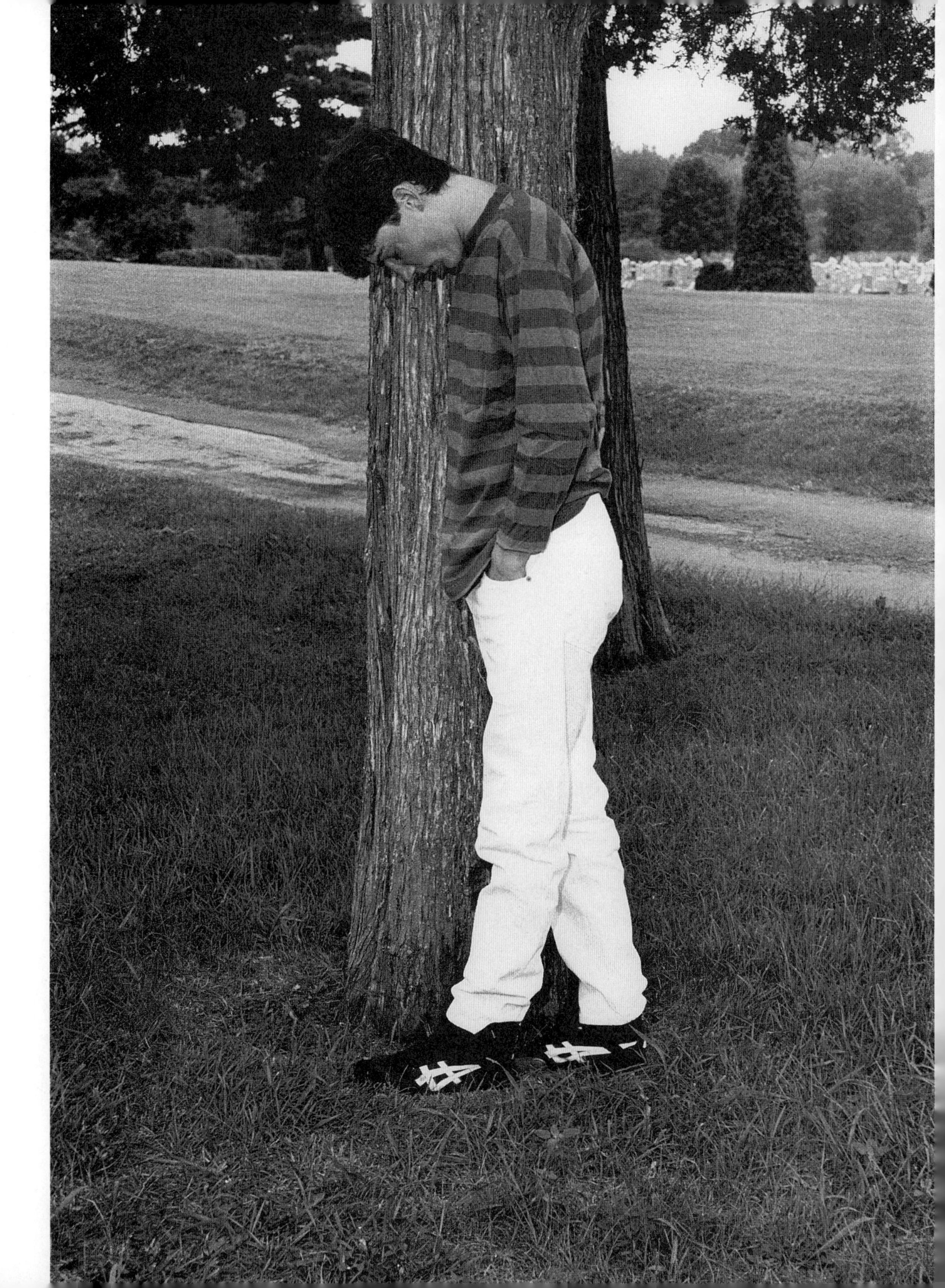

Chapter 9

Suicide

The phenomenon of suicide has existed throughout civilization. Attitudes toward this type of behavior have fluctuated, largely depending upon the historical period, place, and cultural view of death. In ancient Greece, suicide was accepted by many philosophers as a reasonable choice. The Hindu practice of suttee, whereby the wife throws herself onto her husband's funeral pyre to prove her devotion, was abolished by the British in the nineteenth century, but it is still practiced in some parts of India. Suicide has been an expression of maintaining various aspects of personal honor in Japan throughout its history.

According to early Christianity, suicide was regarded as a mortal sin and as a serious offense against society and the state. Until the end of the eighteenth century, people in France who attempted suicide and failed were sometimes hanged. If they succeeded, their bodies were dragged through the streets or thrown onto the public garbage dump. If people living in England during this time committed suicide, they may have had their estates turned over to the crown and probably were buried at crossroads with stakes through their hearts (Colt, 1991).

Attitudes arising from the Age of Enlightenment were more humanistic. Early nineteenth century Romantics considered suicide as rather heroic and poetic. In the twentieth century, suicide in the Western world has been viewed more in terms of a medical–psychological model. Factors which may influence the attitudes of people toward suicide and suicidal behaviors include age, sex, race, and educational level (Marks, 1988–89). In a study of 780 college students' attitudes toward suicide, Deluty (1988–89) found that evaluations of suicide tended to be more favorable when the evaluators were male, when male victims were being judged, when elderly victims were being evaluated, or when terminal cancer was the precipitating factor (p. 315).

Death by suicide remains an enigma despite a vast literature and many perspectives on it. The purpose of this chapter is to discuss a broad overview of the extent of suicide in the United States, the different theories about suicide, the current emphasis on suicide prevention, the impact of suicide on surviving families and friends, and health care professionals' responses to suicide.

Who Commits or Attempts Suicide?

According to 1991 provisional data tabulated by the National Center for Health Statistics, the suicide rate in the United States is 11.4 per 100,000 (p. 17). It currently ranks as one of the 10 leading causes of death (U.S. Bureau of the Census, 1990). The demographic risk factors often associated with suicide include age, sex, race, marital status, affective disorder, alcoholism, lack of social support, history of previous suicidal attempts, and mental illness, although some of these factors are controversial in the literature (Balon, 1987).

The accuracy of statistics about suicide is often questioned. There is still some social stigma attached to suicide, especially with children (Sandoval, Davis, & Wilson, 1987, p. 105). This stigma may lead to underreporting and covering up suicidal behavior. Suicides may be underreported since many deaths that are designated as accidents, such as one-car automobile accidents and drownings, may have been suicide. Wekstein (1979) notes "statistics on suicide are synthetic; that is, they are concocted products and their inaccuracy and unreliability are an open secret" (p. 58). However, statistics can provide some basic information about "who" is involved in suicide and facilitate further inquiry and research into "why." With this in mind, key demographic considerations of age, race, and gender as they relate to suicide are further explored to develop a more complete picture of this phenomenon in the United States.

Age

Data from the Centers for Disease Control, 1986, and the National Center for Health Statistics, 1988 (cited in Centers for Disease Control, 1991) indicate that suicide rates for adolescents 15 to 19 years of age have quadrupled from 2.7 per 100,000 in 1950 to 11.3 in 1988 (p. 633). The reasons for this are multiple and complex. Adolescence marks the transition into adulthood; it is a tumultuous time. Researchers suggest that the fragmentation of family life, the shifts in cultural mores, pressures of parents with high expectations, and problems with interpersonal relationships are contributing factors. An important predictor of suicide is the occurrence and seriousness of a previous attempt (Pfeffer, 1988). Other known risk factors include social isolation, depression, alcohol and other drug use, and access to lethal means to suicide (Centers for Disease Control, 1991).

Homosexuality is also a risk factor. Gibson (1989) notes that "a majority of suicide attempts by homosexuals occur during their youth, and gay youth are two to three times more likely to attempt suicide than other young people" (p. 3–110). American society has historically denied the sexuality of young people. However, sexual orientation is frequently formed by adolesence. It becomes a challenge to confront the issues of adolescent homosexuality and suicide in young people often because of the stigma attached to both categories by society.

According to Heacock (1990), the increase in suicide within the adolescent age group has been greatest among white males, with an increase being noted each year over the past 25 years. Gibbs (1988) notes that suicide rates for African American youth in this age group have also increased, with male rates over four times the rate for females. Although African American youth suicide rates are not as high as white youth suicide rates, suicide remains a significant problem for African American youths as it is one of the leading causes of mortality in the adolescent age group (Smith & Carter, 1986).

A nationwide survey estimating the annual prevalence of suicidal thoughts and behaviors among U.S. high school students was conducted in 1990 (Centers for Disease Control, 1991). Latino and white students reported higher levels of suicidal thoughts and behaviors than African American students, although these differences were not always statistically significant. Latino female students were significantly more likely to have attempted suicide during the 12 months preceding the survey than white or African American female students (p. 634). According to Heacock (1990), Latino adolescent males and females not only share the problems of racial and ethnic discrimination and poverty with African Americans but also have problems related to acculturation and language. These are problems that can cause depression, a known factor in suicidal behavior.

At the other end of the age spectrum, the elderly have a rate of suicide that is more than double that of the general population. By the year 2020, as the percentage of elderly increases dramatically in America, Haas & Hendin (1983) speculate there may also be a dramatic rise in elderly suicides. Currently, elderly white males are the most vulnerable group for suicide in people 65 and over. African Americans and Native Americans have a decrease in suicide rates after age 40 (McIntosh & Santos, 1981).

There are a number of explanations for the high elderly suicide rate, some of which are based on the intense and accelerated rate of changes experienced as people age (La Greca, 1988). These changes include significant life events such as retirement, loss of a spouse, lessening of income, deteriorating health, and loss of friends. However, many elderly people have developed satisfactory coping skills throughout their lives that have helped them deal with such changes in the past. Therefore, an inclusive formulation is difficult to develop for this high elderly suicide rate.

It is also important to consider how elderly people are valued in American society. Many view the elderly as no longer contributing to production and, therefore, as a burden and a drain upon the tax base, requiring social security and health care benefits. Some elderly people may internalize such perceptions, experiencing a loss of self-esteem and meaning in life that could lead to depression and the ultimate response of suicide. Seiden (cited in Nkongho, 1988) suggests one reason for the low incidence of nonwhite elderly suicide may be the extension of traditional values of respect for the elderly in nonwhite cultures, giving these elderly a sense of dignity and worth that prevents them from feeling suicidal.

Race

African American. African American suicide rates, across age groups and gender, are lower than those of whites. The brunt of African American suicide is borne by the 25 to 34 age group, particularly males in that age bracket, although, as noted previously, the suicide rate is increasing among male adolescents. Among African Americans, males commit suicide far more often than females, suicide is higher in urban areas than in rural regions, and the lowest rates of suicide occur in the South where the African American population density is the highest (Group for the Advancement of Psychiatry, 1989).

While many factors in suicidal behavior are present in both white and African American populations—anger, low self-esteem, depression, an inability to express feelings, and difficulties in family structure—Spaights & Simpson (1986) note that some aspects are unique to the African American culture and must be explored. Among these aspects are effects of upward mobility and cultural expectations for males, which include repression of feelings and strict obedience to parents and elders. Young, upwardly mobile African Americans may become isolated from their families, communities, and social institutions. McIntosh (1989) suggests that changes in family and community supports as well as changes in economics and racial prejudice are forces that may contribute to suicide risks.

King (1982) emphasizes the critical contribution of sociological frames of reference in examining African American suicide. He notes that for African Americans, "the issues of racism, oppression, miseducation, unemployment, and a history of dehumanization are central to their social formations. The will to live is clear among Afro-Americans. In the face of this single most critical strength of Afro-American people, what fosters the will not to live, and eventually the choice to die is a significant question" (pp. 232–233). His model of research for inquiry in African American suicide includes looking at the various levels of relationships growing out of the historical social formation of the particular nation, state, community, family, and person (King, 1982, p. 234). Kirk (1986) also discusses African American suicide from a sociopolitical perspective.

Hendin (1982) uses a psychosocial framework to theorize about suicide in African Americans. He notes from his studies of young suicidal African Americans in the ghetto that these young people feel trapped at an early age in an unalterable life situation—trapped by lack of education and job opportunities and by the destructive effects of the ghetto on their own personalities. A sense of despair, a feeling that life will never be satisfying, confronts many African Americans at a far younger age than it does most whites (pp. 92–93).

Clearly these hypotheses require much more extensive research. In addition, none of these theories really explain the marked differences not only between African American and white suicide rates, but between the higher suicide rates of African American men as compared with the lower suicide rates of African American women.

Latinos. There is a serious dearth of publications in the literature on suicidal behavior of Latinos (Zayas, 1989; Heacock, 1990). It is important to remember however, that the Latino population is not homogenous, and what may be characteristic for one subgroup may not be for another. McIntosh (cited in Zayas, 1989) found that Latino suicides were primarily male, young, and, across all age groups, Latinos were half as likely as Anglos to commit suicide. Zayas (1987) suggests that this suicide rate may be attributed to the influence of family honor, solidarity, and support on Latino individuals.

Hoppe & Martin (1986) reported on trends in suicide rates for Mexican Americans and Anglos in Bexar County, Texas, from 1960 to 1980. The results of their study indicated that suicide rates for Anglos increased more than rates for Mexican Americans. Zayas (1989) points out the urgent need for more rigorous clinical research with the fast-growing Latino population in the United States: one research example is the "need to distinguish suicidal behavior based on psychotic processes from suicidal behavior originating in affective disorders based on the stresses of living in a dual cultural context, or in biochemical processes" (p. 53).

Native Americans. The suicide rate for Native American tribes varies widely, from higher to lower, than that of the general population (Shore, cited in Thompson & Walker, 1990). The popular assumption that all tribes have the same health problems and similar patterns of suicide must be questioned. There is tremendous variation in social, economic, and educational factors from one tribe to the next, with resultant diversity in behavior and culture. Levy & Kunitz (1987) suggest that Native American suicide rates often fluctuate with those of surrounding community areas, and that these tribal rates should be compared with the general population living in areas adjacent to reservations.

May (1987) describes emerging general characteristics of Native American suicide: (a) suicide is predominantly among males, aged 15 to 24; (b) women have particularly low rates of suicide in most tribes; (c) tribes with loose social integration that emphasize a high degree of individuality generally have higher suicide rates than those with tight integration (which emphasizes conformity); (d) tribes that are undergoing rapid change in their social and economic conditions have higher suicide rates than those who are not (p. 61).

Several factors have been considered over the years as contributing to destructive behavior in Native Americans. These factors include cultural ambivalence (uncertainty of a sense of belonging to either the majority or minority culture), loss of traditional culture, loss of control over one's life, and a learned pattern of passive survival (Walker & LaDue, 1986). Abuse of alcohol and other drugs have also been implicated as a possible cause of suicide. However, Thompson & Walker (1990) point out that seldom has there been scientific study of these factors to discover whether they are indeed causal. They suggest that statistics on Native American suicide could be greatly enhanced by gathering and reporting data that reflect the mosaic of rates and characteristics of Native American suicide (p. 132).

Asian Americans. The label "Asian American" covers a wide range of people from many countries, with different languages and diverse cultures. Asian Americans include Chinese, Japanese, Koreans, Filipinos, Southeast Asians, Indians, Pakistanis, Sri Lankans, and Pacific Islanders. The most consistent and reliable data on suicide among these groups in the United States are those relating to Chinese and Japanese Americans (Group for the Advancement of Psychiatry, 1989). This discussion will therefore focus on these two groups.

Historically, suicide in Japan has been accepted not only with religious tolerance but with state approval (Colt, 1991). It has been seen as an honorable death, as a way of showing altruism, and as an acceptable solution for certain problems. In a 1980–86 comparison ranking of suicidal rates in 62 countries, Japan ranked 11th and the United States ranked 24th (Diekstra, 1989). However, in the United States, suicide rates among Japanese Americans are generally lower than those of white Americans. There is a minor peak in suicide rates in young adult Japanese Americans and a major peak among the elderly: the age distribution is bimodal (Group for the Advancement of Psychiatry, 1989).

In contrast with Japan, there is no tradition among the Chinese of suicide as a socially acceptable response to difficult circumstances. Rather, the expectations are that troubles are a part of fate that must be borne. Rin (1975) notes that in China "if a suicide occurs out of loyalty to the family, or in order to save face, then the suicide is accepted, but when suicide occurs because of deep unhappiness or mental illness, then people respond with the deepest fear" (p. 246).

Suicide rates among Chinese Americans, though generally lower than those for white Americans, are similarly distributed by age, with peak rates among those aged 65 and over (Group for the Advancement of Psychiatry, 1989). However, there is a high incidence of suicide among older ChineseAmerican women as compared to men, which is different from elderly white Americans. Liu & Yu (1985) in a review of 1980 statistics, found that in every age group starting from 45 years, Chinese women manifest a higher suicide rate than white women (p. 225).

The process of acculturation is relevant to the phenomenon of suicide in Asian Americans. The language barrier can be a major problem for Asian immigrants. Lalinec-Michaud (1988) has noted the remarkable lack of community resources for Chinese immigrants in Canada and stresses the importance of group membership and reinforcing ties with the Chinese community to help in adaptation and acculturation. There is a need for caregivers who understand Asian cultural differences to participate in treatment of Asian Americans. For example, Takahashi (1989) suggests giving more concrete and directive advice, and involving family members in psychotherapy when treating the suicidal Asian patient.

Gender

According to La Greca (1988), "one of the clearest conclusions about suicide is that males commit suicide 2 to 3 times more frequently than females. Females, on the other hand, attempt suicide 3 to 5 times more than males" (p. 232). While these statistics present an overall view of suicide as being a primarily male behavior, this view may not be the only one to consider.

Kushner (1985) notes that if the numbers of those attempting and completing suicide are added together, the rate differential between genders collapses. It may be argued that these two categories cannot be merged because there are differences in intention; those attempting suicide expect to be saved, while those completing suicide generally have a plan that does not allow for intervention. However, official statistics only measure results and not intentions, and those people who intend to kill themselves but by chance survive are not counted as suicides. Despite this discrepancy, official statistics are used to explain motives (Kushner, 1985).

It may be that men are more often completers of suicide than women because of differences employed by the sexes in the lethality of the method of suicide. Statistical reports of the highly lethal use of firearms by more male suicides than female suicides cannot be understood without reference to the cultural context in which suicide occurs (Hendin, 1982, p. 144). "No student of history, particularly of women's history, should be surprised to learn that women have had less access to lethal technology than have men" (Kushner, 1985, p. 551). Method of suicide thus must be considered not only in terms of gender but in relation to culture and to psychosocial factors.

As long as the study of suicide and suicidal behavior continues to focus on completed suicide, it will remain a study of a male issue, excluding the knowledge of cultural, social, and personal factors to be found in women's experiences. Lester (1989) suggests that not only is attempted suicide a more common behavior, it may be more rational and adaptive. It is important that both attempted and completed suicide be studied, for the reality of men and women encompasses both.

Age, race, and gender are only a few of the many variables, including religious beliefs and cultural values of life and death, violence, socio-economic stress, alcohol and other drug use, and affective disorders that may influence this phenomenon. A number of theories have been developed to explain suicide.

Theories of Suicide

Colt (1991) notes that no one knows why people kill themselves and trying to find the answer is like trying to pinpoint what causes us to fall in love or what causes war (p. 39). The motivation for suicide is perplexing and not yet resolved. Attempts to examine and explain the etiology of suicide have been many and varied and have included ethical, familial, interpersonal, and political approaches. The theories discussed here are in the categories of: (a) philosophical, (b) sociological, (c) psychoanalytic, (d) biochemical, and (e) preventionist.

Philosophical

Philosophers have not provided a specific theory of suicide. Their major contribution to the study of suicide has been their willingness to struggle with the issue of self-destructive behavior and the meaning of life and death. Choron (1972) believes that "philosophers seem to have been instrumental in bringing about the permissive and tolerant view of suicide that generally prevails today" (p. 107).

One current philosophical approach, existential suicide, is closely linked to the writings of Camus. He believed that suicide was the only serious philosophical question. For Camus (1955) life is absurd and meaningless. Paradoxically, this also means that death is absurd, and Camus opposes the temptation of suicide. The existential dilemma for the individual is to live in this "absurd state" where one is in constant confrontation with the world. "It is this revolt that gives life its value and confers majesty on it; it is essential to 'die unreconciled and not of one's free will' and to preserve to the bitter end one's integrity and pride" (Choron, 1972, p. 138). Many suicidologists disagree with Camus' premise and believe that lack of meaning in this life is a strong motivation for suicide.

Choron (1972) provides an excellent discussion of "Philosophers on Suicide" (pp. 107–138), which is summarized in Table 9.1. It is particularly

Table 9.1 Philosopher's Position on Suicide

PHILOSOPHER	POSITION ON SUICIDE	RATIONALE
Phythagoras: 582 B.C.	Antisuicide	Belief that the individual must wait for God to release the soul.
Plato: 427–347 B.C.	Antisuicide	Suicide contradicts God's will—believed in the immortality of his true self.
Aristotle: 384–322 B.C.	Antisuicide	Suicide is a cowardly act; contrary to the "right rule of life."
Epicurus: 341–270 B.C.	Antisuicide	"Wise man neither seeks to escape life nor fears the cessation for neither does life offend him nor does the absence of life seem to be evil."
Greek Stoic: 200 B.C.	Neutral	Rational decision on which is preferable in any given situation.
Seneca: 3 B.C.–65 A.D.	Prosuicide	If you like life, live; if you don't, go back where you came from.
Epictetus: A.D. 60–132	Neutral	One can choose to "play or not play."
Montaigne: 1533–1592	Prosuicide	Objected to Church's position: challenged the belief that only despair led to suicide.
Descartes: 1596–1650	Antisuicide	Belief that good in life always outweighs the bad; wanting to die is an error in judgment.
Spinoza: 1632–1677	Neutral	Denied human impulse for self-destruction; suicide is possible only from external pressures.
Voltaire: 1694–1778	Prosuicide	Cited psychological and sociological reasons.
Montesquieu: 1689–1775	Prosuicide	Individual right to choose suicide.
Rousseau: 1712–1778	Prosuicide	Suicide is humanity's natural right; God endowed us with reason and so suicide is "acceptable to God."
Hume: 1711–1776	Prosuicide	Suicide is neutral crime against God or humanity or society. "No one throws away his life as long as it is worth living."

(table continued on next page)

Table 9.1 Continued

PHILOSOPHER	POSITION ON SUICIDE	RATIONALE
Kant: 1724–1804	Antisuicide	Human duty is to self-preservation; therefore suicide is a vice.
Schopenhauer: 1788–1860	Ambivalent	Suicide is vain, foolish act but defends the right of the individual to suicide.
Nietzche: 1844–1900	Prosuicide	To deprive people of the right to die is cruel; suicide is another way to reach "eternal return of the soma."
Hartmann: 1842–1906	Antisuicide	While life is undesirable, it is humanity's duty, through the intellect, to move toward "cosmic redemption," where mankind will decree its own distinction.

interesting to note Spinoza's rejection of a natural impulse to self-destruction, since this is diametrically opposed to Freud's assumption that it is a basic trait of the human psyche. Voltaire used a "sociological approach" and concluded that suicides occurred more frequently in urban areas because city dwellers were more prone to melancholia, because suicidal tendencies were inherited, and because some were motivated by a desire for revenge. Choron (1972) observes: "These conclusions were widely accepted by subsequent students of suicide, and although the first three have been disregarded in recent times, the motive of revenge has been recognized and stressed" (p. 125).

Sociological

Some theories of suicide take into consideration the cultural context of the individual and how the individual relates to that context. These models lay varying emphasis on the individual's adjustment to the social order and the strength of that social order to influence suicide (La Greca, 1988, p. 240). The classic study of suicide in this theoretical area was done by the sociologist Emile Durkheim and was published in his book *Le Suicide* in 1897.

Durkheim (1951) proposed that to understand suicide rates it was necessary to examine social forces rather than isolated individual motives. He claimed that the high suicide rate at the close of the nineteenth century in Europe was related to particular factors in the environment. A major component of his thesis was the capacity of the individual to be adequately integrated into the prevailing social structures such as religion, family, and community. The more an individual was integrated into such social groups, the less likelihood of suicide.

Durkheim categorized suicide into three types according to its social context: (a) egoistic, (b) altruistic, and (c) anomic. In egoistic suicide, the individual feels alienated, has no specific ties to a social group, and is poorly integrated into society. This person is often lonely, unemployed, single or divorced, and has no one person or group to which to belong. Altruistic suicide is the opposite of egoistic suicide. The individual is overly integrated and feels that it is necessary and expected to give one's all to a specific group or organization. The person's own identity, goals, and even life may be sacrificed for a group's beliefs. One form of altruistic suicide is found in terrorism; a person driving a car bomb into an embassy is sure to die, but that death represents the person's commitment to a cause. In anomic suicide, people experience a sense of normlessness, usually occurring in times of sudden change. There is a sense of sudden shifts, the old rules do not apply and there are no new ones to take their place. There is a breakdown of social institutions, and society is unable to provide adequate regulation. On a macro-level, anomic suicide may occur in relation to an event that disrupts a society's equilibrium such as the Great Depression in the United States in the 1930s. On a micro-level, anomic suicide may be precipitated by a death in the family or a painful divorce. In either situation, the person's supports are gone and there is no clear understanding of a normative structure to follow.

Carter (1976) noted that an additional category, egocentric suicide, has been suggested by George De Vos. Egocentric suicide places a greater emphasis on frustration and aggression in contrast to the loss and despair of egoistic suicide (p. 329). Durkheim's theory has functioned as a basis for subsequent sociological investigations into suicide. His theory, which explains suicide rates, cannot be used to understand an individual's psychological motivation for suicide. While all three categories revolve around a person's integration into society, the theory cannot explain why some people who are single, widowed, or divorced killed themselves when most do not (Colt, 1991).

Psychoanalytic

Suicide was the subject of the Vienna Psychoanalytic Society meeting in 1910, thirteen years after the publication of Durkheim's *Le Suicide.* At that time Freud cautioned, "I have an impression that in spite of all the valuable material that has been brought before us, we have not reached a decision on the problem that interests us" (cited in Wekstein, 1979, p. 5). Freud continued to question self-destructive behavior. His classic paper "Mourning and Melancholia," published in 1917, dealt with the dynamics of depression and, in reconstructing the process, explained:

> An object-choice, an attachment of the libido to a particular person had at one time existed; then owing to a real slight or disappointment coming from this loved person, the object-relationship was shattered. The result was not the normal one of a withdrawal of libido from this object and a displacement of a new one . . . . it was withdrawn into the ego. . . . Thus the shadow of the object fell upon the ego and the latter could henceforth be judged by a special agency, as though it were an object, the forsaken object (Freud, 1957, p. 249).

Freud formulated the view that suicide was a form of aggression against an internalized love object. Since the person both loves and hates at the same time, this aggression is markedly ambivalent.

Karl Menninger (1938) elaborated on Freud's theory of aggression turned inward. He felt that any suicide is driven by three conscious or unconscious wishes: the wish to kill, the wish to be killed, and the wish to die. Psychoanalytically, suicide can be seen as murder in the 180th degree (Shneidman & Mandelkorn, 1967, p. 3). There currently has been additional emphasis placed on the importance of the feelings of helplessness, hopelessness, and dependency in self-destructive behavior (Stuart & Sundeen, 1991, p. 465). These feelings, when severe, are characteristics of depression; severely depressed individuals are at risk for suicide.

The psychoanalytic approach assumes that vicissitudes of instinctual drives and unconscious motivation give rise to suicidal behavior. It is the most obvious choice to illustrate individual-oriented approaches to suicide and much of contemporary nursing, psychiatry, psychology, and social work have benefited in their development of theoretical frameworks from the early work of Freud and other psychoanalysts. However, Hendin (1982) states that "it has been evident for several decades that a truly psychosocial approach, not an amalgam of Freud and Durkheim, but an approach that includes the examination of the psychodynamics of suicide of differing social groups, is required for any deeper understanding of the significance of suicide in a society" (p. 18). It becomes important then to understand the psychic, social, cultural, and physiologic factors that interact to produce self-destructive behavior.

Biochemical

Historically, physicians, in an attempt to understand suicide, searched for its cause within the body itself. In doing so, a medical model for suicide as a disease was formed, separating it from being considered a moral problem. Suicide was attributed to climate, change of seasons, heredity, insanity, constipation, and numerous other causes depending upon the diagnosing physician. Treatments varied as much as causes and included cold plunge baths, bleeding, and cupping. In 1838, Jean-Etienne Esquirol, a physician, wrote that suicide was not a disease *per se* but a symptom, and that the treatment of suicide belongs to the therapy of mental illness (Colt, 1991, pp.184–185). The psychiatric theory of suicide today makes a similar assumption that most people who kill themselves suffer from a mental or emotional disorder (La Greca, 1988).

Current research in the physiological study of suicide indicates promising findings in the biochemical area. There is developing evidence that suicidal behaviors may be associated with abnormalities in the serotonergic system. Serotonin is a neurotransmitter that carries chemical messages between neurons in the brain, affecting how people feel and think. Numerous reports indicate that low levels of a serotonin metabolite (a breakdown product of serotonin) called 5- hydroxyindoleacetic acid (5-HIAA) have been found in the cerebrospinal fluid (CSF) of suicidal patients with psychiatric diagnoses, including depressive illness, personality disorder, schizophrenia, and alcoholism (Stanley & Stanley, 1988).

In an overview of current trends in biological suicide research, Traskman-Bendz, Asberg, Nordstrom, & Stanley (1989) report that self-destructive behavior is associated with disturbances in serotonin turnover: in completed suicides, studies of brain regions and CSF indicate a dysfunction of the serotonergic system. There has also been some evidence of certain endocrine functions, particularly the release of cortisol and thyrotropin, associated with suicidal behavior (Shneidman, 1989; Traskman-Bendz, Asberg, Nordstrom, & Stanley, 1989).

Clearly much more research needs to be done to determine more exact relationships between low serotonin and suicidal behavior. However, it is possible that behavioral markers of suicide may be combined with biological markers to predict suicide for certain populations of patients (Stanley & Stanley, 1988). Such a possibility holds great promise for prevention.

Preventionist

Farberow, Shneidman, & Litman are generally associated with analyzing suicide from a prevention perspective. The Suicide Prevention Center in Los Angeles was established in 1958 by these men to "save lives, to integrate with other agencies within the community and to obtain systematically organized data that can be employed in research designs" (Farberow, Shneidman, & Litman, 1965, p. 7). They concluded from their research at the center that the majority of suicides have a recognizable presuicidal phase. In reconstructing events preceding a death by means of a psychological autopsy to help answer "why," "how," and "what," they concluded that suicidal behavior is often a form of communication. Farberow & Shneidman (1965) used the phrase, "a cry for help," to underscore "the messages of suffering and anguish and the pleas for response that are expressed by and contained within suicidal behaviors" (p. xi).

Shneidman (1983) also believes that any suicide is colored with ambivalence: "to cut one's throat and cry for help—in the same breath"

(p. 82). His taxonomy of death-related behavior includes intentioned, unintentioned, and subintentioned death.

In intentioned death, the individual takes a direct active role in bringing about death. Intentioned suicide is subdivided into four categories. First, the "death-seeker" commits suicide "in such a manner that rescue is realistically unlikely or impossible" (Shneidman, 1983, p. 82). Second, the "death-initiator" believes death will occur soon and precipitates the event. Shneidman (1983) uses the example of "older hospitalized persons in the terminal stage of fatal illness . . . with remarkable and totally unexpected energy" who succeed in killing themselves (p. 83). Third, the "death-ignorer" believes that life will continue in some other fashion. The final category is the "death-darer," the person who tempts fate by engaging in risky methods such as Russian roulette.

Unintentioned death occurs when the individual plays no significant role in precipitating death. Although one might assume that in this category, everyone would prefer not to die, Shneidman suggests that there are different attitudes. The "death-welcomer" is glad that death will occur; the "death-acceptor" is resigned to his or her fate; the "death-postponer" endeavors to forestall death; the "death-disdainer" does not believe death will occur; and the "death-fearer" is fearful and fights the notion of death.

"The subintentional death is one in which the person plays some partial, covert, subliminal or unconscious role in hastening his/her own demise" (Shneidman, 1983, p. 87). This category is the most provocative, for Shneidman contends that the individual allows suicide to occur and that this behavior is "unconscious." He (1983) identifies several types of behavior on a "continuum of expectation and possibility of death" (pp. 88–89). The "death-darer" and the "death-chancer" play a game to court death with odds calculated in their favor. The "death-hastener" unconsciously brings about or exacerbates a physiological imbalance. The individual who has a destructive life-style, such as alcohol, drug, or dietary abuses, or who refuses to follow medical orders for a specific condition, is considered to be a death-hastener. A "death-facilitator" will passively make death easy. Shneidman cites unexpected deaths in hospitals and refers to the work of Weisman & Hackett (1961, 1962; Weisman, 1972) to support this category. The "death-capitulator" plays a psychological role, usually through fear, in terminating life. Voodoo deaths fall into this category. Finally, the "death-experimenter" lives on the brink of death, "usually by excessive use of alcohol or drugs—seemingly wishing a chronically altered, usually befogged state of consciousness" (Shneidman, 1983, p. 89). Wolfgang (1968) describes a form of suicide by murder. The individual purposively chooses a superior adversary and thus brings about her own death. Shneidman includes this "victim-precipitated" homicide as another form of subintentional death. A current example of this has been described by Seiden (cited in Williams, 1982); a teenager brandished a gun, knowing it was unloaded, in front of police officers, prompting the officers to shoot him in apparent self-defense (p. 10). However, this type of interpretation must be looked at carefully to avoid blaming the victim for the brutal acts of another. The issues regarding subintentional deaths for health care professionals and for society at large are multiple. Should these deaths be accepted as suicides? Are they preventable? What modality of intervention would be most effective?

Critiques of Theoretical Approaches

Charmaz (1980) criticizes the preceding theoretical approaches because they tend to separate suicidal individuals from the context of their experience. She believes that the psychoanalytic view eliminates the individual's capacity to understand; that Durkheim's theory is only a preliminary set of ideas; and that the preventionist approach is a form of social control (pp. 241–249). For her, the suicidal crisis is a crisis of self within a specific social structure. It is crucial to understand how the multiple variables are "subjectively experienced, acted upon and become a source of interaction with others" (Charmaz, 1980, p. 262). Suicidal individuals experience increasing social isolation as they experience hopelessness, helplessness, and failure.

Charmaz's discussion is thought provoking and defines gaps and discrepancies in current approaches and theories of suicide. Systemic and attitudinal changes are slow processes; in the meantime, the suicidal crisis requires immediate action. The health care practitioner feels compelled to act in the here and now. The life that is saved today is the life that matters. Shneidman (1989) comments that "suicide is enormously complicated, but it is not totally random and it is amendable to some prediction . . . and to effective therapeutic intervention: that is reason for prevention" (p. 35).

Suicide Prevention

Prior to the 1950s and the advent of the Los Angeles Suicide Prevention Center, suicide was still a taboo word and little attention was focused on it as a problem to be treated. Concern over suicide became more highly formalized in the 1960s: The National Institute of Mental Health founded a national coordinating effort on suicide prevention (La Greca, 1988). Suicide prevention centers developed throughout the country, as did other organizations such as Samaritans, a national and international organization that runs a 24-hour, 7-day-a-week crisis hotline.

Suicide Prevention Centers

The prevention centers, many of which also now have the name "crisis intervention" included in their titles to reach a greater number of high-risk callers, came under close scrutiny in the 1970s. A number of studies have indicated no evidence that suicide prevention centers affect community suicide rates (Lester, 1974; Dew, Bromet, Brent, & Greenhouse, 1987). Both Hillman (1964) and Szasz (1986) question the ethics involved in suicide prevention, maintaining people have a right to take their own lives. However, the continued existence of these suicide prevention/crisis intervention centers does indicate that they are meeting community needs. Results of a study comparing suicide rates in counties that added these prevention centers between 1968 to 1973 with counties that did not indicated an association of centers with the reduction of suicides in young white females (Miller, Combs, Leeper, & Barton, 1984).

Calls for help to these centers' "hot lines" involve not only suicide but also can include rape, wife-battering, child abuse, elder abuse, HIV/AIDS, substance abuse, and homelessness. The effectiveness of the centers may need to be evaluated in terms other than decreasing suicide rates in the community. The establishment of a caring connection between the high-risk caller and the person answering the "hot line" at the center may be the basis for deterring the caller from destructive behavior to self or others. As the United States becomes increasingly pluralistic, crisis centers will need to plan intervention in a variety of modes. People of color will comprise one-third of the nation by the year 2000 (American Council on Education, 1988). Cultures differ widely with regard to their attitudes towards suicidal behavior and the acceptability of programs that speak openly and frankly about it. Therefore, Diekstra (1989) suggests that to have even a modest chance of enduring success of prevention, "programs designed to reduce that behavior must be oriented not only to the individual . . . but also to the levels of the family, school, workplace and other large scale organizations, as well as the larger community context" (p. 18).

Individual Suicide Prevention

There are a number of common myths surrounding suicide which are important to dispel in order to assess whether an individual is thinking about committing suicide. Table 9.2 presents a myth and fact sheet developed from the discussion of Farberow, Shneidman, & Litman (1965, pp.12–13) about the mistaken notions of suicide.

What are the prodromal clues for suicide—the distress signals, the cues, the "cries for help"? The following indicators may help in assessing suicide risk in an individual; they are summarized from the works of Litman (1966), Aquilera & Messick (1982), Hoff (1989) and Stuart & Sundeen (1991).

- **Verbal communication**. Statements may be direct: "I wish I were dead," or indirect: "My family will be better off without me."
- **History of suicide attempts**. The majority of people who kill themselves have made previous suicide attempts.

Table 9.2 Facts and Myths about Suicide

Myth:	People who talk about suicide won't commit suicide.
Fact:	Suicide threats must be taken seriously. Many people who commit suicide have given warnings of their intentions.
Myth:	Suicide happens without warning.
Fact:	Suicidal people give clues, warnings and indication of intent. Alertness to these clues is essential.
Myth:	Improvement after a suicidal crisis means that the risk is over.
Fact:	Most suicides occur within 90 days of the emotional crisis when the person appears to recover. Improvement is equated with increased energy. Physicians, relatives and others should be especially cautious and watchful.
Myth:	Suicide and depression are synonymous.
Fact:	Although depression does remain the best indication of potential suicide, there are other reasons for suicide.
Myth:	All suicidal persons are insane.
Fact:	The majority of suicides are unhappy and temporarily overwhelmed. It is circular reasoning to say that suicide is an insane act, and therefore suicidal persons are insane.
Myth:	Suicide is a single disease.
Fact:	Suicide is expressed in various forms and shapes. An accurate taxonomy or classification has not yet been developed.
Myth:	Suicide is immoral.
Fact:	Behavior and customs are neither external nor universal.
Myth:	Suicide can be controlled by legislation.
Fact:	Legislation may have opposite effects: people will be sure they'll be successful to escape punishment and after unsuccessful attempts will be fearful to seek help.
Myth:	Suicide is inherited.
Fact:	Suicide does not run in families.
Myth:	Suicide is the "curse of the poor" or a "disease of the rich."
Fact:	Suicide cuts across all strata—it is "democratic."
Myth:	Suicidal people are fully committed to dying.
Fact:	Most suicidal people are ambivalent. Intervention by proper assessment of distress signals can prevent suicide.

- **Unexplained change in behavior**. People communicate by actions such as giving away important personal possessions, taking daredevil chances, becoming reckless drivers, and having an irregular work attendance.
- **Depression**. Symptoms of depression can be psychological, physiological, or social and can include loss of appetite, weight loss, early wakening, loss of energy and interest in usual pleasures, social withdrawal, and severe feelings of hopelessness and helplessness.
- **Physical illness**. An estimated 75 percent of all suicides see a doctor within four months of taking their lives (Colt, 1991, p. 325). This does not necessarily mean that they are ill but that they may often use physical complaints as a way of seeking help from a physician. It is important that physicians take the time to explore how the person is feeling when no physical basis can be found for the chief complaint. This may be the person's last attempt at seeking relief for her despair. People who are experiencing a disabling illness or one that is unresponsive to treatment can be considered at risk for suicide, as are people who receive a diagnosis of an illness that may be life threatening such as cancer or HIV.
- **Response to recent loss**. Common precipitating stresses for suicide are losses or threat of losses: the death of a loved one; divorce or separation; loss of a job, money, prestige or status; loss of health; forced retirement.
- **Drinking and other substance abuse**. Alcohol and other drugs can increase impulsive behavior and impair judgment. A person under the influence of PCP (phencyclidine) may feel invincible and walk in front of a moving vehicle or jump out a window. Agencies and individuals involved in treating alcoholics and substance abusers should be alert to the risk of suicide among their clients and should be trained to identify and deal with an increased risk of suicidal behavior (Diekstra, 1989, p. 23).

People may experience one or more of these prodromal indicators and not be suicidal. However, if these prodromal indicators are present, it is important to assess and evaluate the individual's suicidal potentiality. Goldberg (1987) suggests that it is helpful to engage the person in a series of escalating questions that create a more meaningful interaction and may help to overcome some of the person's resistance (p. 447). In the assessment interview, it is important for caregivers to convey a legitimate caring and concern for the person's distress as well as to convey an acknowledgment of that person's strengths.

A number of assessment tools have been developed to assess suicidal potentiality, including the *Assessment of Suicidal Potentiality* from the Los Angeles Suicide Prevention Center. Whether caregivers use such tools or not, the following data need to be included and evaluated in the assessment:

- **Suicide plan**. Include queries about lethality of method, availability of method, and specific organization of plan, including time and place. Obviously, someone indicating having bought a gun to shoot herself tomorrow is at high risk, as are people who set specific deadlines.
- **Severity of symptoms**. Assess the level of distress. Is there severe agitation, a sense of helplessness combined with a frantic need to do something? Is there psychotic thinking—"the voices are telling me to hurt myself?" Is there hopelessness that worsens when offered help?
- **Resources and communication**. Does the person have any available support systems—family, friends, agencies, employment, therapist? What is or has been the person's communication with these support systems? Are they available to help? Is the person financially stable?
- **Precipitating stress**. This should be evaluated from the person's standpoint. Remember that people can perceive meaning, degree, and intensity of stress quite differently. The loss of a pet who may have been an elderly person's only love object may be devastating to that person. Determine if this is a special anniversary date of a significant event in the person's life.
- **Reaction of significant other**. Is the person supportive, show feelings of concern, recognize need for help?

Intervention can be primary, secondary, and tertiary. In the primary stage, the assessment is made and appropriate action should be taken. If lethality is low, support from family or friends may be sufficient. High lethality requires referral to a mental health practitioner, mental health center, or crisis center. During this stage it is particularly important that the potentially suicidal person is "heard." Since the individual rarely reveals spontaneously that she is contemplating suicide, caregivers should be aware of the prodromal clues of suicide and feel comfortable enough to question the patient. Caregivers may feel that talking about suicide to people who are upset may encourage them to attempt it. This is another myth surrounding suicide. Hoff (1989) notes that "suicide is much too complex a process to occur as a result of a caring person asking a question about suicidal intent" (p. 179). After the evaluation has been made, the caregiver should continue to be available to supply direct support and to assist the suicidal individual in following through on appropriate recommendations.

In caring for the dying patient, statements such as "I can't go on" or "I wish this were over," or actions such as writing a will are commonplace. They should not be ignored, however, as possible prodromal clues. Time should be taken to explore the intent of the communication. It frequently represents a "cry for help," a plea not to be abandoned and forgotten because of the terminal status. It also may be a form of symbolic communication, conveying emotional and spiritual pain and an attempt to make sense of inner experiences (Dugan, 1987).

Secondary intervention may include a variety of modalities, including individual or group therapy, electroconvulsive therapy, medications, and hospitalization. A traditional practice in the hospital is to place a highly suicidal individual on one-to-one, 24-hour observation and to remove all potentially harmful objects. Carter (1976) questions the efficacy of this behavior, as "the ego of the depressed patient may be lowered further" (p. 340). She underscores the philosophy of suicide prevention centers—that "one must convey to the suicidal person that someone cares deeply" (p. 341). Hospitals may not always prevent suicide. Reynolds & Farberow (1976) note that even at the finest hospitals, patients find ways to kill themselves through use of nails, windows, high places, plastic bags, coat hangers, and accumulated medication.

Tertiary prevention or postvention takes place if a suicide has been completed; it is a form of crisis intervention and its intent is to enable the survivor-victims to cope and to reduce the aftereffects of the traumatic event in their lives.

Impact of Suicide on Survivors

Shneidman (1983) believes that "in the case of suicide, the largest public health problem is neither the prevention of suicide nor the management of suicide attempts but the alleviation of the effects of stress in the survivor-victims of suicidal death whose lives are forever changed and who, over a period of years, number in the millions" (p. 33). Death by suicide is traumatic and stigmatizing for survivors (Kovarsky, 1989). They must deal with feelings of guilt, shame, anger, and ambiguity. The recent emphasis on suicides being "preventable" casts an additional burden, as survivors question "why" they were not able to prevent the act, or whether they "drove" the individual to suicide. Survivors also have to deal with the initial inquiry around the circumstances of the death, sometimes they are even suspected of murder.

Charmaz (1980) analyzes the social responses to suicide that "set in motion a chain of destructive events" (p. 272). Stigma fosters the development of shame; survivors question their capability to have prevented the event; lack of social support heightens guilt and inhibits grief, which culminates in the mourning being distorted and aborted.

A study of funeral directors' observations on survivors' and others' responses to suicide indicated that suicide was viewed as producing more shame and embarrassment, greater difficulty in coping with the death, and greater likelihood of guilt feelings and unanswered questions about the death in the surviving family (Calhoun, Selby, & Steelman, 1988–89). Kovarsky's (1989) study of bereavement in parents who had lost a child to an accidental or suicidal death indicated that losses from suicide place survivors at a higher risk for disturbed grief and loneliness reactions (p. 93).

Children are particularly traumatized by the suicide of a parent. They feel rejected, abandoned, and responsible for the suicide. Families often respond to the stigma of suicide by creating a story for the children to explain the death. This family myth does not protect the child and contributes to further distortion. The family may also respond to a parental death by not talking about it at all, leaving the child to continually wonder what happened. Adults who experienced the suicide of a parent when they were children have described how painful that experience was for them (Bergson, 1982; Hammer, 1991).

For Cain (1977), the legacy of suicide for survivors includes reality distortion, tortured object-relations, guilt, disturbed self-concept, impotent rage, identification with the suicide, depression, self-destructive search for meaning, and incomplete mourning. However, Wrobleski & McIntosh (1988) concluded from their study of suicide survivors that there is no reason to believe that the grief process of suicide survivors is that different from those of survivors of other causes of death. Van der Wal's (1989–90) study, which reviewed empirical studies on survivors of suicide, also does not support the idea that these survivors show more pathological reactions and a more complicated and prolonged grief process than other survivor groups. Future research is indicated to clearly resolve the differences, if any, in the grief of survivors of various causes of death. While the literature on the grieving process of survivors of suicide may not yet provide a definitive description of that process, the proliferation of self-help groups among this population indicates that there are some special needs. Wrobleski (1984–85) writes that "until the day that taboo and stigma have been removed from suicide, suicide survivors will continue to have unique problems that need to be addressed by separate support groups" (p. 183). Self-help groups provide suicide survivors with the support that is often not available from family and friends.

Many of these self-help support groups across the country are called Survivors of Suicide. Others may be called Heartbeat, Seasons, or Friends for Survival. Because new groups are constantly forming, while others disband, it can be helpful to contact either the American Association of Suicidology (2459 South Ash, Denver, CO, 80222) or the American Suicide Foundation (1045 Park Avenue, New York, NY, 10028) for a continuously updated directory of suicide survivor groups in a particular area.

Ideally, every community should have special bereavement counseling programs or self-help groups to help survivors of suicide. Techniques for providing such help are essentially the same as those used in dealing with any other crisis. A survivor should be helped to; (a) express feelings appropriate to the event, (b) grasp the reality of the suicide, and (c) obtain and use the help necessary to work through the crisis (Hoff, 1989, p. 239). Professional help may or may not be necessary. Community resources that can also assist include police, clergy, and funeral directors.

Shneidman (1983) describes the postvention work of Alfred Herzog in Philadelphia with parents of adolescent suicides. His work delineates three psychological stages of postvention care: (a) resuscitation—working with the family in the first 24 hours, (b) rehabilitation—consultation with the family for the first six months, and (c) renewal—tapering off of sessions and the mourning process from six months on (p. 34).

The Health Care Professional's Response to Suicide

If suicide has such a devastating effect on family and friends, how is the health care team affected? Do they respond in a similar fashion? If so, are support systems available for them?

Research indicates that staff reaction to a patient's suicide is similar to that of family and friends. Early research on psychiatrists' responses to suicide was done by Litman (1965), who concluded after interviewing over 200 therapists that fears concerning blame, responsibility, and inadequacy were part of their reactions. Light (1972) did an analysis of psychiatrists' responses based on his observed reactions to five suicides over a two-year period, a sample of 366 suicide cases, and the attitudinal studies of 80 to 100 therapists not involved in a suicide. He suggests from this analysis that therapists experience guilt, heightened love, loss, and anger.

More recent research supports the important impact of a patient's suicide on therapists' personal and professional lives. The results of a national survey of psychologists (n = 365) indicated those who had experienced a patient's suicide reported feelings of anger and guilt and having intrusive thoughts about suicide (Chemtob, Hamada, Bauer, Torigoe, & Kinney, 1988, p. 419). Several studies done on the responses of psychiatry trainees to the suicide of a patient, either their own or a colleague's, suggest reactions similar to seasoned clinicians (Brown, 1987; Sacks, Kibel, Cohen, Keats, & Turnquist, 1987). It is important that educational training programs assist these trainees through these crises and provide them with the support for continued personal and professional growth.

Dunne (1987) suggests that if a patient's suicide occurred in the context of a treatment team, all team members may have had close relationships with the deceased and will feel a sense of loss. Their professional identities may be threatened in that they "allowed" this to occur, and they may experience guilt. Staff members all experience a sense of failure. They will need time to mourn and to work through feelings of anger and fear. Kayton & Freed (1967), comparing staff reactions on a group of units after a suicide, found that after varying intensities of insecurity, the main reaction of the staff on the units was a form of overcompensation, a need to help the other patients. These investigators believe that the initial response of staff "suggested a similarity to a traumatic neurosis" (p. 187). Hodgkinson (1987) suggests that the longer term consequences of the suicide on staff are more difficult to determine and may represent the interaction of the pre-existing staff dynamics with the stress of the suicide (p. 388). Thus if staff were having difficulty discussing conflicts and disagreements before the suicide, this difficulty may be extended and escalated after the suicide.

In order for staff to observe their own reactions to a patient's suicide and to deal with their own depressed, anxious feelings, it is important for them to talk about these responses with each other (Vogel & Wolfersdorf, 1987). Informal peer contact may be the most important initial support, and the rituals of death may be supportive in terms of releasing feelings (Hodgkinson, 1987). If staff support groups have been meeting regularly, staff should be encouraged to attend these. Focus at these meetings may be on the staff's work with the patient as well as the sharing of concerns, fears, and feelings. As intense feelings emerge, it is suggested by several researchers that a suicide review conference be held (the psychological autopsy discussed earlier in this chapter) by an outside consultant to reconstruct the suicide and its antecedents (Light, 1972; Cotton, Drake, Whitaker, & Potter, 1983). The review may also serve as a mode to reaffirm the staff's sense of worth.

Patients will also be deeply affected by a suicide from their group membership. They may be frightened that it could happen to them and angry at staff for allowing this to happen. They may have feelings of guilt that they should have known about this and prevented it. It is important then that a community meeting be held for all staff and patients to attend. Patients need this opportunity to discuss the event with staff and for staff to share information with patients (Vogel & Wolfersdorf, 1987). Such a meeting may facilitate the grieving process. Dunne (1987) suggests the following general guidelines to lessen the impact of a suicide death on a treatment service: (a) avoid the birth and proliferation of rumors, (b) provide for the appropriate expression of emotional responses (patients), (c) take special precautions with previously suicidal patients, (d) return to routine as quickly as appropriate, but do not promote denial of affect (pp. 186–188).

SUMMARY ❧

The preceding delineates in some small measure the complexity of suicide as a biopsychosocial phenomenon and stresses the dimension of suicide as a public health concern. Although the etiology of suicidal behavior continues to elude us, research in the biochemical area of causation is revealing possible relationships between physiological changes and behavior. Throughout history, some societies have responded to suicide in cruel ways. Bodies of people who died by suicide have been dragged through the streets, impaled on stakes, left at public crossroads, and refused burial. Their property was confiscated. While attitudes have changed considerably, there are contradictory data about the predominant attitude of society toward suicide today.

More research is needed to refine and define statistics related to suicidal behavior. Specific research on suicidal behavior is indicated for various ethnic groups such as Mexican Americans and Korean Americans rather than simply research under the broad categories of Latinos and Asian Americans. The phenomenon of attempted suicide in women and men needs further exploration, as does the high rate of suicide in the elderly. While any suicide is tragic, the fact that adolescent suicide has risen dramatically over the past three decades is probably more dramatic because it is particularly devastating to survivors and because it represents an enormous loss of human potential (Williams, 1982).

There is some debate on the effectiveness of suicide prevention centers and if they significantly lower suicide rates. However, such centers continue to exist, often combining suicide prevention with other crisis interventions. More public education is required to sensitize everyone to "cries for help." This multidimensional issue requires an interdisciplinary approach that also includes significant others, family, and community resources.

Caregivers should be alert to the needs of suicide survivor-victims. Survivors need the opportunity to express feelings in a nonjudgmental environment. Since the stigma of suicide often dominates responses to the survivor, special efforts should be made to identify and encourage environmental supports. Caregivers must also be aware of their own attitudes and emotional responses to suicidal patients and to death by suicide. Hopefully, as it becomes more acceptable to discuss suicide as a public health concern, it will be possible to learn more about suicide as a part of all our humanity.

LEARNING EXERCISES ❧

1. Is suicide ever justifiable? If so, under what conditions? Would you be willing to assist someone to commit suicide? Why or why not?
2. Role play with other members of the class what you might say to a friend who is indicating suicidal thoughts.
3. Read Sylvia Plath's *The Bell Jar.* If you had been a health professional consulted by Plath, how might you have intervened?

4. Explore what is available in your community for suicide prevention. Do all people have access to these services? How well are they advertised?

AUDIOVISUAL MATERIAL ❧

Going On: The Aftermath of Suicide. 29 minutes/videocassette. Films for the Humanities and Sciences. Box 2053, Princeton, NJ, 08543.
Through interventions with survivors, this video helps those who have experienced the death by suicide of a family member or friend to cope. Discussion focuses on understanding common physical and emotional symptoms of survivors and how to cope with these.

Teen Suicide: Who, Why, and How You Can Prevent It. 45 minutes/videocassette/includes teacher's notes and text. Educational Audiovisual, Inc., 17 Marble Avenue, Pleasantville, NY, 10570.
This program sensitively focuses on prevention of teenage suicide. It heightens awareness of the reasons behind suicide and encourages prevention.

The Inner Voice In Suicide. 32 minutes/videocassette/1984. The Glendon Association, 2049 Century Park East, Suite 3000, Los Angeles, CA, 90067.
Susan, a 38-year-old woman is interviewed by a psychologist about the thought processes that preceded her recent serious suicide attempt. Through the interview process, the viewer is helped to understand motives and causative factors in suicide.

Ernie And Rose. 29 minutes/videocassette and 16 mm film/1983. Filmakers Library, Inc., 124 East 40th Street, New York, NY, 10016.
Suicide among the elderly is rising steadily. In this video, Ernie and Rose, two elderly men who are sharing a house and caring for each other in their old age and infirmities, live out the last days of their lives together. How they come to terms with their deaths is beautifully portrayed.

REFERENCES ❧

American Council on Education, in association with the Education Commission of the States. (1988). *One-third of a nation.* Washington, DC: Author.

Aquilera, D. C., & Messick, J. M. (1982). *Crisis intervention: Theory and methodology* (4th ed.). St. Louis: C. V. Mosby.

Balon, R. (1987). Suicide: Can we predict it? *Comprehensive Psychiatry. 28* (3), 236–241.

Bergson, L. (1982, November 14). Suicide's other victims. *New York Times Magazine.* pp. 101–105.

Brown, H. N. (1987). The impact of suicide on therapists in training. *Comprehensive Psychiatry. 28* (2), 101–112.

Cain, A. (1977). Survivors of suicide. In S. Wilcox & M. Sutton (Eds.). *Understanding death and dying: An interdisciplinary approach* (pp. 229–233). Port Washington, NY: Alfred Publishing.

Calhoun, L. G., Selby, J. W., & Steelman, J. K. (1988–89). A collation of funeral directors' impressions of suicidal deaths. *Omega: Journal of Death and Dying. 19* (4), 365–373.

Camus, A. (1955). *The myth of Sisyphus and other essays.* New York: Random House.

Carter, F. M. (1976). *Psychosocial nursing* (2nd ed.). New York: Macmillan.

Centers for Disease Control. (1991, September 20). Attempted suicide among high school students, 1990. *Morbidity and Mortality Weekly Report. 40* (37), 633–635. Washington, DC: U.S. Department of Health and Human Services/Public Health Service.

Charmaz, K. (1980). *The social reality of death.* Reading, MA: Addison-Wesley.

Chemtob, C. M., Hamada, R. S., Bauer, G., Torigoe, R. Y., & Kinney, B. (1988). Patient suicide: Frequency and impact on psychologists. *Professional Psychology: Research and Practice. 19* (4), 416–420.

Choron, J. (1972). *Suicide.* New York: Scribners.

Colt, G. W. (1991). *The enigma of suicide.* New York: Summit Books.

Cotton, P. G., Drake, R. E., Whitaker, A., & Potter, J. (1983). Dealing with suicide on a psychiatric inpatient unit. *Hospital and Community Psychiatry. 34*, 55–59.

Deluty, R. H. (1988–89). Factors affecting the acceptability of suicide. *Omega: Journal of Death Dying. 19* (4), 315–326.

Dew, M. A., Bromet, E. J., Brent, D., & Greenhouse, J. B. (1987). A quantitative literature review of the effectiveness of suicide prevention centers. *Journal of Consulting & Clinical Psychology. 55* (2), 239–244.

Diekstra, R. F. (1989). Suicide and the attempted suicide: An international perspective. *Acta Psychiatrica Scandinavica. 80* (suppl. 354), 1–24.

Dugan, D. O. (1987). Death and dying: Emotional, spiritual, & ethical support for patients & families. *Journal of Psychosocial Nursing & Mental Health Services. 25* (7), 21–29.

Dunne, E. J. (1987). A response to suicide in the mental health setting. In E. J. Dunne, J. L. McIntosh, & K. Dunn-Maxim (Eds.), *Suicide and its aftermath: Understanding and counseling the survivors* (pp. 182–190). New York: Norton.

Durkheim, E. (1951). *Suicide.* New York: Free Press.

Farberow, N., & Shneidman, E. (1965). Preface. In N. Farberow & E. Shneidman (Eds.), *The cry for help* (pp. xi–xiii). New York: McGraw-Hill.

Farberow, N., Shneidman, E., & Litman, R. (1965). The suicide prevention center. In N. Farberow & E. Shneidman (Eds.), *The cry for help* (pp. 6–18). New York: McGraw-Hill.

Freud, S. (1957). Mourning and melancholia. In J. Strachey (Ed. & Trans.), *The standard edition of the complete psychological works of Sigmund Freud* (Vol. 14, pp. 237–258). London: The Hogarth Press.

Gibbs, J. T. (1988). Conceptual, methodological, and sociocultural issues in Black youth suicide: Implications for assessment and early intervention. *Suicide and Life-threatening Behavior. 18* (1), 73–87.

Gibson, P. (1989). Gay males and lesbian youth suicide. In Alcohol, Drug Abuse, and Mental Health Administration, *Report of the secretary's task force on youth suicide: Volume 3: Prevention and interventions in youth suicide* (pp. 3–110 – 3–142). DHHS Pub. No. (ADM) 89–1621. Washington, DC: Superintendent of Documents, U.S. Government Printing Office.

Goldberg, R. J. (1987). The assessment of suicide risk in the general hospital. *General Hospital Psychiatry. 9* (6), 446–452.

Group for the Advancement of Psychiatry: Committee on Cultural Psychiatry. (1989). *Suicide and ethnicity in the United States.* Report No. 128. New York: Brunner/Mazel.

Hammer, S. (1991). *By her own hand: Memoirs of a suicide's daughter.* New York: Soho Press.

Haas, A., & Hendin, H. (1983). Suicide among older people: Projections for the future. *Suicide and Life-threatening Behavior.* (13), 147–154.

Heacock, D. R. (1990). Suicidal behavior in Black and Hispanic youth. *Psychiatric Annals. 20* (3), 134–142.

Hendin, H. (1982). *Suicide in America.* New York: W. W. Norton.

Hillman, J. (1964). *Suicide and the soul.* New York: Harper & Row.

Hodgkinson, P. E. (1987). Responding to in-patient suicide. *British Journal of Medical Psychology. 60* (4), 387–392.

Hoff, L. E. (1989). *People in crisis: Understanding and helping* (3rd ed.). Redwood City, CA: Addison-Wesley.

Hoppe, S. K., & Martin, H. W. (1986). Patterns of suicide in Mexican Americans and Anglos, 1960–1980. *Social Psychiatry. 21* (2), 83–88.

Kayton, L., & Freed, H. (1967). Effects of suicide in a psychiatric hospital. *Archives of General Psychiatry. 17*, 187–194.

King, L. M. (1982). Suicide from a "Black Reality" perspective. In B. A. Bass, G. E. Wyatt, & G. J. Powell (Eds.), *The Afro-American family: Assessment, treatment, and research issues* (pp. 221–230). New York: Grune & Stratton.

Kirk, A. (1986). Destructive behaviors among members of the Black community with a special focus on males: Causes and methods of intervention. *Journal of Multicultural Counseling and Development. 14* (1), 3–9.

Kovarsky, R. (1989). Loneliness and disturbed grief: A comparison of parents who lost a child to suicide or accidental death. *Archives of Psychiatric Nursing. 3* (2), 86–96.

Kushner, H. I. (1985). Women and suicide in historical perspective. *Signs: Journal of Women in Culture and Society. 10* (3), 537–552.

La Greca, A. J. (1988). Suicide: Prevalence, theories, and prevention. In H. Wass, F. Berardo, & R. Neimeyer (Eds.), *Dying: Facing the facts* (2nd Ed., pp. 229–255). New York: Hemisphere Publishing Corporation.

Lalinec-Michaud, M. (1988). Three cases of suicide in Chinese-Canadian women. *Canadian Journal of Psychiatry. 33* (2), 153–156.

Lester, D. (1974). Effect of suicide prevention centers on suicide rates in the United States. *Health Services Report. 89*, 37–39.

Lester, D. (1989). The study of suicide from a feminist perspective. *Crisis. 11* (1), 38–43.

Levy, J. E., & Kunitz, S. J. (1987). A suicide prevention program for Hopi youth. *Social Sciences and Medicine. 25* (8), 931–940.

Light, D. (1972). Psychiatry and suicide: The management of a mistake. *American Journal of Sociology. 77* (5), 821–838.

Litman, R. (1965). When patients commit suicide. *American Journal of Psychotherapy. 19*, 570–576.

Litman, R. (1966). Acutely suicidal patients: Management in general medical practice. *California Medicine. 104*, 168–174.

Liu, W., & Yu, E. (1985). Ethnicity, mental health, and the urban delivery system. In L. Maldonado & J. Moore (Eds.), *Urban ethnicity in the United States* (pp. 211–247). Beverly Hills, CA: Sage.

Marks, A. (1988–89). Structural parameters of sex, race, age, and education and their influence on attitudes toward suicide. *Omega: Journal of Death and Dying. 19* (4), 327–336.

May, P. J. (1987). Suicide and self-destruction among American Indian youths. *American Indian and Alaska Native Mental Health Research. 1* (1), 52–69.

McIntosh, J. L. (1989). Trends in racial differences in U.S. suicide statistics. *Death Studies. 13* (3), 275–286.

McIntosh, J. L., & Santos, J. R. (1981). Suicide among minority elderly: A preliminary investigation. *Suicide and Life-threatening Behavior. 11,* 151–166.

Menninger, K. (1938). *Man against himself.* New York: Harcourt Brace.

Miller, H. R., Combs, D. W., Leeper, J. D., & Barton, S. N. (1984). An analysis of the effects of suicide prevention facilities on suicide rates in the United States. *American Journal of Public Health. 74* (4), 340–343.

National Center for Health Statistics. (1991, September 27). *Monthly Vital Statistic Report: Provisional Data from the National Center for Health Statistics. 40* (6), 16–17. Washington, DC: U.S. Department of Health and Human Services/Public Health Service/Centers for Disease Control.

Nkongho, N. O. (1988). Suicide in the elderly: A beginning investigation. *Journal of the National Black Nurses' Association. 2* (2), 47–55.

Pfeffer, C. R. (1988). Risk factors associated with youth suicide: A clinical perspective. *Psychiatric Annals. 18* (11), 652–656.

Rin, H. (1975). Suicide in Taiwan. In N. L. Farberow (Ed.), *Suicide in different cultures* (pp. 239– 254). Baltimore, MD: University Park Press.

Reynolds, D. K., & Farberow, N. L. (1976). *Suicide: Inside and out.* Berkeley, CA: University of California Press.

Sacks, M. H., Kibel, H. D., Cohen, A. M., Keats, M., & Turnquist, K. N. (1987). Resident response to patient suicide. *Journal of Psychiatric Education. 11* (4), 217–226.

Sandoval, J., Davis, J. M., & Wilson, M. P. (1987). An overview of the school-based prevention of adolescent suicide. *Special Services in the Schools. 3* (3–4), 103–120.

Shneidman, E. (1983). *Deaths of man.* New York: Aronson.

Shneidman, E. (1989). Approaches and commonalities of suicide. In R. Diekstra, R. Maris, S. Platt, A. Schmidtke, & G. Sonneck (Eds.), *Suicide and its prevention* (pp. 14–36). Leiden, The Netherlands: E. J. Brill.

Shneidman, E., & Mandelkorn, P. (1967). *Suicide—It Doesn't Have to Happen* (American Association of Suicidology pamphlet). Los Angeles, CA: Neuropsychiatry Institute, University of California.

Smith, J. A., & Carter, J. H. (1986). Suicide and Black adolescents: A medical dilemma. *Journal of the National Medical Association. 78* (11), 1061–1064.

Spaights, E., & Simpson, G. (1986). Some unique causes of Black suicide. *Psychology: A Quarterly Journal of Human Behavior. 23* (1), 1–5.

Stanley, M., & Stanley, B. (1988). Reconceptualizing suicide: A biological approach. *Psychiatric Annals. 18* (11), 646–651.

Stuart, G. W., & Sundeen, S. J. (1991). *Principles and practice of psychiatric nursing* (4th ed.). St. Louis: C. V. Mosby.

Szasz, T. (1986). The case against suicide prevention. *American Psychologist. 41* (7), 806–812.

Takahashi, Y. (1989). Suicidal Asian patients: Recommendations for treatment. *Suicide and Life-threatening Behavior. 19* (3), 305–313.

Thompson, J. W., & Walker, R. Dale. (1990). Adolescent suicide among American Indians and Alaska natives. *Psychiatric Annals. 20* (3), 128–133.

Traskman-Bendz, L., Asberg, M., Nordstrom, P., & Stanley, M. (1989). Biochemical aspects of suicidal behavior. *Progress in Neuro-psychopharmacology and Biological Psychiatry. 13* (supplement), 535–544.

U.S. Bureau of the Census. (1990). *Statistical abstract of the United States* (110th ed). Washington, DC: U.S. Government Printing Office.

Van der Wal, J. (1989–90). The aftermath of suicide: A review of empirical evidence. *Omega: Journal of Death and Dying. 20* (2), 149–171.

Vogel, R., & Wolfersdorf, M. (1987). Staff response to the suicide of psychiatric inpatients. *Crisis. 8* (2), 178–184.

Walker, R. D., & LaDue, R. (1986). An integrative approach to American Indian mental health. In C. B. Wilkinson (Ed.), *Ethnic psychiatry* (pp. 143–149). New York: Plenum.

Weisman, A. (1972). *On dying and denying.* New York: Behavioral Publications.

Weisman, A., & Hackett, T. (1961). Predilection to death. *Psychosomatic Medicine. 23,* 232–256.

Weisman, A., & Hackett, T. (1962). The dying patient. *Forest Hospital Publications. 1,* 16–21.

Wekstein, L., (1979). *Handbook of suicidology: Principles, problems, and practice.* New York: Bruner/Mazel.

Williams, J. (1982, April 25). Young suicides—tragic and on the increase. *New York Times,* p. 10E.

Wolfgang, M. E. (1968). Suicide by means of victim-precipitated homicide. *Journal of Clinical and Experimental Psychopathology. 20,* 335–349.

Wrobleski, A. (1984–85). The suicide survivors grief group. *Omega: Journal of Death and Dying. 15* (2), 173–184.

Wrobleski, A., & McIntosh, J. L. (1988). Problems of suicide survivors: An exploratory investigation. In E. Chigier (Ed.), *Grief and bereavement in contemporary society* (Vol. 1, pp. 158–169).

Zayas, L. H. (1987). Toward an understanding of suicide risks in young Hispanic females. *Journal of Adolescent Research. 2,* 1–11.

Zayas, L. H. (1989). A retrospective on the "suicidal fit" in mainland Puerto Ricans: Research issues. *Hispanic Journal of Behavioral Sciences. 11* (1), 46–47.

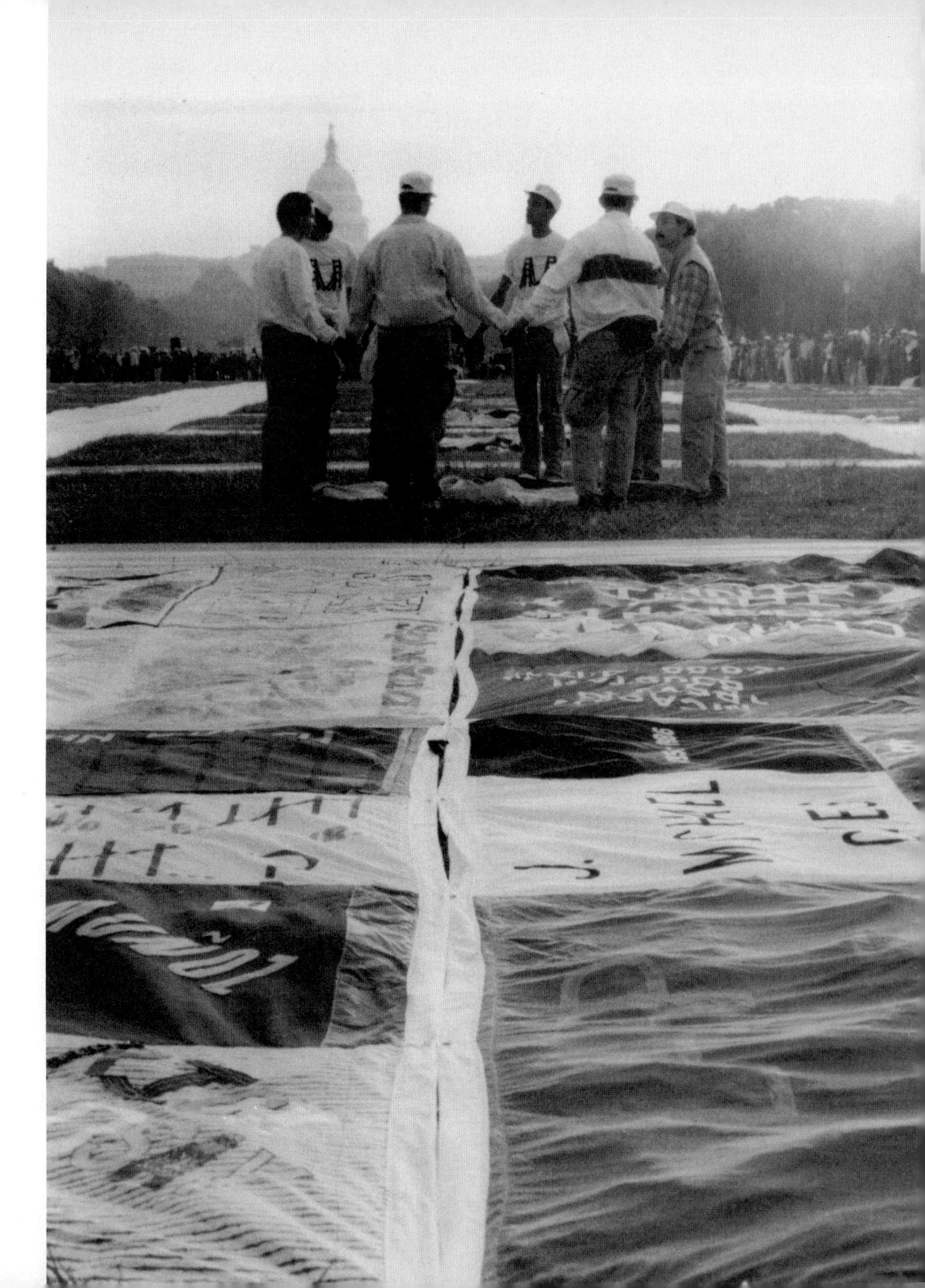

Chapter 10

Grief and Bereavement

When most people get married, they believe that they will live together with the one they love for the rest of their lives. When they die, they will die together. However, most married couples will not die together; one of the couple, usually the wife, will experience grief and bereavement. Despite this likelihood, people are not prepared for the grief they will feel.

This chapter focuses on the process of grief and bereavement, examines the problems associated with becoming a widow or widower, and reviews the roles of caregivers with the bereaved. Both the loss of a spouse, and the loss of child are discussed.

First, grief and bereavement must be distinguished. Bereavement is the actual state of the deprivation caused by the loss. Grief is a psychological state characterized by mental anguish. It is the response of emotional pain to the loss.

Grief

When people grieve, they experience opposite behaviors and feelings: "We find anger and apathy, weight loss and weight gain, preoccupation with or suppression of memories of the deceased, and removal versus treasuring their possessions" (Stroebe and Stroebe, 1987, p. 8). It is a time of great ambivalence.

> The bereaved may be desperately lonely, yet shun company; they may try to escape from reminders of their loss, yet cultivate memories of the dead; they complain if people avoid them, embarrassed how to express their sympathy, yet rebuff that sympathy irritably when it is offered (Marris, 1974, p. 28).

The ambivalence comes from a desire to return to the past, yet to reach out to the future. During a period of grief, the present may be meaningless.

Why do people grieve? Three major theories are the psychoanalytic model represented by Freud (1959), the attachment model developed by John Bowlby (1971, 1975, 1980), and the stress model developed from the works of Selye (1976) and Holmes and Rahe (1967).

Psychoanalytic Model. For Freud the grieving process allows persons to break their ties with the lost object. When people lose a person they love, the libido, or our mental energies, are still directed towards the deceased. Since a person only has a limited amount of libidinal energies, these energies have to become detached from the lost object. The person focuses on the deceased, which brings back memories, and finally begins to realize that the lost object no longer exists. Because of the extra energy needed to do this, the bereaved goes through a powerful process. The goal of the grief work is completed when the bereaved severs the attachment to the deceased and "the ego becomes free and uninhibited again" (Freud, 1959, p. 245).

Attachment Model. Developed by John Bowlby, attachment theory conceptualizes grief as a form of separation anxiety. Grieving is an attempt to reestablish ties and is not a process of withdrawing from them. There is a searching for the deceased. Obviously, this search is extremely frustrating. Eventually, this frustrated search for the deceased lessens. Bowlby developed his theory from his studies of children who had been separated from their mothers. Children reacted to the separation first with tears and anger, but they were still hopeful that their mothers would return. These feelings then turned to despair, with hope and despair alternating. Finally, there was a fading of the memory of the mother.

When a loved one dies, people have the same feelings as a child separated from his mother. In grief, persons are continuously trying to find the lost object, going through periods of anger, yearning, and despair. Eventually the search for the deceased lessens. But Bowlby believes these feelings are necessary if people are to recover from grief. Although the two theories posit different dynamics underlying the grief, the results are similar: there is intense pain and an intense focus on the deceased.

Stress Theory. The loss of a loved one is viewed as a major stressful event:

> While depression models (e.g., psychoanalytic model and attachment theory) construe bereavement in terms of loss and focus on the emotional reaction, stress models view bereavement as a stressful life event, that is, as an experience that overtaxes the coping resources of the individual (Stroebe, 1989, p. 77).

On the Holmes-Rahe scale of stressful events, the death of a spouse is ranked the highest in stress of any event, meaning that the death of a spouse requires the "most intense readjustment" to a person's life (Stroebe, 1989, p. 84). The stress a person has because of a death may then lead to a number of various physical and emotional disruptions.

The Grief Process

Grief consists of a number of phases: shock and numbness, intense grief (which consists of yearning, anger, guilt, and disorganization) and finally reorganization. (Other theorists have posited more stages; however, their stages may be subsumed under the three already mentioned.) "Phases" rather than "stages" are used in describing the grieving process since the term "stage" is more likely to imply a sequential process. Rather, "phases" allow us to look at grief as "a succession of clinical pictures which blend into and replace one another" (Parkes, 1986, p. 27).

Shock and Numbness. The most immediate reaction to a death is generally a feeling of numbness. The bereaved cannot believe that the death has occurred. It is a time when feelings are not yet admitted to consciousness. This stage works as emotional anesthesia, for to allow the feelings of grief at this point would be totally overwhelming. This is why the bereaved may appear to be doing so well at funerals. They may not break down; they may greet everyone with a handshake and say: "I'm so glad you could come. Doesn't he look lovely?" Yet on closer examination, the bereaved is saying exactly the same thing to everyone. He or she is acting as an automaton. People admire those bereaved who act with dignity at funerals, and do not break down. They are exhibiting the first stage of grief.

The numbness of the bereaved may fool others into believing that they are doing well. After a few hours or a few days, however, the numbness should wear off, and the bereaved will enter the next stage.

Intense Grief. The intensity of the grief is not necessarily related to the degree of love felt for the individual who has died; rather, it is related to the degree of feelings, both negative and positive, one had toward the dead person.

C. S. Lewis (1961), chronicling his grief over the death of his wife, expresses the feelings that occur in this stage:

> No one ever told me that grief felt so like fear. I am not afraid, but the sensation is like being afraid. The same fluttering in the stomach, the same restlessness, the yawning. I keep on swallowing.
>
> At other times it feels like being mildly drunk, or concussed. There is a sort of invisible blanket between the world and me. I find it hard to take in what anyone says. Or perhaps, hard to want to take it in. It is so uninteresting. Yet I want the others to be about me. I dread

> the moments when the house is empty. If only they would talk to one another and not to me. . . .
>
> And no one ever told me about the laziness of grief. Except at my job—where the machine seems to run on much as usual—I loath the slightest effort. Not only writing but even reading a letter is too much. Even shaving. What does it matter now whether my cheek is rough or smooth? They say an unhappy man wants distractions—something to take him out of himself. Only as a dog-tired man wants an extra blanket on a cold night; he'd rather lie there shivering than get up and find one. It's easy to see why the lonely become untidy; finally, dirty and disgusting (pp. 1–2).

In the first phase of intense grief, there is continued pining and searching for the deceased. The thoughts and behavior of the bereaved are focused on the lost person. There is a perceptual set for the lost person; the bereaved believes in the person's presence. The bereaved's thoughts are constantly concerned with the deceased, and attention is directed toward objects associated with the lost person.

Hallucinations are not uncommon. For example, in one study, 46.7 percent of 293 bereaved people had post-bereavement hallucinations (Rees, 1975), including both visual and auditory hallucinations; 11.6 percent of those studied stated that they spoke with the deceased. The majority of the bereaved found the hallucinations helpful, although some of them questioned their own sanity. Rees reported some of the reactions:

> I think she's in my present house. I find hearing her breathing disturbing, but I like the feeling she is in the house.
>
> I feel him guiding me.

There is also anger and guilt. Anger will be reflected by irritability and bitterness. It may be directed at all those nearby, the doctors who took care of the deceased, at God, and at the deceased. The bereaved are angry at the deceased for causing such pain. Young survivors are angry because they are left alone to raise the children. Older bereaved ask what happened to the retirement plans they made together.

The bereaved may be angry at God: If God were a just God, how could He have taken my spouse? She was such a good person, while there are so many bad persons still alive.

Anger is also directed at oneself in terms of guilt. The bereaved go through many "if only I hads." An example of this comes from author Robert Anderson (1974) over the death of his wife:

> I made the discovery of the very small lump in my wife's breast. I had no idea what it was. I said nothing until a solicitation from the Cancer Society listed the warning signals of cancer. For years after, I cursed my own ignorance and the negligence of all the doctors who had never taught my wife breast self-examination. For years, with hot flashes of anger and guilt, I went over and over those weeks of delay. Why didn't I mention even in passing the small lump in her breast? My brother is a doctor; why didn't I check with him? A simple phone call. For years I rewrote compulsively that scene in my head, playing it differently—I mention the lump to my wife; we go to the doctor; we are in time, and my wife is alive (p. 10).

During intense grief the bereaved will lapse into despair. They are disorganized. Apathy and aimlessness are two predominant feelings. There is a sense of futility and emptiness, and a loss of patterns of interaction. These feelings of despair may come and go as the bereaved start to reorganize their lives. As they take each step, such as finding a new friend, or a job, the depression begins to lift until the final phase, reintegration, occurs.

Reintegration. Reintegration, or recovery, has occurred when the bereaved are functioning normally again. A sense of continuity in life must be reestablished. As Marris (1974) points out, this is done, "not by ceasing to care for the dead, but by abstracting what was fundamentally important in the relationship and rehabilitating it" (p. 34). It is giving up the deceased without giving up what the deceased meant to the bereaved.

A Cleveland surgeon, Dr. George Crile (1969), depicts the final stage of grieving, a little more than a year after his wife had died:

> I still live in the same house. Many of the same birds, the wood ducks and the swan, are still in our back yard. Many of the relics that Jane and I collected in our travels are about our house. But there are no ghosts. Memories that were for a time inexpressibly sad have once again become a source of deep pleasure and satisfaction.
>
> Since we know nothing of death except that it comes to all, it is not unreasonable to be sad for the person who has died. The sorrow that I once felt for myself, in my loss, now has been transformed to a rich memory of a woman I loved and the ways we traveled through the world together (p. xxiii).

One never totally gets over the grief. On special occasions, such as birthdays or anniversaries, the depression may reoccur. The memories continue to exist, but they may become good memories.

The Symptomatology of Grief and Bereavement

Throughout the process of grieving, the bereaved may suffer from various physical symptoms. Normal grief is normal only in a statistical sense, since grief is such a different state from what we consider healthy (Engel, 1961).

Much of what is known about the symptomatology of grief stems from the work of Erich Lindemann (1944). In 1942, a nightclub in Boston, the Cocoanut Grove, caught fire: 499 people died; 200 survived. Many of the survivors, although physically well, kept complaining of physical symptoms such as shortness of breath, insomnia, and loss of appetite. One of the psychiatrists treating the survivors was Lindemann. He proceeded to study 101 bereaved persons, including the survivors of the fire, and recorded his observations. He found that "acute grief is a definite syndrome with psychological and somatic symptomatology" (p. 141). Within grief, there was (1) somatic distress, especially respiratory disturbances; (2) preoccupation with the image of the deceased while feeling emotionally distant from others; (3) guilt; (4) hostile reactions; and (5) loss of patterns of conduct.

Stroebe and Stroebe (1989) list the symptoms of grief as described in Table 10.1.

Table 10.1 List of Grief Symptoms

SYMPTOM	DESCRIPTION
A. Affective	
Depression	Feelings of sadness, mournfulness, and dysphoria, accompanied by intense subjective distress and "mental pain." Episodes (waves) of depression may be severe and are sometimes (but not always) precipitated by external events (locale, receiving sympathy, reminders of shared activities, anniversaries, meetings, etc.). Feelings of despair, lamentation, sorrow, and dejection predominate
Anxiety	Fears, dreads, and forebodings such as fear of breaking down, of losing one's mind or going mad, of dying, fear of being unable to cope without spouse, separation anxiety, fear about living alone, financial worries, and worries about other matters previously dealt with by spouse
Guilt	Self-blame and self-accusation about events in the past, notably about events leading up to death (feeling that more could have been done to prevent death). Guilt feelings about behavior toward partner (should have treated differently, made different decisions)

(table continued on next page)

Table 10.1 Continued

SYMPTOM	DESCRIPTION
Anger and hostility	Irritability toward family, in child rearing, with friends (feeling they lacked understanding for and appreciation of the deceased, and about the bereaved's grief). Anger about fate, that death has occurred, anger toward the deceased spouse (e.g., about being left alone, not provided for), toward the doctors, nurses of spouse
Anhedonia	Loss of enjoyment of food, hobbies, social and family events, and other activities which had previously been pleasurable even if the spouse were not actually present. Feeling that nothing can be pleasurable without spouse
Loneliness	Feeling alone even in the presence of others, and periodic bouts of intense loneliness, notably at the times when spouse would have been present (evenings, weekends) and during special events that they would have shared
B. Behavioral manifestations	
Agitation	Tenseness, restlessness (atypical), jitteryness, overactivity often without completing tasks (doing things for the sake of the activity), searching behavior (looking for spouse, even though they "know" this is useless)
Fatigue	Reduction in general activity level (sometimes interrupted by bouts of agitation mentioned above); retardation of speech and thought (slowed speech, long latencies); general lassitude
Crying	Tears and/or watery eyes, general expression one of sadness (drooping of sides of mouth, sad gaze)
C. Attitudes toward self, the deceased, and environment	
Self-reproach	See A: Guilt
Low self-esteem	Feelings of inadequacy, failure, and incompetence on one's own, without spouse; worthlessness
Helplessness. hopelessness	Pessimism about present circumstances and future, loss of purpose in life, thoughts of death and suicide (desire not to go on living without spouse)

(table continued on next page)

Table 10.1 Continued

SYMPTOM	DESCRIPTION
Sense of unreality	Feeling of "not being there," of "watching from outside," that events in the present are happening to someone else
Suspiciousness	Doubting the motives of those who offer help or advice
Interpersonal problems	Difficulty in maintaining social relationships, rejection of friendship, withdrawal from social functions
Attitudes toward the deceased	*Yearning* for deceased, waves of longing, calling out for him/her, intense pining
	Imitation of deceased's behavior (e.g., manner of speaking, walking), following deceased's interests, pursuits
	Idealization of deceased; the tendency to ignore any faults, exaggerate positive characteristics of spouse
	Ambivalence: alternation of feelings about deceased
	Images of deceased, often very vivid, almost hallucinatory; firm conviction of having seen/heard spouse
	Preoccupation with the memory of the deceased (both with sad and happy memories) and need to talk, sometimes incessantly, about deceased, to the exclusion of interest in any other topic
D. Cognitive impairment	
Retardation of thought and concentration	Slowed thinking and poor memory; see also B: Fatigue
E. Physiological changes and bodily complaints	
Loss of appetite	(Occasionally, overeating) accompanied by changes in body weight; sometimes, a considerable loss of weight
Sleep disturbances	Mostly insomnia, occasionally oversleeping; disturbances of day/night rhythm
Energy loss	See B: Fatigue

(table continued on next page)

Table 10.1 Continued

SYMPTOM	DESCRIPTION
Bodily complaints	These include headaches, neckache, back pain, muscle cramp, nausea, vomiting, lump in throat, sour taste in mouth, dry mouth, constipation, heartburn, indigestion, flatulence, blurred vision, pain on urination, tightness in throat, choking with shortness of breath, need for sighing, empty feeling in abdomen, lack of muscular power, palpitations, tremors, hair loss
Physical complaints of deceased	Appearance of symptoms similar to those of the deceased, particularly of those symptoms of the terminal illness (e.g., heart fluttering if loss were from heart attack); the bereaved may be convinced of having the same illness that afflicted the deceased
Changes in drug taking	Increase in the use of psychotropic medicines (tranquilizers, etc.) in alcohol intake, in smoking
Susceptibility to illness and disease	Particularly infections (lowering of immunity), also those relating to lack of health care (cancer, tuberculosis, etc.), and stress-related diseases (e.g., heart conditions)

Reprinted with permission from *Bereavement and Health* by Wolfgang Stroebe and Margaret Stroebe. New York: Cambridge University Press, 1989.

Physical health has been shown to deteriorate during bereavement whether measured by visits to physicians, medications taken, or report of symptoms by the widowed. For example, Parkes' study (1964) of the case records of 44 widows showed each patient saw her general practitioner on the average of 2.2 times every six months during the 18 months before her husband's death. It rose to 3.6 times during the first six months following bereavement. Wiener et. al. (1975) found similar results in their study of the elderly bereaved. They further found that the bereaved were much more likely to be taking medication five to eight months after the death than a control group of nonbereaved elderly. Bowling and Cartwright (1982) found in their study of 352 elderly British widows and widowers that they reported experiencing eight symptoms (including breathlessness, indigestion, headaches, backaches, and rheumatism) to a greater extent than a comparable group of nonbereaved. The most common symptom was rheumatism. Parkes and Weiss (1983) in the analysis of the Harvard Bereavement Group (49 widows and 19 widowers in the Boston area) reported more ill health than the control group, particularly those resulting from "nervous tension" such as sweating, palpitations, and dizziness.

Besides being related to ill health, is grief related to death? Do people die of broken hearts? Although grief is not listed as a cause of death on a death certificate, epidemiological studies have shown that widows and widowers have a higher mortality rate than married people of the same sex and age. This finding cuts across different cultures and across history (Stroebe and Stroebe, 1989, p. 151). In a study of 4,486 widowers aged 55 and over, Young, Benjamin, and Wallis (1963) found an increase in the death rate of 40 percent during the first six months of bereavement. Seventy-five percent of these deaths were attributed to heart disease, particularly coronary thromboses and arteriosclerotic heart disease. Since then, numerous studies [as discussed by Osterweis et al. (1984), Parkes (1986), Stroebe & Stroebe (1989), and Haig (1990)] have confirmed that the bereaved are at a higher risk in terms of mortality. For example, Mellstrom (as discussed by Parkes (1986) and Stroebe and Stroebe (1989)) found in his study of all 360,000 people who were widowed in Sweden between 1968 and 1978 that widowers had a shorter life expectancy of one and one-half years than other men; and widows a shorter life expectancy of six months than nonbereaved women.

Jones [as discussed by Haig, (1990)] in a 10-year longitudinal study of almost 22,000 widows and widowers found that the widowers experienced a mortality rate ten percent greater than nonbereaved men.

As concluded by Osterweis et al. (1984) and Stroebe and Stroebe (1989), in their extensive reviews of studies, bereavement does indeed lead to a higher death rate. In order to explain this, five hypotheses were proposed as discussed by Epstein et. al. (1975), Rees (1972), and Stroebe and Stroebe (1989):

1. *The selection hypothesis:* The healthy among the widowed tend to remarry and select themselves out, leaving the widowed population with higher death rates. However, since the death rate is highest for those most recently bereaved, those who remarry would have to do so quickly. This is generally not the case.
2. *The homogamy or mutual choice of poor riskmates hypothesis:* Here, it is presumed that the unfit marry the unfit. Although individuals with similar physical disabilities may marry each other, it is unlikely that this hypothesis is true since the large increase in mortality occurs so rapidly after the death of a spouse.
3. *The joint unfavorable environment hypothesis:* The survivor and spouse shared an unfavorable environment so that what led to the death of the deceased will lead to the death of the other. However, except for a study by Ciocco done in 1940, which showed a tendency for married couples to die of tuberculosis, no other study has been able to document a relationship between causes of death in spouses.

4. *The non-grief-related, behavior-change hypothesis:* Because the deceased spouse is no longer there, the survivor may be more likely to skip meals, to skip medicine, and generally not to take care of himself. This may be true for the elderly widower, who may have been cared for by his wife, but it is not generally true of widows.
5. *The desolation-effects hypothesis:* The effects of grief, including feelings of hopelessness, may result in physical vulnerability. The death of a spouse has been shown to cause the greatest amount of stress, which may then result in death.

This last hypothesis seems best to explain the statistical relationship between grief and death. People may indeed die from "broken hearts."

Pathological Grief Reactions

> My mother sits home alone day after day. All she does is watch television or read in between visits to Dad's grave, two, three times a week. That's what she seems to live for—those visits when she kneels down and talks to him—as if he were there, listening. Once in a while she'll go to a movie with us, or for a drive. Or let a friend come visit. But not often. I don't know. Is she losing it? (Dersheimer, 1990, p. 31).

Is the woman described above having a normal reaction to the death of her spouse? Or is what she is exhibiting abnormal? Would it be considered normal at any time? At a month after the death? A year? Two years? It is very difficult to answer these questions, since it is not yet known what constitutes normal grieving outcomes for everyone (Osterweis et. al., 1984). Yet studies have shown that about 15 percent of those who are bereaved seem to exhibit some prolonged grief reactions (Zesook et. al. (1982) and Parkes and Weiss (1983).

Horowitz et al. (1980) provide a definition of abnormal or pathological grief as: "The intensification of grief to the level where the person is overwhelmed, resorts to maladaptive behavior, or remains interminably in the state of grief without progression of the mourning process towards completion . . ." (p. 1157).

The patterns exhibited by persons suffering from abnormal grief reactions exaggerate the normal aspects of grief (Marris, 1974)—"the impulse to escape from everything connected with bereavement, the worsening of physical health, the despair or refusal to surrender the dead. And in each, counterbalancing impulses have been suppressed. The process of normal grief seems to be a working out of conflicting impulses: while in abortive grief patterns, the conflict is never resolved" (p. 28). The depression, panic, guilt, and ill health that are felt in these distorted forms of grief do not differ in kind, but rather in duration and intensity, from normal grief reactions (Parkes, 1972, p. 117).

Patterns of abnormal grief reactions include:

1. *Delayed Grief:* Here, the bereaved feels little sorrow and continues on with life. The bereaved will act very busy and will be very calm. This may last a few weeks or even longer. Suddenly, the grief may be triggered by the loss of some object such as a wristwatch, or it may occur when the circumstances surrounding the death are recalled. A person with a very severe reaction to a recent death may be grieving for a death that occurred years ago. For example, Lindemann (1944) discusses a woman who grieved intensely for her mother, but who actually was engrossed in fantasies concerning her brother, who had died twenty years before.
2. *Inhibited Grief:* The bereaved never feels the grief. Wortman and Silver (1989) question the validity of categorizing this as a form of pathological grief; the necessity and the inevitability of all people to feel distress when bereaved is not borne out in the literature. Perhaps, only if other symptoms develop, including such physical conditions as ulcerative colitis, asthma, or rheumatoid arthritis, should this be viewed as a pathological form of grieving.
3. *Chronic Grief:* The grieving continues; the person can never get beyond the intense yearning for the person, the anger, the guilt, and the despair. Raphael (1983) describes a man still actively grieving his wife after three years:

> Alan K. was fifty-five when his wife Mary died from carcinoma of the breast . . . . The word of her death left him stunned. He did not see her body after death and went through the funeral in a "state of shock." When he went home to the empty house he felt he had lost his "whole life." He cried for her repeatedly. He reminisced constantly over their marriage, idealizing what had been a reasonable but average relationship.
>
> Three years later the picture was unchanged. He was angry with the world that such a good woman should die. He seemed unable to look after himself (pp. 209–210).

Bereavement may be prolonged when society does not recognize a person's right to grieve as in the case of gay men who have experienced the death of their lover by AIDS. Doka (1989) has called this *disenfranchised grief.*

Who is most likely to have a poor outcome? Although theorists list over ten variables that affect the outcome of the bereavement (including age, sex, social class, prior grief experiences, religiosity, personality of the bereaved, type of relationship, timeliness, mode of death, cause of death, and quality of social supports) the evidence clearly supports only the following:

1. Men have more difficulty adjusting than women.
2. Younger bereaved persons are at greater risk than the older bereaved.
3. Overdependent and ambivalent relationships generally lead to poor outcomes.
4. Social support and perceived social support are important in defining those bereaved who are at high risk.

For the other variables, the evidence relating them to bereavement outcome is either scanty or contradictory.

Anticipatory Grief

When people expect the death of someone close, they begin to experience their grief in advance. It is assumed that anticipatory grief offers the survivor time to work through a large portion of the trauma normally associated with loss. However, research findings do not necessarily bear this out. Rather, studies of the bereaved have found contradictory results when examining the adaptational value of anticipatory grief. Many of the studies find anticipatory grief to be helpful and adaptive [for example, Parkes and Weiss (1983), Raphael and Maddison (1976), and Vaclon et. al. (1982)]; some studies found that anticipatory grief could have negative consequences for the bereaved [for example, Gerber et. al. (1975), Schwab et. al. (1975), and Rando (1983)]; and some did not find any relationship between anticipatory grief and the grief reaction [for example, Bornstein et. al. (1973), Clayton et. al. (1973); and Maddison (1968)].

Why are the findings contradictory? The answer, in part, is that the studies define anticipatory grief differently, examine different age groups, and measure outcome at a different time. A number of studies confound the effects of an untimely death, where the deceased is young, or a traumatic death, where death was caused by violence or an accident, with the effects of sudden death. As pointed out by Rando (1986):

> The sudden death of an elderly individual under natural circumstances, of course, would be expected to elicit different reactions than the sudden and violent death of a younger person; however, such important variations have heretofore been insufficiently accounted for in the literature (p. 8).

There is also an assumption in the studies that a forewarning of the loss is the same as anticipating grief. The definition of anticipatory is generally based upon the amount of time a person was ill prior to dying. This does not mean that the survivor actually grieved in anticipation; the bereaved may have denied the oncoming death.

Rando (1986) posits that the contradictory findings may be explained by her study showing that there is an optimal length of time for a person to experience anticipatory grief. Either sudden death or short illnesses or very long illnesses may both lead to poor bereavement outcomes. This was further confirmed by Sanders (1983), who showed that the situations that had the best outcome were those where the deceased had an illness lasting less than six months as compared to those where the deceased either died suddenly or was ill for a longer period of time.

Another reason for the contradictions is that anticipatory grief is not inherently positive or negative, especially in terms of the ambivalence that is felt when a loved one is dying. As Aldrich (1974) points out: "A period of anticipation may provide a mourner with an opportunity to carry out grief work in advance of loss, but at the same time it complicates the working-through process by giving the hostile component of ambivalence a more realistically destructive potential" (p. 7). If the patient is not to be told that he is dying and a closed or mutual pretense awareness exists, it becomes difficult to work out the ambivalent feelings. Furthermore, throughout anticipatory grief, the survivor must maintain hope; if not, the survivor is viewed as not having loved the person. Anticipatory grief may lead survivors to feel that they gave up hope too early.

Anticipatory Grief of Parents

Anticipatory parental mourning has been defined as "a set of processes that are directly related to the awareness of the impending loss, to its emotional impact and to the adaptive mechanisms whereby emotional attachment to the dying child is relinquished over time" (Futterman & Hoffman as cited in Tietz, McSherry, & Britt, 1977, p. 417). These series of processes are interwoven, and, as defined by Futterman and Hoffman (1973), consist of: (a) acknowledgment—a growing realization by parents that their child's death is inevitable; hope and despair alternate as this realization deepens; (b) grieving—beginning as intense undifferentiated responses and feelings, but these eventually become less acute; (c) reconciliation—the development of some perspective by parents about their child's impending death; recognition that the child's life has been worthwhile, and that life will continue after the child dies; (d) detachment—while still offering love and security to the dying child, parents begin to reinvest in relationships that will continue after the child dies; (e) memoralization—development of a positive mental image of the child that will endure after her death; thinking of the child in generalities rather than in terms of specific behaviors (pp. 130–131).

Although anticipatory grief may be helpful, it may also result in family members separating from the child before the child has died. This can occur when the dying process extends over a long time, or if the child has an unexpected late remission. Parents may be upset to find that they have withdrawn from their child before the actual death. Both they and the child may need support from staff so that isolation of the child does not occur.

Caregivers' Role

During the period of anticipatory grief, patients and all involved in their care, including the health care team, need as much support as possible. This period is particularly stressful for everyone. Both the patient and family are attempting to cope with uncertainties that lead to ambivalence, anger, and guilt. Family members can become preoccupied with their own grief and withdraw from the patient. Sometimes family members are at various levels of acceptance or have conflicting attitudes that isolate one family member from another. This is particularly difficult if the patient is a child, as the lack of understanding of one parent toward another can adversely affect their entire future. Premature mourning and the concomitant withdrawal of the family isolates the patient. This behavior frustrates the health care team if they cannot understand the underlying dynamics. At the same time, they are also struggling with their sense of impotence and having to shift from curing to caring. Their anger can just as easily be projected onto the family for "not caring" when they are actually unable to deal with their own feelings about "not curing."

The use of groups to help families discuss what must be faced and how to accomplish this is an extremely effective method of promoting better understanding during this period. It is particularly beneficial if members of the health care team can participate, or at least are informed of, the process. Lebow (1976) hypothesized that it is more desirable to encourage greater family involvement during the period of anticipatory grief. She postulated that while each family member was threatened by a sense of loss, each could be helped to enhance awareness and understanding of his relationship to others. She suggested six adaptational tasks: (1) remaining involved with the patient; (2) remaining separate; (3) adapting to role changes; (4) bearing the effects of grief; (5) coming to some terms with the reality of impending loss; and (6) saying good-bye. Obviously, tasks 1 and 2, which sound mutually exclusive, require understanding and creative therapeutic intervention. These techniques, however, need not be complex. For example, a family member can be encouraged to include the patient in all family decisions and communications. Often family members will convey to staff what they feel a patient needs, and must gently be reminded to ask the patient's preference. Similarly, family can be given "permission" by staff not to visit. At the Victoria General Hospice program, one day is set aside as "relatives' day off."

Instead of asking whether anticipatory grief is adaptive for all bereaved, studies should be addressing the questions: For whom is anticipatory grief adaptive? What is the optimal length of time for anticipatory grief? Under what conditions is anticipatory grief helpful? What was the nature of the relationship between the deceased and the bereaved?

Grieving the Death of a Child

The death of a child, no matter what age, is one of the most traumatic experiences a family will ever have to endure. In the initial phase of numbness and shock, parents may not be able to believe what has happened. The child's death is an unreal experience that may be denied. Parents may be flooded with feelings of anger, guilt, rage, and frustration. The most important response caregivers may give at this point is one of caring, of availability to listen and be with the parents. Parents may also need practical help in decision making such as whom to notify about the death and arranging for a funeral home.

The numbness and shock may persist as a protective shield for days or weeks, but gradually it will give way to a period of intense grief. This time is painful and depressing. Grieving family members may find that they are isolated from the community while their child is dying and for a time after the child's death. Friends and relatives may avoid the family, perhaps even more so if the child is dying from a disease, such as AIDS, that society fears. Parents, however, often want to talk about the child's death, and they want company. Single parents may feel particularly alone. One single parent wrote . . . "I had no one to share the experience with; no one to even enter my house of silence" (Wyler, 1988, p. 301). Thus, at a time when a family needs the most support from friends and community, the least is offered, and the family mourns alone.

In a small study of five families grieving the death of a child, Nolfi (1977) found that three of the mothers expressed an intense need to talk about the child and the death; their husbands, however, were unable to speak about it and even refused to allow the child's name to be mentioned (p. 77). Each parent reacts to the death of a child in their own way. This seems axiomatic, but parents do need to understand that their partners, while experiencing feelings of grief and loss, may express these feelings in unique ways. Thus, while one parent talks and cries about the loss, the other may suffer in silence. Fathers are often put in the role of the strong and silent one, even if they have painful and sad feelings and would like to express these (Miles, 1985). One parent may have a need to cope with grief by sexual intimacy, whereas the other parent may find this aspect of the relationship of little interest at this point.

Parents also may not be in the same phase of grieving at the same time. A mother, often because of her usually closer and more continuous contact with the dying child, may have worked through anticipatory grieving feelings and be more in a stage of detachment than a father who may still be experiencing tremendous feelings of anger and guilt. Generally, difficulties between parents arise when one parent expects the other to respond to grief in the same way and at the same time (Miles, 1985). Parents may need help in understanding that they may have different responses to the death of their child, and that each response of the other person is his individual way of grieving.

During this period of intense grieving, parents may experience physical distress, including poor appetite, insomnia, irritability, muscular aches and pain, and digestive problems. Caregivers can help bereaved parents try and maintain appropriate eating, sleeping, and exercise patterns. Some parents may turn to the use of drugs and alcohol to avoid the pain of grieving. There is a real danger of such use changing into abuse, which can lead to addiction. If substance abuse occurs, caregivers need to refer the person to an appropriate treatment center for help.

At this point in the grieving process reorganization becomes more evident as parents begin to feel that life does indeed still contain some pleasures, some degree of comfort. They are able to enjoy aspects of living that they enjoyed prior to the child's death such as sports, watching television, reading a good book, taking a vacation. Parents may feel guilty about "having fun" and may need reassurance that it is quite acceptable to begin to enjoy life again.

Miles (1985) notes that "it is important to remember, however, that reorganization is not recovery, for parents say that they never recover from the loss of a child" (p. 234). For many people, the pain of grief can still be evoked years after a child's death—that pain may be less sharp and not last as long, but it can still be there. The death of a child changes a parent:

> The self after the resolution of the death of child is different than the self was before the death. Such psychic reorganization provides elements for a new self; this can be a rich development in the life of the bereaved parent . . . Reformed inner representations of a dead child provide the parent with the personal qualities not available before. All ends are also new beginnings. Just as parenthood is a developmental phase, so is parental bereavement (Klass & Marwit, 1988–89, p. 47).

People who have experienced the death of a child may or may not agree with the above idea of bereavement as a developmental phase in life; however, the dying and death of a child affects all family members.

Role Changes After the Death of a Spouse

Once the bereaved begin recovering from their grief, they are still faced with being widows or widowers. They are now single again, yet they are not single. The rules of behavior for a husband or a wife are clear in our society. What are the rules for the widow or widower? Widowhood is generally viewed as a temporary state, but a temporary state on the way to what? Where do you go from being a widow or widower? When do you stop being a widow or widower and become a single person? It is difficult to answer these questions since being a widow or widower, after the intense grief has passed, is an undefined role in our society.

Widows and widowers face specific problems in no longer being married and in being alone in a couples-oriented society. In Helen Lopata's (1979) study of widows, over 50 percent agreed with the statement: "One problem of being a widow is feeling like a fifth wheel." Younger widows may be perceived as a sexual threat by many of their friends; 37 percent of the women in Lopata's study agreed that other women are jealous of a widow when their husbands are around.

An attractive widow in her 40s, interviewed by one of the authors, reported how her relationship with her sister-in-law changed after her husband's death. While the widow's husband was alive, she always greeted her brother-in-law and sister-in-law with a hug and kiss. Now, when she started to kiss her brother-in-law, the sister-in-law gave her a dirty look.

Dating and sex become issues for the bereaved. Widows, especially, are not supposed to have any interest in sex. For example, a young widow interviewed by Kreis and Pattie (1969) reported: "My husband and I had a good sex life. Since he passed away, I've lived like a virgin. My minister was evasive when I mentioned my sense of frustration. He gave me that, 'Now, now, my dear,' but I got his message: 'Respectable women shouldn't have such desires, it isn't nice'" (p. 71).

When does it become all right for a woman to begin dating again? And when is it all right to have sex again? Although some would argue that the answers are best left to the individual, some societal guidelines would help alleviate the guilt the widow or widower may feel when beginning to date. As one widow asked, "When is it all right for me to take off my wedding band?"

Widows and widowers of different ages face specific problems. Lopata (1979, pp. 382–383) discusses the difficulties encountered by widows of various age groups:

Ages 30 to 54. With the death of the spouse, the income of the family will probably fall substantially. There are probably children who must be taken care of, yet there is a lack of inexpensive day-care.

Ages 55 to 65. Since the widow is not likely to have dependent children, she is not eligible for Social Security benefits, and she may be destitute. It is also harder for her to reenter the job market if she has not worked outside the home in a number of years. Although she may want to date and eventually remarry, there is a paucity of eligible males.

***Ages 65+*.** Here, the widow may be left relatively isolated. One effect of this may be that she is deprived of being touched. Although many studies have documented that touch deprivation in infants may have many negative effects, including death, there are no such studies of the elderly. What are the effects of touch deprivation in the elderly? We do not know. Yet it may be just as hurtful to the elderly as to infants.

Widowers, too, face a number of problems in dealing with their new role. The younger widower with children must find appropriate care for them that he can afford. He must now become more aware of his children's social and emotional needs, and become able to meet them. As Gerber (1975) points out: "His (the younger widower with children) awareness of how dependent he was on his spouse for maintaining the emotional level of the family is obvious only after the death" (p. 3).

The older widower may not be prepared to take care of himself. His wife was responsible for the housework, the cooking, and the cleaning, and the widower may not feel competent to do these jobs. Since the older widower may have retired, he in effect no longer has the two primary roles in our society; worker and spouse. As a result, he may begin to feel worthless.

The one major advantage a widower has over a widow is that it is easier for him to remarry because there is a 5-to-1 ratio of widows to widowers (Campbell, 1987, p. 1). Many of the widowers are aware of this ratio. As one, aged 72, answered in response to a query concerning his plans, "I think I'll go down to Miami and look over the beach for a future mate."

Caregivers' Roles with the Bereaved

Although studies indicate that the bereaved represent a higher-risk population with regard to physical and emotional illness and even death, relatively few programs are available to provide support through this difficult period. Everyone assumes that the grieving individual will "get over it." Certainly this is true for the vast majority. The question is not so much whether the individual will "get over it," but rather how the health care team and the community can facilitate grief work and provide support to enhance her continued growth and development. Our sophisticated, technologically oriented culture promotes the development of elaborate schemes and programs, yet the obvious often escapes our attention. The bereaved person often needs someone who will be able to sit and listen. This sounds simplistic, but we often feel pressured to give advice and counsel to escape our own feelings of helplessness. This "rush to help" often prevents us from hearing what the bereaved individual says is needed. Our cultural emphasis on competency, strength, and adequacy prevents the bereaved from experiencing the emotions necessary for appropriate resolution of grief.

Simos (1977) notes that repetition is necessary for the mastery of loss. The bereaved require repeated opportunities to verbalize their feelings in an attempt to make sense of their loss, to ask the unanswerable whys before acceptance of the loss can occur. One father (Hullinger, 1980), in discussing his response to his daughter's death, explained: "I needed the opportunity to talk over and over and over, to repeat and repeat and repeat. And to have somebody able to listen to that" (p. 2). This process begins as soon as the individual is told that death has occurred.

Currently the majority of deaths occur in institutional settings. The health care team, pressured by the demands of the setting and their own sense of failure, often allocates little time with family members after a patient has died. Even when death is expected, the family will respond with shock, numbness, and dismay. Physicians, nurses, and social workers often experience impatience with this response, and a common reaction is to withdraw while muttering, "But she knew he was dying." Some member of the health care team should remain available to assist family members as they incorporate the initial shock. Often this is perceived as a social work task, since the social worker is not responsible for ongoing, direct patient care. If possible, provision should also be made for a room where privacy is insured. Whether or not they were present at the exact moment of death, family members usually require reassurance that "everything was done."

Each family member has an individual response to death, and the caregiver must carefully observe and respond to these needs. A few common themes do emerge during this period: (1) ambivalence about seeing the person immediately following death; (2) how to tell other family members; and (3) beginning preparation for funeral arrangements. Family members will look to the caregiver as the "expert," and will require assistance in working through and arriving at decisions that are most meaningful for them. During the first few weeks following the death, family members usually have the support of their extended family and friends. While not essential, if members of the health care team have had an extended, intensive relationship with the deceased and family, attending the funeral or memorial service has salutary effects for everyone. The family welcomes the recognition of their needs and the respect for their dead, and the caregiver has an opportunity to "say good-bye."

To help facilitate the grieving process, the bereaved may get involved in grief counseling. Worden (1982) discusses four tasks that the bereaved must complete and the corresponding four goals for grief counseling:

Task	*Goal*
1. To accept the reality of the loss.	1. To increase the reality of the loss.
2. To experience the pain of grief	2. To help the counselee deal with both expressed and latent affect.

3. To adjust to an environment in which the deceased is missing.	3. To help the counselee overcome various impediments to readjustment after the loss.
4. To withdraw emotional energy and reinvest it in another relationship.	4. To encourage the counselee to make a healthy emotional withdrawal from the deceased and to feel comfortable reinvesting that emotion in another relationship.

In order to accomplish these goals, Worden presents a number of guidelines for the counselor: (1) Help the survivor actualize the loss by allowing the survivor to talk about the loss; (2) Help the survivor identify and express feelings. It is important to allow the bereaved to express anger, guilt, anxiety, helplessness, and sadness; (3) Assist living without the deceased by helping the survivor make decisions; (4) Facilitate emotional withdrawal from the deceased by encouraging the bereaved to form new relationships; (5) Provide time to grieve by recognizing that grieving takes time and that certain dates, such as birthdays and Christmas, may be especially difficult; (6) Interpret normal behavior by reassuring the bereaved that what they are going through is not "craziness"; (7) Allow for individual differences; (8) Provide continuing support; (9) Examine defenses and coping style, particularly those that may be hurtful such as using alcohol; (10) Identify pathology and refer—some people may need more intensive therapy and the counselor should make sure that these people are referred appropriately. By following these principles, the counselor can help the bereaved come to terms with the loss and go on with his life.

The bereaved may choose to become part of a self-help group. One example is the Widow-to-Widow program developed by Phyllis Silverman (1972, 1977b; Silverman et. al., 1974, 1986). These programs are run by volunteers who are widowed and who are willing to use their experience to help others. "Those who participate in a Widow-to-Widow program are learning to deal with the transition as a means of preventing problems at a later date. They learn to cope, to find hope and to look forward to a future" (Silverman, 1977a, p. 270).

SUMMARY ❧

Most of us are ill prepared for experiencing grief. Grief consists of different phases: shock and numbness, intense grief, and reorganization. Associated with grief are various physical symptoms. The mortality rate of the bereaved is higher than the mortality rate of similar married men and women.

People may experience anticipatory grief. However, researchers have found contradictory results as to whether the effects of anticipatory grief are positive or negative.

The bereaved must face various other problems, depending upon their age and sex. Therapeutic intervention by a professional or a self-help group may help the bereaved come to terms with their grief.

LEARNING EXERCISES ❧

1. Make a survey of services in your community for the bereaved. What do your findings indicate about treatment of the bereaved?
2. Would you prefer to die before your spouse? Explain your response.
3. With regard to anticipatory grief—would you prefer for someone you love to die a sudden death or after a long-term illness?
4. Reexamine what your family's financial status would be if you or your spouse died. For example, do you have adequate life insurance?

AUDIOVISUAL MATERIAL ❧

A Family Again. 47 minutes/videocassette/1989. Coronet/ MTI Film and Video, 108 Wilmot Road, Deerfield, IL, 60015.
Dramatization of a family going through the grieving process after the death of their oldest daughter. The video shows the difficulties of family members helping each other to grieve.

A Family in Grief: The Ameche Story. 26 minutes/videocassette/1987. Research Press, Box 3177, Dept. 84, Champaign, IL, 68121.
The Ameche family shares their feelings and thoughts six months after their 22-year-old son (and brother) died.

The Pitch of Grief. 30 minutes/videocassette/1985. Fanlight Productions, 47 Halifax Street, Boston, MA, 02130.
In depth interviews with four grieving adults show the process of bereavement.

The Rebellion of Young David. 26 minutes/videocassette/1986. Beacon Films, P.O. Box 575, Norwood, MA, 02062.
A widower learns to express his grief through his relationship with his growing son.

REFERENCES ❧

Aldrich, C. K. (1974). Some dynamics of anticipatory grief. In B. Schoenberg, A. C. Carr, A. Kutscher, D. Perez, & I. Goldberg (Eds.), *Anticipatory grief.* New York: Columbia University Press.

Anderson, R. (1974). Notes of a survivor. In S. Troup & W. Green (Eds.), *The patient, death and the family.* New York: Scribners.

Bornstein, P. E., Clayton, P. J., Halekas, J., & Robins, E. (1973). The depression of widowhood after thirteen months. *British Journal of Psychiatry, 122,* 561–566.

Bowlby, J. (1971). *Attachment and loss (Vol 1): Attachment.* Hammondsworth: Pelican Books, 1971.

Bowlby, J. (1975). *Attachment and loss (Vol 2): Loss.* Hammondsworth: Pelican Books, 1975.

Bowlby, J. (1980). *Attachment and loss (Vol 3): Loss: Sadness and depression.* New York: Basic Books.

Bowling, A., & Cartwright, A. (1982). *Life after a death.* London: Tavistock Publications.

Campbell, S. (1987). *Widower.* New York: Prentice Hall.

Ciocco, A. (1940). On mortality in husbands and wives. *Human Biology, 12,* 508.

Clayton, P. J., Halikas, J. A., Maurice, W. I., & Rubias, E. (1973). Anticipatory grief and widowhood. *British Journal of Psychiatry, 122,* 47–51.

Crile, G. (1969). Memorial Service, Kent Road, Cleveland Heights. In A. Kutscher, (Ed.) *Death and bereavement.* Springfield, IL: Charles C. Thomas.

Dersheimer, R. (1990). *Counseling the bereaved.* New York: Pergamon Press.

Doka, K. (1989). *Disenfranchised grief.* Lexington, MA: Lexington Books.

Engel, G. (1961). Is grief a disease? *Psychosomatic Medicine, 23,* 18–22.

Epstein, G., Weitz, L., Roback, H., & McKee, E. (1975). Research on bereavement: A selection and critical review. *Comprehensive Psychiatry, 16,* 537–546.

Freud, S. (1959). *Mourning and Melancholia.* Collected papers (Vol 4). New York: Basic Books.

Futterman, E., & Hoffman, I. (1973). Crisis and adaptation in the families of fatally ill children. In E. J. Anthony & C. Koupernick (Eds.), *The child in his family: Vol 2. The impact of disease and death* (pp. 127–143). Yearbook of the International Association for Child Psychiatry and Allied Professions. New York: Wiley.

Gerber, I. (1975). *The widower and the family.* Paper presented at the Second Annual Interdisciplinary Educational Conference on Bereavement and Grief, Yeshiva University, New York.

Gerber, I., Rusalen, R., Hannon, N., Batter, D., & Arkin, A. (1975). Anticipatory grief and aged widows and widowers. *Journal of Gerontology, 30,* 225–229.

Haig, R. A. (1990). *The anatomy of grief.* Springfield, IL: Charles C. Thomas.

Hollinger, R. (1980). Parents of murdered children need special grief work. *Thanatology Today, 2,* 3.

Holmes, T. H., & Rahe, R. H. ( ). The social readjustment rating scale. *Journal of Psychosomatic Research, 11,* 213–18.

Horowitz, M., Wilner, N., Marmar, C., & Kerupnick, J. (1980). Pathological grief and activation of latent self-images. *American Journal of Psychiatry, 137,* 1157–62.

Klass, D., & Marwit, S. J. (1988–89). Toward a model of parental grief. *Omega: Journal of Death and Dying, 19* (1), 31–50.

Kreis, B., & Pattie, A. (1969). *Up from grief.* New York: Seabury Press.

Lebow, G. (1976). Facilitating adaptation in anticipatory mourning. *Social Casework, 57* (7), 458–465.

Lewis, C. S. (1961). *A grief observed.* New York: Seabury Press.

Lindemann, E. (1944). Symptomatology and management of acute grief. *American Journal of Psychiatry, 101,* 141–148.

Lopata, H. (1979). *Women as widows.* New York: Elsevier North-Holland.

Maddison, D. (1968). The relevance of conjugal bereavement for preventive psychiatry. *British Journal of Medical Psychology, 41,* 223–233.

Marris, P. (1974). *Loss and change.* New York: Pantheon Books.

Miles, M. S. (1985). Helping adults mourn the death of a child. *Issues in Comprehensive Pediatric Nursing. 8* (1–6), 219–241.

Noli, M. W. (1977). Families in grief: The question of casework intervention. In L. Wilkenfeld (Ed.), *When children die* (pp. 75–83). Dubuque, IA: Kendall/Hunt.

Osterweis, M., Soloman, F., & Green, M. (1984). *Bereavement: Reaction's, consequences and care.* Washington, DC: National Academy Press.

Parkes, C. M., (1964). The effect of bereavement on physical and mental health. *British Medical Journal, 2,* 274–279.

Parkes, C. M. (1972). *Bereavement: Studies of Grief in Adult Life.* New York: International Universities Press.

Parkes, C. M. (1986). *Bereavement* (2nd Ed.). Madison, CT: International Universities Press.

Parkes, C. M., & Weiss, R. (1983). *Recovery from bereavement.* New York: Basic Books.

Rando, T. A. (1983). An investigation of grief and adaptation in parents whose children have died from cancer. *Journal of Pediatric Psychology, 8,* 3–20.

Rando, T. A. (1986). A comprehensive analysis of anticipatory grief, perspectives, processes, promises and problems. In T. A. Rando (Ed.), *Loss and anticipatory grief.* Lexington, MA: Lexington Books.

Raphael, B. (1983). *The anatomy of bereavement.* New York: Basic Books.

Raphael, B., and Maddison, D. (1976). The care of bereaved adults. In O. W. Hill (Ed.), *Modern trends in psychosomatic medicine.* London: Butterworth.

Rees, W. D. (1975). The bereaved and their hallucinations. In B. Schoenberg, I. Gerber, A. Wiener, A. Kutscher, D. Peretz, & A. Carr (Eds.), *Bereavement: Its psychosocial aspects.* New York: Columbia University Press.

Schwab, J. J., Chalmer, J. M., Conroy, S., Farris, D., & Markush, R. (1975). Studies in grief: A preliminary report. In B. Schoenberg, I. Gerber, A. Wiener, A. Kutscher, D. Peretz, & A. Carr (Eds.), *Bereavement: Its psychosocial aspects.* New York: Columbia University Press.

Selye, H. (1976). *The stress of life.* New York: McGraw-Hill.

Silverman, P. (1972). Widowhood and preventive intervention. *The Family Coordinator, 21,* 95–102.

Silverman, P. (1977) Bereavement as a normal life transition. In E. Prichard, J. Collard, B. Orcutt, A. Kutscher, I. Seeland, & N. Lefkowitz, (Eds.), *Social work with the dying patient and the family.* New York: Columbia University Press.

Silverman, P., (Ed.). (1974). *Helping each other in widowhood.* New York: Health Sciences.

Silverman, P. (1986). *Widow-to-Widow.* New York: Springer Publishing.

Simos, B. (1977). Grief therapy to facilitate healthy restitution. *Social Casework,* June, *58* (6), 337–344.

Stroebe, W., & Stroebe, M. (1989). *Bereavement and health.* Cambridge, England: Cambridge University Press.

Tietz, W., McSherry, L., & Britt, B. (1977). Family sequelae after a child's death due to cancer. *American Journal of Psychotherapy. 31* (3), 417–424.

Vaclon, M., Rogers, J., Lyall, W., Lancree, W., Sheldon, A., & Freeman, S. (1982). Predictors and correlates of high distress in adaptation to conjugal bereavement. *American Journal of Psychiatry, 139,* 998–1002.

Wiener, A., Gerber, I., Battin, D., & Arken, A. (1975). The Process and phenomenology of bereavement. In B. Schoenberg, K. Berber, A. Wiener, A. Kutscher, D. Peretz, and A. Carr (Eds.), *Bereavement: its psychosocial aspects*. New York: Columbia University Press.

Worden, W. (1982). *Grief counseling and grief therapy*. New York: Springer Publishers.

Wortman, C., & Silver, R. (1989). The myths of coping with loss. *The Journal of Counseling & Clinical Psychology, 57*, 349–357.

Wyler, J. (1988). Grieving alone: A single mother's loss. *Issues in Comprehensive Pediatric Nursing, 12* (4), 299–302.

Young, M., Benjamin, B., & Wallis, C. (1963). The mortality of widowers. *Lancet, 2*, 454–456.

Zesook, S., Devaul, R., & Click, M. (1982). Measuring symptoms of grief and bereavement. *American Journal of Psychiatry, 139*, 1590–1593.

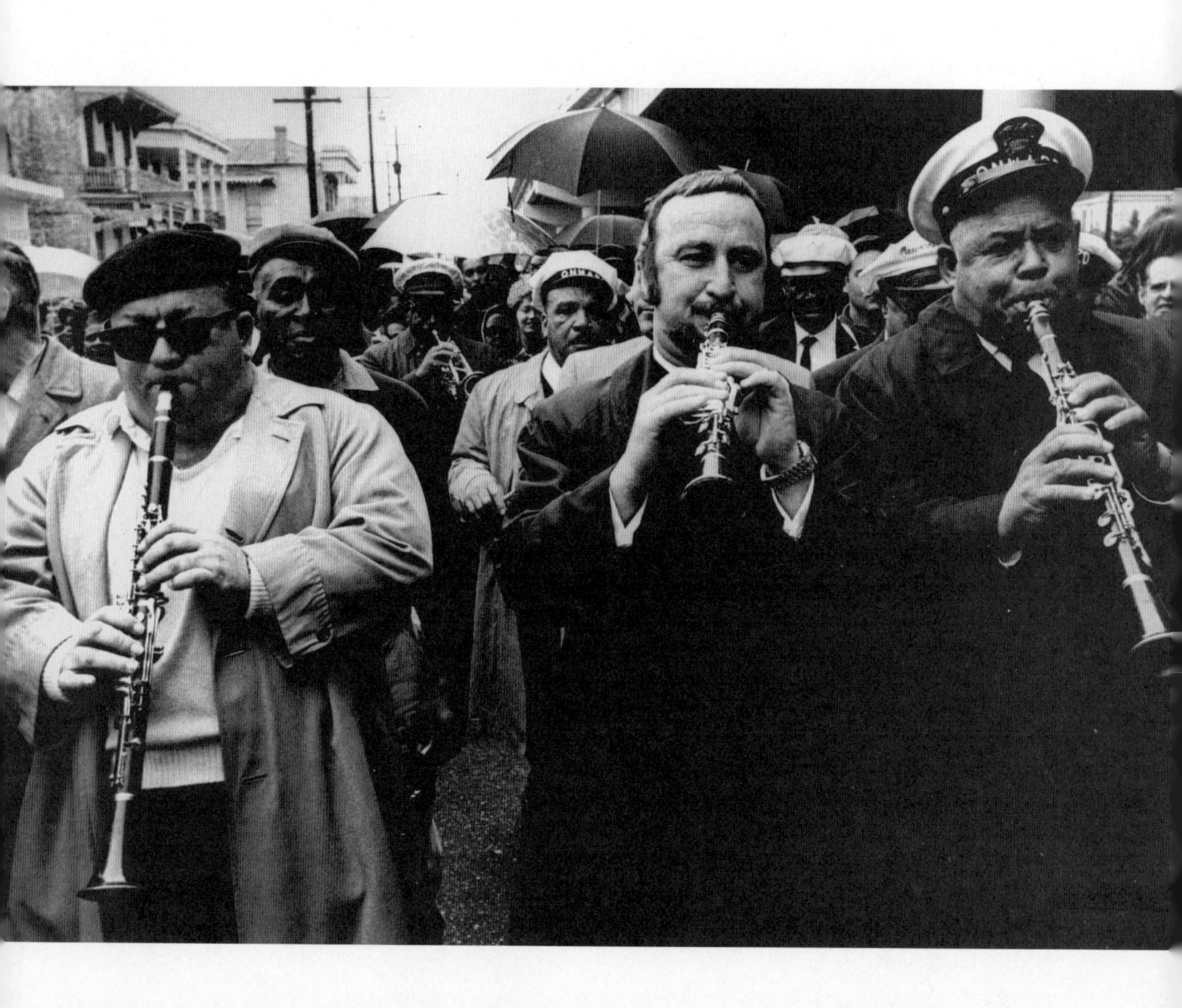

Chapter 11

Funerals

The body of the deceased, lying in a casket, is placed in a reception room of a funeral home where family and friends come to pay their last respects. A ceremony, generally religious, is held eulogizing the deceased. A funeral cortege then leaves the funeral home or place of worship to go to the cemetery where another ritual is held in order to bury the deceased. Friends and family then go and share a meal together.

At the end of life, the funeral ceremony serves as the beginning of the grieving process for the survivors. The funeral serves to reinforce the integration of the community, the family, the religious group, and the ethnic group while helping the bereaved begin their separation from the deceased (Fulton, 1979, pp. 249–253).

This chapter looks at the funeral in American society. Has it become meaningless? How has the funeral industry influenced the American funeral? What is the role of religion?

Functions of Funerals

Paul Irion (1966) asked whether the funeral has value or is only a vestige of our history. Besides the overt or manifest function of disposing of the body, the funeral performs other more covert or latent functions for the bereaved and for the society. For the individual, the funeral performs the following functions:

1. It increases the reality of death. One feeling at the beginning of grief is denial; that the person you love could not have died.

Courtesy of William Ransom/Hogan Jazz Archive, Tulane University Library. Photo by Michael P. Smith.

The final rite of the funeral brings home the reality that death has occurred.

2. The funeral provides "consensual validation" for the mourner (Irion, 1976), since the mourner is joined by others who are also feeling the loss:

> A young man whose career had been joyously and usefully devoted to human service had died. Entering the church for the funeral service, his stricken parents appeared utterly crushed and forlorn.
>
> In the audience were a large number of young people who had known this man and shared his concerns. The speaker talked of the young man's life and what he stood for and went on to say that his ideals and spirit were alive and growing in each of those present . . . The response of the listeners could be seen in their faces; most of all in the faces of the parents . . . (Morgan, 1988, pp. 72–73)

3. As a commonsense function, the funeral provides the bereaved with something to do (Cassem, 1976). It provides specific role behaviors so that the bereaved does not have to think about how she should act. The bereaved must meet with the funeral director, set up the funeral, and follow the appropriate ritual.
   Studies on the effect of participation in funeral arrangements and grief show that, although no relationship was found between participation and adjustment a year after the death, the majority of respondents did report that participation in the funeral arrangements helped with their grief (Doka, 1984–85; Bolton & Camp, 1986–87). For example, one man reported: "It was comforting to be able to talk about her favorite songs and Bible verses, it brought back a lot of memories," (Doka, 1984–85, p. 123).
4. The funeral also provides the bereaved with support during the beginnings of grief by providing a network of relationships to which they may turn.
5. The funeral helps people gain a greater perspective on life and death. It is a time when survivors may affirm their own values since funerals are "a necessary series of interactions which help realize death, a social reality, and the promise that we, too, shall die" (Weissman, 1976, p. xv).
6. The memory of the deceased gets rehabilitated. When an older person, or someone with a long, painful illness, dies, the funeral serves as a reminder of who the person once was (Morgan, 1988,

p. 73). Furthermore, the tributes paid to the deceased, which emphasize the worth of the person, show the bereaved that the deceased is worthy of the pain that is being felt (Cassem, 1976).

The funeral is important for the society because it performs the following functions:

1. The funeral reaffirms the cohesiveness of the family. The joke that people in a family only see each other at funerals stresses this function. It is a time when family members come together in a unit to partake in a ritual. By doing so, they visibly demonstrate the importance of family networks in the society while showing the bereaved that they are not alone.
2. The funeral acts as a mirror of the values and expectations we have of each other (Weissman, 1976). For example, in our society we value self-control, discipline and self-reliance. At funerals, we admire those people who behave in this manner, thus reaffirming certain values in the society.
3. A funeral may reinforce the social order. When well-known persons in positions of power or prestige die, the funeral may become a public event where the people in the society pay homage not only to the deceased but to the position he once held. When John F. Kennedy died, the American people participated in his funeral through television. This not only allowed us to mourn the man but also made us aware of the importance of the presidency.
4. Funerals also reaffirm religious and ethnic identity. The majority of funerals are religious ceremonies; even those people who do not attend a church or synagogue often choose a religious ceremony for their death. Ethnic group identity is also important. For example, although the majority of Irish and Italian people are Roman Catholics, their funerals reflect ethnic differences. An Italian wake and funeral are much more somber than an Irish wake and funeral where there may be a great deal of eating and talking.
5. Funerals serve as rites of passage. They are ceremonies marking the transition from one status to another status (Van Gennap, 1960). There are three phases: separation from the previous status, transition to the new status, and incorporation into the new status. It is a rite of passage both for the deceased and the bereaved. Separation between the deceased and the living is seen at the committal rites, when the deceased is buried. The transition stage occurs during the funeral; it is a way of maintaining a relationship with the deceased. After the funeral,

there are rites to incorporate the newly deceased with the dead. This can occur in prayers said for the soul of the deceased.

The funeral also serves to incorporate a bereaved spouse into the family and the community, although he or she is assuming a new status as widow or widower.

A critique of funerals today is that they no longer have value. Yet as we look at the functions of the funeral, we see how valid the funeral still is both for society and for the individual. Although the whole community may no longer totally participate in the funeral, family and friendship networks do. Funerals provide the bereaved with a sense of community while reestablishing the importance of primary networks to the larger community. Those who say that the funerals of yesterday were worth more because they were simpler and less extravagant are probably idealizing history.

History of the American Funeral

Extravagance in funerals always existed in our country, except for a short time after the Pilgrims settled here. When the Puritans arrived in New England, the dead were buried with an absence of ceremony and a lack of emotion (Stannard, 1977, p. 103). Since the soul was already at its predestined fate, the body was thought of as meaningless. Funeral sermons were no different than other sermons, and were not delivered upon burial. No religious prayers were said for the deceased, for fear that praying for the deceased would lead people to believe the Catholic doctrine of purgatory, rather than the Puritan belief of predestination (Harmer, 1963, p. 70). However, according to Stannard (1977), this lack of ritual lasted for only about two decades. In 1649 the Boston Artillery officers requested:

> one barrell and a halfe of the countryes store of powder to acknowledge Boston's great worthy dew love & respects to the late honoured Govner [John Winthrop], which they manifested in solemnizing his funerall (Shurtleff as cited in Stannard, 1977, p. 110).

These cannon may have symbolized the beginning of extravagant funerals in New England.

For the Puritans in the latter half of the seventeenth century, funerals became very elaborate. The body of the deceased was washed and dressed, and the body was laid out in the home or in the church. Gloves were sent to those people who were invited to the funeral. According to Harmer (1963, p. 70), one Boston minister collected 2,940 pairs of gloves in thirty years, which he then sold for a substantial sum. It was important for coffins to be properly lined and made of good wood. After the burial, a feast was held at the home or church, at which time people were given gold funeral rings to mark their attendance.

The funerals were obviously very costly; "even in the cases of the wealthiest individuals, it was not uncommon for funeral expenses to consume 20 percent of the deceased's estate" (Stannard, 1977, p. 113).

In order to control the giving of gloves and rings, which was becoming a financial burden, government regulations came into effect. In 1721, Massachusetts passed a "law which forbade the giving of scarves, gloves (except six pairs to the bearers and one pair to the minister), wine, rum and rings" (Harmer, 1963, p. 70).

In other colonies, such as New York and Virginia, funerals were just as extravagant if not more so:

> It is said that the obsequies of the first wife of Hon. Stephen Van Rensselaer (of Albany) cost twenty thousand dollars. Two thousand linen scarfs were given, and all the tenants were entertained for several days (Earle, 1977, p. 34).

The poor also had elaborate funerals. The following is a list of expenses for the funeral of one Ryseck Swarb, which was taken care of by the church (Earle, 1977, p. 35):

Funeral Items	**Guilders**
3 dry boards for a coffin	7
3/4 lb. nails	1
Making coffin	24
Cartage	10
Half a vat & an anker of good beer	27
1 gallon rum	21
6 gallons madeira for women and men	84
Sugar and cruyery	5
150 sugar cakes	15
Tobacco and pipes	5
Grave digger	30
Use of pall	10
Wife Jan Lockermans	36
	275

After the American Revolution, funerals continued to be elaborate in the cities, although there were laws limiting the amount that could be spent. However, in the Western territories and in rural areas, funerals were simpler out of necessity. The family was a participant in the funeral ritual. The deceased was washed by the family and viewed in the home. The family wagon served as a hearse. This is the "ideal" funeral envisioned by those who tend to wish for the way things were. However, this occurred for only a proportion of the population and only lasted until the Civil War.

As studied by Farrell (1980), four major changes occurred in the funeral between 1850 and 1920. They were in the care of the body, the container of the body, the places of the funeral, and the funeral procedures.

In the care of the body, embalming came into practice. During the Civil War, families of dead soldiers wanted them brought home for burial. This was an opportunity for embalmers to descend on the battle areas to preserve the remains of the deceased: "The war gave the opportunity for further experimentation, a measure of perfection in the process, and a foothold for a full-time vocation" (Bowman, 1959, p. 117). With embalming came an emphasis on the body for the funeral ritual.

At the same time, casket manufacturers began to create sophisticated products. In 1848 Almond Fisk came up with a casket that would prevent putrefaction—a metallic burial case. The demand for this type of coffin led to its mass production. By 1889, there were 194 coffin factories and one could choose from over 100 casket styles. Gone was the small coffin shop and the demand on local cabinetmakers to make coffins (Harmer, 1963, pp. 91–92).

The funeral itself moved from the family "parlor" to the funeral "parlor." As pointed out by Farrell (1980, p. 173), this came about, not because of the need for space to embalm (funeral directors carried embalming kits with them) nor because of smaller homes. Rather, funeral homes developed because of the push by the funeral director to have "a consolidation of three functional areas, the clinic, the home and the chapel, into a single operational unit" (Farrell, 1980, p. 173).

"With modifications in all the accouterments of the funeral, changes in the funeral itself were virtually inevitable" (Farrell, 1980, p. 177). The funeral service became shorter. An effort was made to "degloom" the funeral (Nichols, 1979, p. 387).

Flowers came into fashion at funerals, though they were strongly opposed. Flowers were viewed as pagan and wasteful. As Haberstein & Lamers (1955) point out, the opposition was to the extensive use of flowers.

Mourning cards became popular. These were cards given to friends at the funeral that expressed hopeful views of death such as the following:

> There is no death. What seems so is transition;
> This life of mortal breath
> Is but the suburb of the life elysian,
> Whose portal we call death.*

The words used in funerals changed (Nichols, 1979, p. 387):

"Undertaker" is now "funeral director."

The "morgue" is the "preparation room."

---

*The Mourning Card of James Pelling; quoted in Haberstein & Lamers, 1955, p. 401.

"Graveyard" is now "cemetery."

A "coffin" is now a "casket."

The "tombstone" is now called a "monument."

Today, we are combining the extravagance of the Colonial funeral with the beautification of the nineteenth century funeral. A major difference, though, is that the undertaker has truly become the "director" of the funeral (Kearl, 1989, p. 272).

The Funeral Industry

The funeral industry is a seven-billion-dollar-a-year business (Kearl, 1989, p. 271). There are approximately 22,000 funeral homes in the United States, ranging from small, family-owned homes to those owned by large conglomerates. The largest company, Service Corporation International, owns 300 funeral homes, 75 cemeteries, 50 flower stores, and a casket manufacturer. They have projected earnings of $28 million on sales of $215 million (Morgan, 1988, p. 47). A small, family-owned funeral home may do less than 60 funerals yearly, with an average profit of about $30,000.

A typical funeral costs about $3,500, with many frequently exceeding $5,000 (Micheli, 1988, p. 143). Included in the funeral prices are removal of the body; use of the hearse and other limousines; arranging for the burial permit, death benefits, newspaper death notices, and religious services; arranging and caring for the flowers; and providing a guest register and acknowledgment cards. There are additional costs for the burial and vault (Consumers Union, 1977, p. 32).

How are the expenses justified? The Funeral Directors Services Association of Greater Chicago (1980) explains that the funeral director charges only about 10 percent above the costs of maintaining a funeral home, salaries of personnel, and merchandise costs. It is considered important to have an elegant, comfortable funeral home. One director told the authors how proud he was of his new funeral home, which had fireplaces in each of the viewing rooms and comfortable Colonial-style furniture. He also pointed out that his business tripled when he moved into the new funeral home. People apparently wanted to have funerals in an attractive setting.

Personnel, the major operating expense, may consist of any number of undertakers, receptionists, and managers, who must be on call 24 hours a day. The costs of an average funeral also must help pay for services provided for the indigent and for the credit extended to those who cannot pay immediately. The funeral director feels that she is performing a service for the community that very few want to do, preparing and taking care of the deceased's body.

There is a great deal of ambivalence concerning the funeral industry. In the 1960s and 1970s, the funeral industry came under major criticism. Jessica Mitford (1963) gave example after example of unethical funeral practices where the bereaved were pressured into spending more than they could afford. In 1978, the *New York Times* found similar abuses. Yet, a Federal Trade Commission study in the 1970s found that during a time period covering ten million funerals, only 1,000 complaints were registered against the funeral industry, a .0001 percent level of consumer complaint (DeSpelder & Strickland, 1983).

A Gallup poll reported by Kearl (1989, p. 278) found that Americans rated funeral directors just above lawyers, politicians, and business executives on honesty and ethical standards. But, studies of clients of funeral homes have shown them to be generally happy with the funeral directors they have used.

Most of the 68 widows and widowers studied by Glick, Weiss, & Parkes (1974) *generally* felt that the funeral director was supportive. Phyllis Silverman, who has worked extensively with widows, reported that widows found the funeral director to be more helpful than the physician or the clergyman (Dempsey, 1975, p. 173). In a study directed at finding out specifically how the bereaved felt about the funeral and the funeral director, Khlief (1975) consistently found that the bereaved thought highly of the funeral director, were satisfied with the funeral costs, and were happy with the presentation of the body.

Fulton's study (1965) of the attitudes of the American public had similar findings; most had positive attitudes toward the funeral director. Many of those with negative attitudes had little direct information about funerals. Fulton concludes that some of the anger we may feel toward the funeral director is anger toward death:

> The guilt generated by desire on the part of the bereaved to rid themselves quickly of the body and by the death itself, the possible confusion and anxiety in the selection of the "right" casket, and the attitude of the funeral director as the constant reminder and associate of death, prompt the public to lash out at him (p. 101).

Funeral Costs

Funeral costs consist of six major parts: professional fees, the coffin, embalming, extras, the vault, and the cemetery (Consumers Union, 1977).

Consumers are protected by the Funeral Rule of the Federal Trade Commission (1982), which went into effect in 1984. This rule provides the consumer with the right to receive telephone price disclosures; a general price list for inquiry purposes; and an itemized statement with the total cost of funeral goods and services. Funeral directors are prohibited from giving inaccurate information regarding embalming, caskets, and body preservation claims.

Professional Services. This is an arbitrary fee generally in the range of $900 for the services of the funeral director. It includes arrangements and supervision of the funeral and a share of the funeral director's overhead.

The Coffin or Casket. The price of the coffin will play a large part in determining the price of the funeral and the profits of the funeral director. Generally, the greater the price of the coffin, the higher the profit for the funeral director. Coffins may be arranged in the selection room so that the consumer will not purchase the cheapest one. Wilber Krieger developed the approach in his book Successful Funeral Management (as discussed in Consumers Union, 1977, pp. 72–75; and Mitford, 1963, pp. 24–26). It is a method of arranging coffins so that the consumer will generally spend slightly above the average; the coffins are divided by price into four quartiles. In the "Avenue of Approach" are those caskets that sell for more than the median, in the third quartile; to the left is an aisle called "Resistance Lane," which has the cheapest caskets on the left and most expensive ones on the right. The contrast between the two sets is so great that the buyer usually ends up purchasing a casket for slightly above the average price. The "carefully planned strategy of the display room allows as much freedom of choice as a loaded gun" (Consumers Union, 1977, p. 74).

Embalming. Embalming involves replacing the blood of the deceased with formaldehyde in order to preserve the body. This allows the body to be displayed in an open coffin. The major rationale for embalming and restoration is that it allows viewing of the body. There is much debate as to whether this is psychologically helpful. Some thanatologists believe that viewing the body gives people a chance to say goodbye to the deceased. It is claimed that it also facilitates realization of the death, since the bereaved are seeing the deceased laid out in the coffin. Others believe that viewing the body places too much emphasis on the "lifeless shell" and not on who the person actually was. Since the goal of restoration is to make the deceased as lifelike as possible, viewing may actually postpone the reality of death. The findings of Parkes (1972, pp. 152–153) illustrate the debate. Eight widows viewed the corpses of their husbands. Three had unpleasant memories of it, while four were pleased. (One expressed no reaction.) They referred to how peaceful the corpse looked. Similar findings appeared in a study of Boston widows and widowers (Glick, Weiss, & Parkes, 1974). Half the widows and a quarter of the widowers were upset by viewing the corpse; the others were not.

Embalming is not mandated by state law except under certain circumstances—if the body is to be transported on a common carrier or, in some states, if death occurs from a communicable disease or if burial does not take place within a certain time limit. Many states consider refrigeration an alternative to embalming.

One undisputed fact is that embalming is important for the funeral industry. It is not important in and of itself; embalming is not a major funeral cost. It is important because it permits viewing of the body and all the extra expenses associated with it.

Extras. Extras include burial clothes, flowers, limousines, out-of-town transportation of the body; that is, anything that is not part of the casket, the embalming, or the cemetery. These items can add hundreds of dollars to the total.

Vaults. Vaults are containers that enclose the coffin in the ground. They are not required by law, although they may be required by cemeteries since they keep the ground from collapsing when the coffin disintegrates. Vaults may be purchased either through the cemetery or the funeral director; they are generally less expensive when purchased through the cemetery.

Cemetery Costs. Cemetery expenses of about $1,500 include the plot itself, the grave marker, and opening and closing the burial plot.

The following is an actual bill for a funeral in 1990 in Rockland County, a suburb of New York City:

Poplar casket	$875
Enclosure, pine	100
Removal of body	185
Embalming	200
Use of funeral home—two days	345
Arrangements, supervision	800
Use of hearse	205
Use of limousine	185
Acknowledgment cards	60
Twelve transcripts of death certificate at $5	60
Gratuities	40
	$3,055

The preceding was considered a modest funeral for the community, not including cemetery charges.

Why do Americans spend so much on funerals? According to Pine & Phillips (1971), "monetary expenditures have taken on added importance as a means for allowing the bereaved to express (both to themselves and others) their sentiments for the deceased" (p. 138). Extravagance at funerals may be a way of assuaging guilt. As a widower quoted in Taylor (1979) remarked: "Her death left unfinished business between us and it comforted me to spend more than I could afford on the funeral" (p. 379). An expensive funeral is a way to communicate love; it may be an attempt to gain social status; or it may be another indication of our standard of living (Irion, 1966, pp. 55–56). As noted previously, one function of the funeral is to reinforce values, and one American value is consumption. How different is going into debt for a funeral from going into debt for a vacation or a car? It is the American way (Jackson, 1963, p. 85).

For those who wish to lower the costs of funerals, memorial societies help to provide an alternative. Memorial societies are nonprofit organizations formed by consumers that assist people in "achieving simplicity, dignity and economy" in their funerals. They do not conduct funerals but help people in arranging them. According to Consumers Union (1977, pp. 214–219), there are three different types of memorial societies. A *contract society* has a contract with at least one undertaker to provide society members with funerals at less than regular costs; the undertaker makes a profit by having a higher volume. A *cooperating society* has an understanding between the undertaker and the society to provide lower-cost funerals, but there is no formal agreement. An *advisory society* acts as an information center. Anyone may join a memorial society for a fee of about $15.

The Religious Funeral

Even though religion may not be as important in people's lives as it once was, it is still important in death. The nonreligious funeral is still in the minority. Each religion has its own structure and beliefs concerning death.

Catholicism

Although there are ethnic differences, the Roman Catholic funeral generally follows a specific ritual. The first part of the ritual, the wake, is the vigil before the funeral. Generally lasting two days, it is the time when the community, friends, and colleagues come to pay their respects. Flowers are sent and cards are left, announcing that prayers are being said for the deceased. The casket may be open or closed. In the evening, a priest will hold a wake service that will include prayers and readings from the Bible. The rosary may also be said.

The funeral is incorporated in the Mass. A procession by the family will bring the casket to the church from the funeral home. "The casket is covered with a white pall, symbolic of the white robe of baptism. The priest himself wears white vestments, emphasizing the joy of faith that overcomes the sadness of death" (Butler, 1974, p. 106). The paschal candle, representing the new life of Christ, is lighted and placed at the casket. The service consists of prayers, Bible readings, a homily that may include references to the deceased, the Eucharist prayer (which includes a celebration of Christ's death and resurrection, and an offering of the sacrifice), and Communion. A eulogy is not given. The rite of commendation ends the Mass, the last farewell before the body is buried.

The funeral procession proceeds to the cemetery, where a public committal rite is held. The family then returns home. A month after the death, a month's Mass is celebrated. Anniversary Masses are celebrated every year on the anniversary of the death.

For the dying, there is the ritual of anointing. Prior to the Second Vatican Council in 1973, extreme unction, or the last rites, were administered to those who were very near death. Today, the ritual of anointing is performed on anyone considered seriously ill. This allows both the dying person and the family to participate in the ritual. At death, the Viaticum (a special type of Communion) is given. If sudden death occurs, the priest leads the family in prayers.

Catholics believe in life after death. However, before entering the kingdom of heaven, the soul must be purified, and the mystery of love perfected in purgatory. The living offer prayers that the period in purgatory will not last too long, that the soul will not suffer greatly, and that God will take the soul to heaven. The funeral rites celebrate the passage from death to life and the deceased's entering "the fellowship of saints." (For further discussion, see Butler, 1974; and Nowell, 1972).

Judaism

The Jewish system of mourning is based upon the halakah, a detailed system of law that specifies behavior after a death. When death occurs, immediate plans are made for burial. There is a tearing of the mourner's clothes, *terrah,* to symbolize grief. Years ago, every Jewish community had its holy society, the *Chevra Kadisha,* whose charge it was to care for the body of the deceased and to prepare it for the funeral. Today, funeral directors have generally taken over these arrangements. The body is ritually cleansed so that it may enter God's presence in purity. Then, whether rich or poor, since in death all are equal before God, the body is dressed in a white linen shroud.

The presence of a casket at the funeral is required to emphasize the rite of separation; however, viewing is considered disrespectful. The funeral service generally takes place at the funeral home and is officiated by a rabbi. Appropriate psalms are said to give comfort to the bereaved and to glorify the dead. The prayer "El Molay Rachamim" is said, which asks God to have compassion on the soul of the deceased. "The eulogy of the dead (*Hesped*) is usually included in the service to recognize not only that a death has occurred but that a life has been lived" (Grollman, 1974, p. 126).

There is a procession to the cemetery where the burial service is ended. Kaddish, a prayer praising God and praying for the establishment of God's kingdom on earth, is said. The prayer of condolence is also recited: "May the Lord comfort you among all the other mourners of Zion and Jerusalem."

When the mourners arrive home, it is customary for them to wash their hands to ritually cleanse themselves. Neighbors and friends bring food, including hard-boiled eggs, which symbolize the continuation of life. The Shiva period begins; it lasts for seven days. As signs of mourning, the bereaved do not wear leather, and they sit on low stools and cover all mirrors so that they may not be concerned with vanity. A seven-day candle is lighted representing the soul of the deceased.

After Shiva, the bereaved may return to normal activity, but they must avoid places of entertainment for 30 days. This ends the mourning period, except when a parent has died. Then mourning proceeds through the following 11 months, during which Kaddish is said at daily services.

Commemoration of the cemetery plaque is called the unveiling. It occurs after the 30 days of mourning, but before the first anniversary of the death. Every year the anniversary of the death is commemorated by lighting a candle and reciting Kaddish. Memorial prayers are also said at synagogue four times per year: Yom Kippur, Shemini Atzeres, the eighth day of Passover, and the second day of *Shavons.*

Grollman (1974) discusses some concepts Jewish people have regarding death.

1. Death is inevitable.
2. The human spirit does not die: "Man is immortal; in body, through his children; in thought, through the survival of his memory; in influence, by virtue of the continuance of his personality as a force among those who come after him; and ideally, through the identification with the timeless things of spirit" (p. 131).
3. There is some belief that the soul will be rewarded or punished depending upon the life that was led.
4. The dead will be resurrected with the coming of the Messiah.
5. The soul may enter a new body and begin a new life.

Jewish people vary in their beliefs about the last three concepts:

> There are many thoughts, yet none is declared authoritative and final. The tradition teaches, but at the same time seems to say there is much we do not know and still more we have to learn. And even then, only God can completely discern the mysteries of life and death (Grollman, 1974, p. 135).

(For further discussion, see Grollman, 1974; and Riemer, 1974.)

Protestantism

There are many differences among Protestants regarding funerals because of all the various denominations. In order to get a picture of the Protestant funeral, Irion (1966) sent a questionnaire to 160 ministers representing ten major denominations. The following pattern emerged: After the body is prepared by the undertaker, it is first viewed by the family.

Then there is public visitation, which may be a few hours or all afternoon and evening. The funeral is usually held on the afternoon of the third day after the death, in the chapel of the funeral home. One-third of the 2,000 funerals conducted by the ministers questioned by Irion took place in church. Scriptures are read and prayers are said. Generally the scripture passages reflected four themes: "the Christian hope for resurrection, the sustaining power of God, the Christian understanding of death, and the Christian understanding of life" (p. 16). Prayers involved intercession for the bereaved and thanksgiving to God. A funeral sermon is preached that might include references to the deceased.

After the funeral service, there is a procession to the cemetery where a brief committal service is held to signify the breaking of the ties with the dead. Then the bereaved return home. In some communities, a supper may be served by friends and neighbors. One alternative to the traditional service is the memorial service where the casket is not present.

Jordan (1974) presents a good discussion of the Protestant theology of death. As does the funeral ritual, Protestant theology varies from denomination to denomination, from a belief in no afterlife to a belief in reincarnation. However, most beliefs in an afterlife focus on resurrection and immortality. In resurrection, the being enters a new dimension of eternal life; in immortality, the soul continues its existence after death. There are also different views of heaven and hell. Hell is defined by some as a realm of everlasting torment; others do not believe in the existence of hell at all. Heaven is seen as involving communion with God, saints, and other persons. For some, heaven allows for spiritual development, while for others it is a place of passive rest.

Despite the variations, Jordan points out commonalities with which most Protestants agree:

- Death is a mystery, and we cannot fully comprehend the meaning surrounding death.
- Death is a corporate event in the fellowship of believers.
- The impact of death is realized and experienced in the community of faith, and it calls forth the caring resources of the congregation to the bereaved.
- The religious resources and rituals of the faith group are significant to the bereaved in dealing with the death event (p. 83).

Alternatives to the Traditional Funeral

Besides the traditional funeral and burial, there are alternatives for disposition of the body, including cremation, direct disposition, and donation of the body to medical science.

Cremation

Cremation occurs after the funeral ritual unless there is direct cremation—an immediate disposition of the body. In the United States, few people have chosen this alternative. Although cremation has existed throughout history, cremation did not develop in the United States until 1876, when the first American crematory was set up by a Washington physician, primarily for sanitary reasons. But cremation never really became popular. In 1976 only slightly more than seven percent of the dead in the United States were cremated (Consumers Union, 1977, p. 157).

The body is cremated in the container in which it was brought to the crematory. This container may be a regular wooden casket, or it may be pressed wood or cardboard. Generally, the crematory requires a container made from an inflexible material. Once the body has been incinerated, the ashes of the bones are left. These cremated remains are placed in an urn, or a special container, and special care taken that the ashes are properly labeled. Urns may be deposited in a columbarium, a structure attached to a crematory that has recesses in the walls for keeping the cremated remains; they may be buried, or they may be kept on one's mantle.

Most religions in the United States do not oppose cremation, including most Protestant denominations. In a study of 1,100 clergy, the majority of Protestant (61.3 percent) and Catholic clergy (70.2 percent) were neutral towards the practice of cremation. Only the majority of Jewish clergy (78.5 percent) were opposed (Minton, 1981).

Orthodox Judaism prohibits cremation because of the belief in resurrection of the body with the coming of the Messiah. Conservative Judaism is also opposed to cremation, but permits the burial of cremated remains in a Jewish cemetery. Reform Judaism allows cremation.

Two advantages of cremation are that the remains take up less space and that it can be cheaper than burial: a vault is not needed; a coffin is unnecessary; and there are no grave-opening and -closing fees. (However, the funeral service may still be expensive.) The disadvantages are that it is not as familiar a method of disposal, and it does not provide a site to go to in remembering the dead.

As Irion (1966) points out, though the values of cremation and burial may be the same:

> The rapid dissolution of the body indicates with considerable clarity that death has occurred, that relationships have been ended, that things can never again be as they have been in the past (pp. 207–208).

Direct Disposition

The body is transferred directly to either the crematory or the burial ground. It may either be followed by a memorial service or a grave-side committal service. Expenses are low because there is no viewing or embalming.

Donation of the Body to Science

Another choice is to leave one's body to medical science. The Uniform Anatomical Gift Act, approved in 1968 by the National Conference of Commissioners on Uniform State Laws, serves as the basis for legislation in all states for allowing people to leave their bodies, or any part thereof, to medical or dental schools without requiring permission of next of kin. The following is typical of the form that must be completed by a potential donor:

I, ______________________________, in the hope that I may
(Print or Type Your Name Here)

help others, hereby make this anatomical gift, if medically acceptable, to take effect upon my death. I give my entire body for the purposes of transplantation, therapy, medical research or education. Signed by the donor and the following two witnesses in the presence of each other.

______________________ Signature of Donor	______________________ Date of Birth of Donor
1. ______________________ Signature of Witness	2. ______________________ Signature of Witness
______________________ Address (Street and Number)	______________________ Address (Street and Number)
______________________ City, State and Zip Code	______________________ City, State and Zip Code

There is no guarantee that the medical school will accept the body. Also, once the medical school is finished with the body, the final disposition must still be arranged, although the medical school will assume responsibility.

Except for Orthodox and Conservative Judaism, religions approve of donating one's body to a medical school.

SUMMARY ❧

The value of the funeral ritual has been criticized, yet it still performs a number of valuable functions both for the individual and for society. The funeral has been criticized because it has become an extravagant affair; however, throughout our history, funerals have generally been extravagant. Today funeral costs include the funeral director's professional fees, the coffin, embalming, extras, the vault, and the cemetery plot. The funeral industry has been attacked for unethical practices, yet the bereaved tend to find the funeral director helpful.

Religion is still very important in terms of determining funeral ritual. Catholicism and Judaism both have very specific rituals, whereas Protestantism differs by denomination.

In addition to the standard funeral and burial, people may choose to dispose of their bodies through cremation, donation to medical science, or a direct disposition. However, relatively few people in the United States have chosen these alternatives.

One can summarize the chapter by saying that the funeral is not only a vestige of history but is also of contemporary value.

LEARNING EXERCISES ❧

1. Speak to a clergyman about the funeral rites in his religion.
2. Call three funeral homes and ask about their prices. Were they willing to give you the information? How did the prices compare?
3. Debate whether the funeral is a vestige of the past or has present-day value.
4. Fill out the form "Suggestions on Those Who Plan My Funeral" (at end of chapter). Discuss this with members of your family.

AUDIOVISUAL MATERIAL ❧

Eulogy. 25 minutes/videocassette/1986. IFEX Films, 201 West 52nd Street, New York, NY, 10019.
Through the writing of a eulogy, a man and his wife comes to terms with the life and death of his brother.

A Plain Pine Box. 15 minutes/film. United Synagogue of America, Committee on Congregational Standards, 155 Fifth Avenue, New York, NY, 10010.
A sensitive film on traditional Jewish funeral and burial customs in the United States. Each part of the process is explained, emphasizing its symbolic significance and benefit to the mourners.

The National Funeral Directors Association (11121 West Oklahoma Avenue, Milwaukee, WI, 53227) has a number of videos on funerals, including *Hospice and the Funeral Director,* and *Why Study Death?*

REFERENCES ❧

Bolton, C., & Camp, D. (1986–87). Funeral rituals and the facilitation of grief work. *Omega: Journal of Death and Dying, 17,* 86–87.

Bowman, L. (1959). *The American funeral.* Westport, CT: Greenwood Press.

Butler, R. (1974). The Roman Catholic way in death and mourning. In E. Grollman (Ed.), *Concerning death: A practical guide for the living.* Boston: Beacon Press.

Cassem, N. (1976). The first three steps beyond the grave. In V. Pine, A. Kutscher, D. Peretz, R. Slater, R. DeBellis, R. Volk, & D. Cherico (Eds.), *Acute grief and the funeral.* Springfield, IL: Charles C Thomas.

Consumers Union. (1977). *Funerals: Consumers' last rights.* New York: Norton.

Dempsey, D. (1975). *The way we die.* New York: McGraw-Hill.

DeSpelder, L., & Strickland, A. (1983). *The last dance. Encountering death and dying.* Palo Alto, CA: Mayfield Publishing.

Doka, K. (1984–85). Expectation of death, participation in funeral arrangements, and grief adjustment. *Omega: Journal of Death and Dying, 15,* 119–129.

Earle, A. M. (1977). Death ritual in colonial New York. In C. Jackson (Ed.), *Passing, the vision of death in America.* Westport, CT: Greenwood Press.

Farrell, J. J. (1980). *Inventing the American way of death.* Philadelphia, PA: Temple University Press.

Federal Trade Commission. (1987). Consumer guide to the FTC funeral rule. Reprinted in L. Carlson. *Caring for your own dead,* 314–317. Hinesburg, VT: Upper Access Publishers.

Fulton, R. (1965). The sacred and the secular. In R. Fulton (Ed.), *Death and identity.* New York: John Wiley.

Fulton, R. (1979). Death and the funeral in contemporary society. In H. Wass (Ed.), *Dying, facing the facts.* Washington, DC: Hemisphere.

Funeral Directors Service Association. (1980). The funeral: what determines the cost. In J. Fruehling (Ed.), *Sourcebook in death and dying.* Chicago: Marquis Professional Publications, 1982, 347–350.

Glick, I., Weiss, R., & Parkes, C. M. (1974). *The first year of bereavement.* New York: John Wiley.

Grollman, E. (1974). The Jewish way in death and mourning. In E. Grollman (Ed.), *Concerning death: A practical guide for the living.* Boston: Beacon Press.

Haberstein, R., & Lamers, W. (1985). *The history of American funeral directing.* Milwaukee, WI: Bulfin Printers.

Harmer, R. M. (1963). *The high cost of dying.* New York: Collier Books.

Irion, P. (1966). *The funeral: Vestige or value?* Nashville, TN: Abingdon.

Irion, P. (1976). The funeral and the bereaved. In V. Pine, A. Kutscher, D. Peretz, R. Slater, R. DeBellis, R. Volk, & D. Cherico (Eds.), *Acute grief and the funeral.* Springfield, IL: Charles C Thomas.

Jackson, E. (1963). *For the living.* Des Moines, IA: Channel Press.

Jordan, M. (1974). The Protestant way in death and mourning. In E. Grollman (Ed.), *Concerning death: A practical guide for the living.* Boston: Beacon Press.

Kearl, M. C. (1989). *Endings. A sociology of death and dying.* New York: Oxford University Press.

Khlief, B. (1975). Attitudes to the funeral, funeral director and funeral arrangements. In O. Margolis, H. Raether, & A. Kutscher (Eds.), *Grief and the meaning of the funeral.* New York: MSS Information.

Micheli, R. (1988). Paying for the big chill. *Money Magazine,* December, 143–148.

Mitford, J. (1963). *The American way of death.* New York: Simon & Schuster.

Minton, F. (1981). Clergy views of funeral practices. In J. Fruehling (Ed.), *Sourcebook in death and dying.* Chicago: Marquis Professional Publications, 1982, 159–169.

Morgan, E. (1988). *Dealing creatively with death. A manual of death education and simple burial.* Burnsville, NC: Celo Press.

New York Times, April 23, 1978, *1,* 51.

New York Times, April 24, 1978, *1,* B9.

New York Times, April 25, 1978, *1,* 20.

Nichols, C. (1979). Mortuary Operation as a career. In J. Fruehling (Ed.), *Sourcebook in Death and Dying.* Chicago: Marquis Professional Publications, 1982, 384–399.

Nowell, R. (1972). *What a modern Catholic believes about death.* Chicago: Thomas More Press.

Parkes, C. M. (1972). *Bereavement.* New York: International Universities Press.

Pine, V., & Phillips, D. (1971). The cost of dying: A sociological analysis of funeral expenditures. In F. Scott & R. Brewer (Eds.), *Confrontations of death.* Corvallis: Oregon State University.

Riemer, J. (Ed.). (1974). *Jewish reflections on death.* New York: Schocken Books.

Stannard, D. (1977). *The puritan way of death.* Oxford: Oxford University Press.

Taylor, C. (1979). The funeral industry. In H. Wass (Ed.), *Dying, facing the facts.* Washington, DC: Hemisphere.

Van Gennap, A. (1960). *The rites of passage.* Translated by M. Vegedom & G. Caffee. Chicago: University of Chicago Press.

Weissman, A. (1976). Why is a funeral. In V. Pine, A. Kutscher, D. Peretz, R. Slater, R. DeBellis, R. Volk, & D. Cherico (Eds.), *Acute grief and the funeral.* Springfield, IL: Charles C Thomas.

SUGGESTIONS TO THOSE WHO PLAN MY FUNERAL

National Selected Morticians

Use this form wisely. Consider well your entries. Be moderate. Be clear. Remember that you can neither explain nor change your comments after you are gone.

Do not feel compelled to complete this form in full. Keep in mind that you may harm your family by trying to give too much guidance. Help those you love to help themselves.

About My Family and Friends:

These persons should be notified of my death as soon as possible:

Name Relationship Address Telephone Number

____

____

____

____

The following persons because of age, infirmity, or other reasons should be notified personally by their clergyman, a friend, or an associate:

____

____

____

My clergyman is ____________________
My physician is ____________________
My lawyer is ____________________
My funeral director is ____________________

About Personal Data: The following information will be needed for official certification. Accuracy is very important. Claims, benefits, and legal procedures may be involved. This will become a permanent record and could be important to your family many generations hence.

Full Name: ________________________________
First Middle Last

Also any other name, if commonly used ____________

Usual residence: ____________________________
Street number or location if rural

City: ______ County: ______ State: ______ Length of Residence: ______

Birth date: ____________ Birthplace: __________________

Usual occupation: __________ Kind of business or industry: __________

Employer: ____________________ Retired? __________

Spouse: __________________ Birthplace: ____________
Full maiden name

Father: ______________________ Birthplace: __________
Full name

Mother: ______________________ Birthplace: __________
Full maiden name

Social Security Number: ______________________

If ever employed by a railroad, list company and dates:

____

If ever in Armed Services, Service Serial Number: __________

Dates of Service: ______________________

If in Service under any other name: ______________________

Attach a listing of biographical information, family relationships, church, fraternal, vocational, professional, club, or union affiliation, etc. Although not necessarily required, this might be useful.

About My Estate:

I have ☐ I have not ☐ executed a will.

If "yes" it is dated: __________ and will be found: __________

My executor is: ______________________

My bank is: ______________________

I have Safety Deposit Box No. __________ in __________
Bank

It is held jointly with ______________________

Valuable papers not in this box will probably be found: __________

____
(or attach separate notations, if advisable.)

About the Ceremonies:

This form is intended to convey suggestions only. Except as hereinafter provided, your comments will be treated as suggestions only, not binding instructions. Unless otherwise indicated, your family will assume that this is only for their information, that you have not dictated firm decisions, and that they are free either to confirm, or not confirm, your suggestions. It will be ONLY in connection with items that you ENCIRCLE AND INITIAL that it will be considered that your instructions shall prevail insofar as may be possible under the applicable laws.

Unless in conflict with the legal rights of others, I desire that the

preferences of ______________________
name

my __________ shall be given special consideration in connection
relationship

with the ceremonial arrangements. If not possible, I designate

____ under the
name relationship

same conditions.

My preferred clergyman: ____________________

Alternate, if necessary: ____________________

My preferred funeral director: ____________________

Alternate, if necessary: ____________________

I prefer to have the ceremony held at ____________________

____
(church, funeral home, residence or other location)

I desire that final disposition shall be:

☐ Burial in ____________________
Cemetery

Where I do ☐ Do not ☐ Have space.

If you do, describe: ____________________

Where is the cemetery lot certificate? ____________________

☐ Entombment ____________________ Where? ____________________

☐ Cremation . . . Disposition of cremated remains: ____________________

I do ☐ do not ☐ desire to comment on the costs or qualities of caskets, vaults, funeral services, et cetera.

If you do, make appropriate notations: ____________________

____

____

Outline as much detail of the funeral service as you feel necessary. Avoid such terms as "usual" or "customary." Such terms can be meaningless. You might want to suggest such things as scripture, music, or other ceremonial details. If lodge, or other semi-secular services are to be considered, make a notation—but DO NOT specify such preferences UNLESS FULLY DISCUSSED with your family and your clergyman.

____

____

____

You might note here the "little" things which could make a big difference: (Clothing, hairdresser, glasses, bearers, flowers, or anything else) ______

____

____

If you are considering donating tissue or organs from your body for medical research, you should first discuss this thoroughly with your family, your doctor and your funeral director. Ordinarily, such wishes cannot be fulfilled unless preparations are made IN ADVANCE. In any event, your comments on the funeral are still appropriate. Donation does not usually interfere with the body being present for services.

I have ☐ or have not ☐ made payment of any costs. If yes, attach copy of receipt or a notation as to where it will be found.

In subscribing to all the foregoing, I state that I have set forth these suggestions only in a spirit of helpfulness. I recognize that it is impossible for me to anticipate accurately all the circumstances that might affect my funeral. Therefore, excepting only such things as I may have encircled and initialed, the effect of which has already been listed in this folder, I specifically direct that the preferences of my family shall prevail.

Date ______________________________ Signature ______________________________

Copies of this form should be given to persons who will be available and able to act at any time. An extra copy is attached for this purpose. Relatives, close friends, or your clergyman might be considered. If your selection of funeral director is definite, he should have a copy since he or an associate must be constantly available. DO NOT put it in your safety deposit box.

Reprinted with permission from National Selected Morticians, Evanston, Illinois.

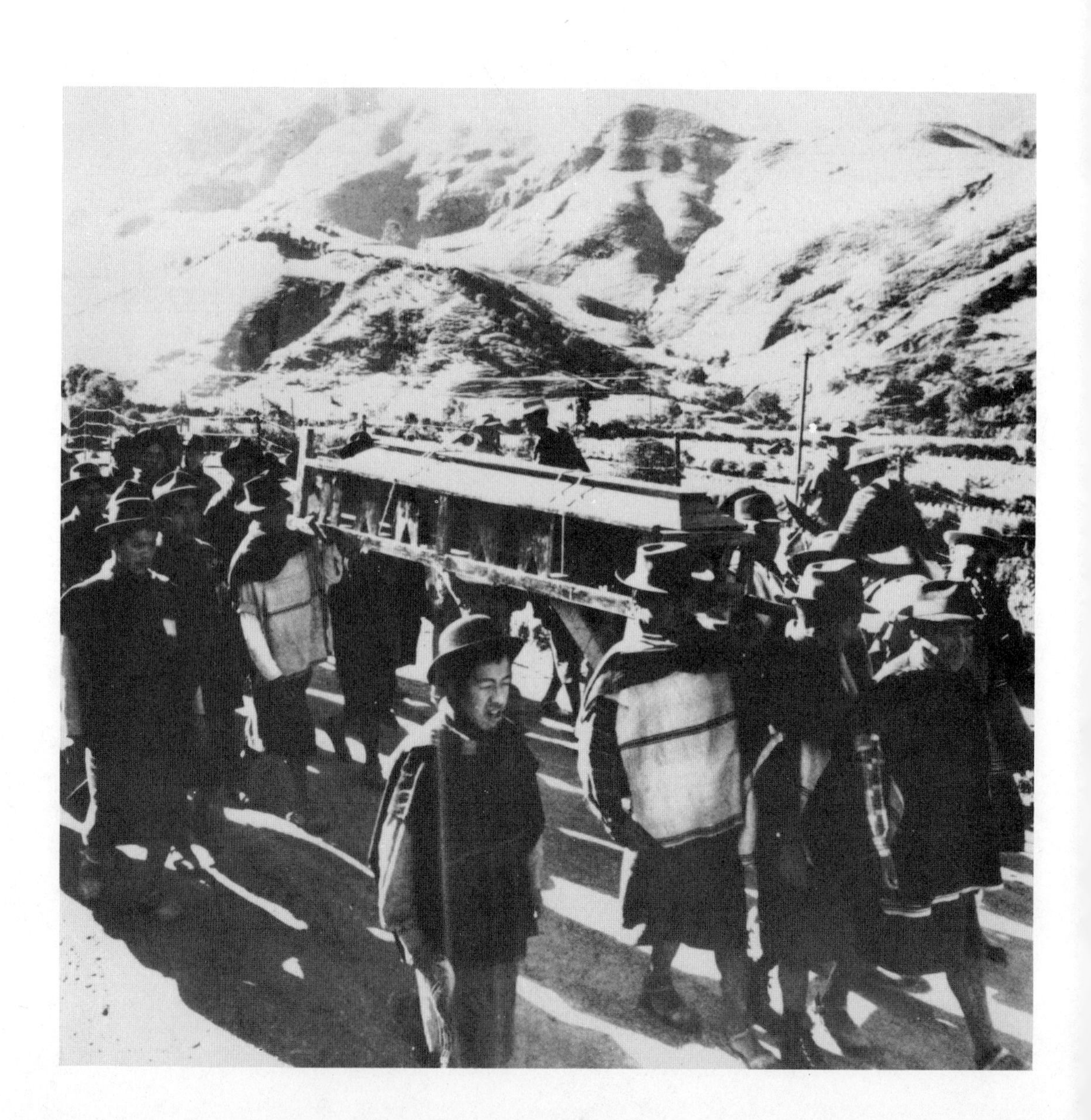

Chapter 12

Death from a Cross-cultural Perspective

Serena Nanda

"Today is a good day to die, for all the things of my life are present."
—Crazy Horse, leader of the Oglala Sioux

Death is universally regarded as a significant event both for the individual and the social group. Every culture provides for its members a way of thinking about death and of responding to it. In all cultures, death is set off by ritual and surrounded by culturally patterned beliefs and social institutions. It is surrounded by an atmosphere of the sacred and approached with intense emotions. This sacredness and intensity of feeling make it difficult to see the role culture plays in shaping not only the beliefs and practices regarding death and dying but also the emotions elicited by these events. Because death is a universal phenomena, but is responded to in different ways in different cultures, we can use our cultural knowledge to understand a society's response to death and also use our knowledge of death beliefs and practices as a way of understanding a society.

This is true for our own society as well as other societies. In the United States, death is probably the most intensely experienced of all human crises, yet also the least talked about. This, in itself, is an indication of our anxiety about it. Indeed, this culturally shaped anxiety about death may partly explain why it is so rarely a focus of our studies of other cultures in spite of its universality and its social and ritual importance almost everywhere in the world (Palgi and Abramovitch, 1984, p. 385).

This chapter attempts to put beliefs, practices, and emotions regarding death and dying in the United States in a cross-cultural perspective, comparing the major dimensions of death, as it is experienced in our own culture, with those of other societies. Many of the most problematic ethical problems of our society raise problems of life and death: the abortion controversy, assisted suicide, the AIDS epidemic. A comparative approach can help us look at our own responses to death and dying more objectively, allowing us to think about alternative responses that might help individuals—and our society—deal with death and dying in a more adequate way.

Death Beliefs

The universality of beliefs and rituals that center on death and the fate of the human soul attest to a human preoccupation with the dying and decaying human body. These diverse beliefs and rituals suggest that all human societies attempt to control death by symbolically imposing order on the universe and thus giving purpose to life. The belief that death is not the end of the person, but rather a passage from the world of the living to another world, or spirit realm, is one found in many cultures. This belief offers an active role to dead persons, viewing them as potential enemies that require propitiation or as potential guardians. In our own society, the influence of a biomedical perspective shapes our belief that death occurs "because our genetic structure requires that people die." And yet we, like other cultures, are uncomfortable with the notion that death means the end of all individual awareness. Honoring the dead by carrying out some of the wishes the individual made in life, suggests that we are ambivalent "about the ability of the dead to remain aware of what we, the living, are doing for them" (Kalish, 1980, p. 2).

Most cultures, however, are much more explicit about their belief that death is but a transition from one social status to another, and that the dead remain in touch with the living (van Gennep, 1960). A society in which conversations between the living and the dead are an important element in everyday life is the Gikuyu of East Africa. Jomo Kenyatta, in *Facing Mt. Kenya* (1965) points out that the term "communion with ancestors," rather than "ancestor worship," most accurately describes the relationship of the living and dead in this society. Because the Gikuyu believe that the spirits of the dead can be pleased or displeased by the behavior of the living and can act accordingly, in a beneficent or spiteful manner, the ceremony of communing with the ancestral spirits is observed constantly in Gikuyu society.

The dead also play important roles in guiding the society of the living. In his fictionalized account of the Ibo of West Africa, Chinua Achebe (1959) describes the traditional importance of the ancestors who are represented in masquerades and who act as judges in the town councils whereby disputes are settled and wrongdoers brought to justice.

In societies where concepts of time are different than our own, and where past, present, and future are merged, beliefs about the continuous relationship of the dead with the living pose no intellectual problem. A dramatic example of this kind of belief is the Dreamtime of the indigenous peoples of Australia. The Dreamtime is that long-ago time when the ancestors created all the animate and inanimate things of the cosmos, including the aboriginal people themselves. In all the important Australian ceremonies, the Dreamtime is recreated through the telling of legends and ritual performances. The Australians believe that each person's spirit came from a clan pool of spirits, entering their mother's womb at the time of conception and returning to the common pool after death. In order to pay this debt of creation to the ancestors, the Australians commemorate the events of the Dreamtime in their great initiation ceremonials. During these performances, the participants believe that they become the totemic ancestors. The Dreamtime is thus both temporal and eternal, forever connecting the living with their historical and legendary ancestors (Elkin, 1964).

A similar belief, connecting the living and dead, exist among the Central Inuit of the Arctic. Here, the name of the last person to die in a settlement is given to the first child born thereafter, and the child is considered the reincarnation of the dead person (Boaz, quoted in Mauss, 1979, p. 28).

Beliefs about death as the passage from one social world to another vary in picturing what the afterworld looks like. In some cases, it is described as an earthly paradise, providing humans with all that they lack in this world. In other cases, the afterworld closely resembles life on earth. Among the Tikopia of Polynesia, for example, the soul makes courtesy visits to ancestral spirits guided by the same rules of etiquette that hold on earth. And, unlike the Christian belief that all souls will be equal in Heaven, in Tikopian belief, the souls of the dead keep their earthly status. The system of clan dwellings, the special position of chiefs and ritual leaders, and the role of the married and the unmarried all broadly reflect Tikopian society. This reproduction of the social system reinforces the belief that not only the individual, but, more importantly, the society will continue even after its present members have died (Firth, 1967).

The social and psychological functions of these widespread beliefs are not difficult to understand. Societies regard themselves as ongoing systems, and the death of any member threatens the very existence of society. As Robert Hertz (1960, p. 78) so eloquently writes, "When a man dies, society loses in him much more than a unit; it is stricken in the very principle of its life, in the faith it has in itself." Death is perceived as antisocial, even unnatural. Society refuses to consider death irrevocable. Death is not seen as simply an end to life; it is also the beginning of a new existence. Thus, the idea of death is linked with that of resurrection–separation followed by a new integration.

Beliefs in an afterlife can be seen as meeting the threat that death makes to the social system. Such beliefs speak to the contradiction that exists between, on the one hand, the continuity of the social system as a system of norms, groups, and beliefs and, on the other hand, the impermanence of its personnel—the conflict between the mortality of the human body and the immortality of the larger social body. In Western thought, life is identified with individuality and death is threatening because it ends this differentiation. Hence the importance of grave monuments that identify us as individuals. Indeed, even science is influenced by this cultural anxiety: archaeologists use grave-goods and skeletal data to reconstruct as many of the individual features of the dead as possible, and the current concern of physical anthropologists with the survival of genes also is related to the Western interest in the transmission of individualizing features from generation to generation. As one scientist has commented "As an ideology of death . . . [this] seems distinctly bizarre." (Humphreys, 1981:6). Certainly, from a comparative, cross-cultural and historical perspective, contemporary Western beliefs, which emphasize the discontinuities between past and present, the separation of the living and the dead, and the integrity of the individual soul and personality at the expense of the continuation of the community and the universe, stand nearly by themselves. Other societies emphasize continuity—between past and present, living and dead, individual and community. The differences between ourselves and other societies in this regard are manifest in the contrast between attitudes toward death in our own and other societies.

Attitudes toward Pain, Death, and Dying

Very little has been written about the response to pain in other cultures, about the attitudes of actual individuals to death and dying, or about the milieu of the dying person and how this affects their attitudes toward death. A small amount of psychological and anthropological work done in the United States indicates that there are important cultural dimensions both in the experience of pain and in the emotional and behavioral responses to it (Wolff & Langley, 1977). Zborowski's work, as discussed in Chapter 5, indicates that the experience of, and response to, pain are tied up with attitudes toward sickness, health, the medical profession, and the commitment to emotional restraint as a cultural value.

A cultural dimension to pain experiences has been noticed in the case of Alaskan Native Americans, who are reported to tolerate extreme pain very calmly for brief periods, provided it is accompanied by the hope of fast relief and recovery, but tolerate pain very poorly if the prognosis is unknown (Wolff & Langley, 1977). A study of Samoan patients with severe burns in a United States hospital found them extraordinarily stoical in the face of their great pain, and the emotional trauma usually observed in severe burn cases of American patients was absent both among the Samoan patients and their families (Ablon, 1973).

Among Hindus, the attitude toward pain is related to the attitude toward death, which itself is influenced by such religious beliefs as karma (fate). Just as the quality of one's life is shaped by one's deeds in previous lives, so the quality of one's death is believed to be affected by how well one has behaved in this life. Those people who can look back on their own lives with the conviction that they have acted rightly, can accept the fact of death. Unlike in the United States, where every effort is made to prolong life, even if that involves permanent, debilitating, and agonizing pain, with little hope of cure, in India, older persons are taught to prepare positively for death, and to prefer an early death to a long life of pain and suffering. Death is openly talked about among family members, and the acceptance of death's inevitability permits older people to prepare for it emotionally and spiritually (Vatuk, 1990, p. 82).

For Hindus, being psychologically prepared for death distinguishes a good death: "It's like if you start getting ready for a holiday a long time before the holiday . . . for this journey we start renouncing our things . . . in the world and people around you—you have less and less attachment towards the family, towards belongings, and more and more . . . [toward] religious giving. We have to be dead and living, not living dead. People who worry about death are living dead because they are so worried thinking about it. People who are not thinking about it, who are all ready for it, will never . . . die . . . the body dies, the soul just takes over the next form . . ." (Firth, 1989:69). Part of the preparation of death for Hindus is that the family of the dying person wishes to be by their side, chanting from religious scripture, and when death takes place in a hospital, preparing for death runs counter to the reluctance of Western hospital personnel to say someone is dying. This reluctance of Westerners to face death and the absence, in our culture, of explicit norms about preparing for death is, undoubtedly, part of the reason why there is so little cross-cultural information on dying, as opposed to cultural information on death. As one anthropologist notes, the anthropological literature focusses on "the bereaved and on the corpse, but never on the dying" (Palgi and Abramovitch, 1984, p. 385). The few available descriptions of dying in other cultures are contradictory. An early historian of medicine, Henry E. Sigerist, making reference to "primitive societies," distinguishes between the injuries and disabilities (such as skin diseases) that nevertheless allow the affected individual to keep up with normal life, and serious illness, accompanied by fever, that occasions complete isolation of the sick person from the group. Describing the Kubu of Sumatra, he says: "The sufferer from such illness can no longer take part in the life of the tribe. Sickness isolates him so completely that he is left helpless and in pain, even by his relatives. He is shunned, as death is shunned . . . the sick man is dead to society even before his physical death" (Sigerist, 1977, p. 380).

While it is true that in some societies bereavement begins before an individual has died, we cannot take Sigerist's view as characteristic of all "primitive" societies. Among the Cubeo of South America, for example, the dying do not appear to be shunned, although they are apparently not treated with any great concern, either. Goldman (1979, p. 185) describes the dying of a headman who had been ill for several weeks. The medicine men had given up on him, and his death was therefore expected. Once this acceptance occurred, the dying man was treated indifferently by his community. When at last the old man's time seemed near, as indicated by the difficulty of his breathing, his wife took up a death watch at his hammock. It was only after the man died that the society mobilized itself by beginning the mortuary ritual. Goldman reports that for neighboring tribes, those who are believed to be fatally ill with no hope of recovery may even be buried alive. In cases of voodoo death among the aboriginal tribes of Australia, it is also reported that once those who believe themselves bewitched refuse to take nourishment and show signs of decline, they are considered taboo and are isolated from the group out of fear.

On the other hand, Turnbull's (1961) description of an old woman's death among the Pygmy foragers of the Ituri forest in Africa suggests that among technologically simpler peoples, the dying person may be a focus of concern and warmth. The Pygmies express various degrees of illness by saying that someone is hot, with fever, ill, dead, completely dead, absolutely dead, and, finally, dead forever. When someone is ill, the women relatives will wail, but this is more of a ritual than spontaneous expression of grief. When someone "really dies," both kin and friends of the deceased burst into uncontrollable expressions of grief. Turnbull heard this wailing one evening when Balekimito, an old woman who was the mother of the best hunter in the group, was carried into her son's camp. Turnbull (1961) writes:

> "She had been ill for some time, but as she was an old woman nobody had thought much of it. She had been ill before and not died completely, not even just died, but now she had died completely and absolutely . . . and her son was running up and down, his face streaked with tears, beating himself on the head with his fists and crying that his mother was going to die forever. (p. 42)

The woman, in fact, was not yet dead; however, the room was filled with wailing men, women, and children. People waited both inside and outside her hut for the end, for her to die forever.

It is possible that the long dying process that is characteristic of some diseases in our own society is not frequent in these other cultures, which are nonurbanized and nonindustrial. Among the !Kung, who still live by hunting and gathering in the Kalahari Desert in southern Africa, such degenerative diseases as hypertension and coronary heart disease are unknown. People mainly die from accidents or respiratory ailments, and those who live into old age remain vigorous and alert—senility is unknown. The !Kung attitude in general is one of gratitude to the old for having worked to raise their children properly, and the old are generally treated very well, even when they are blind and totally dependent on the group. Researchers do point out, however, that this is more likely to be true for those old people with close relatives than otherwise, a point that parallels our own society with regard to hospital care (Fried & Fried, 1980, p. 155).

Among the LoDagaa of West Africa, whose mortuary ritual has been extensively described (Goody, 1962), the end of a person's life also takes place in the midst of the kin group. When a man is about to die, his brothers send young boys to tell others living in nearby villages. The dying man should be attended in his last hours by his sisters, his wives, and his sons. For the moment of his death, he should be sitting up, preferably in the arms of a close kinswoman. It is considered sinful for a man to die lying down, as if he were a slave with no one to take care of him. In such cases a payment must be made to the Earth priest, who then moves the corpse into the proper position. In this context, Goody quotes an informant, "If I suddenly got ill . . . my mother's sister would come to see me. If one of my matriclan doesn't come when I'm ill, to turn me over when I need it, who is there to help me? I'll die with my head on my mat." Because death is a matter of public concern, it is immediately marked by the wailing of women to inform the immediate neighbors, while the playing of xylophones spreads the news farther away. Messengers are sent out to inform kin in distant villages.

In Islam, too, the dying person should ideally be surrounded by friends and relatives. Islam imposes responsibilities on persons who know their death is imminent: they must ask forgiveness and forgive others; they must pay off their debts or arrange to have them paid by others, or ask creditors for forgiveness. A dying person must also make a will. They must also take care of their bodies in certain ways, they must clean their teeth and bodies and put on clean clothes. They dying person must recite the Quran, and remember God and ask his forgiveness. It is the responsibility of those near the dying person to remind them of these duties, as well as performing other duties, such as the recitation of the *Kalima* (profession of faith) until the person expires (Muwahidi, 1989, p. 47).

What seems apparent from these few examples of dying in other cultures is that whether the dying person is treated indifferently or with great care, he or she dies in the milieu of the community. At the moment of death, if not during the long illness that may precede it, the community responds to what is a matter of public, nor merely private, concern. Dying people in other cultures die in the midst of life going on around them. The surviving kin take an active part in death rituals, unlike the passive role to which kin are relegated in our own society, and must frequently be at the dying person's side to perform the proper rituals to facilitate the deceased's journey to the afterworld. Responses to the dying person may thus be viewed as responses both to a personal loss and to the loss experienced by the society at large. Grief reactions in other cultures appear to be directed effectively toward both consoling the bereaved persons closest to the deceased and toward reintegrating the society around the loss of the dead person.

Grief Reactions: Common Cross-Cultural Experiences

Because people everywhere build long-term, interdependent relationships that produce feelings of attachment and caring, the end of these relationships produces emotional distress and disorganization in every culture. In spite of cultural differences, then, there are some universal, or at least very widespread, individual and social reactions to death. In all cultures, as in the United States, people react to death with expression of emotions—sadness, emptiness, fear, and anger.

Of all the expressions of grief associated with death, crying, or "wailing," is the most common (Rosenblatt, Walsh, & Jackson, 1976). The intensity of emotion expressed in some nonWestern societies may seem shocking to Americans, where outward "bearing up" and emotional self-restraint are important values in funeral behavior. In the following scene among the Warramunga of Australia, a group of participants and spectators was leaving the area where a totemic ceremony had just been celebrated, when a piercing cry suddenly came from the camp where a man was dying:

> At once the whole company commenced to run as fast as they could while most of them commenced to howl. . . . Some of the men . . . sat down bending their heads forward . . . while they wept and moaned. . . . Some of the women . . . were lying prostrate on the body, while others were standing or kneeling around, digging the sharp ends of their yam sticks into the crown of their heads, from which the blood streamed down over their faces, while all the time keeping up a loud, continuous wail. Many of the men, rushing up to the spot, threw themselves upon the body. . . . To one side three men began wailing loudly . . . and in a minute or two another man of the same [totemic group] rushed on to the group yelling and brandishing a stone knife. Reaching the camp, he suddenly gashed both thighs deeply, cutting right across the muscles, and unable to stand, fell down into the middle of the group. The (dying) man did not actually die until late in the evening. As soon as he had given up his last breath, the same scene was re-enacted, only this time the wailing was still louder,

> and men and women, seized by a veritable frenzy, were rushing about cutting themselves with knives and sharp-pointed sticks, the women battering one another's heads with fighting clubs. (Durkheim; quoted in Huntington & Metcalf, 1979, pp. 29–30)

This emotion, however sincerely felt, is nevertheless a ritual norm structured by kinship relations to the deceased.

Every culture has norms about the kinds and intensity of emotions that are appropriate at death. While some religious traditions, such as Islam, censure loud wailing at death, because it contests the idea of God's omnipotence and wisdom, many cultures other than our own, permit, or even encourage intense emotional expressions of grief, which have a positive cathartic effect on the survivors closely related to the deceased. Among the Toraja of Indonesia, death is highly culturally elaborated and traditional expressions of grief, including music, funeral chants, and crying and wailing are an essential part of a Toraja funeral. Feelings of sadness, longing and pain are expected to be very intense and enduring at the death of a close relation, and the grief over a death may be expected to lead to insanity, severe illness, or even death. The funeral rites are designed to allow for the expression of such feelings. Vigorous crying, wailing, calling out to the dead, and even fainting from grief is expected not only by those close to the deceased, but by others, for whom the funeral recalls the deaths of their own loved ones. But with the conclusion of the funeral, it is expected that the grief will also diminish, and in subsequent revisiting of the gravesite, the culturally approved emotion is that of happiness at meeting again with one's ancestors (Wellenkamp, 1988, p. 490).

Sociologist Emile Durkheim viewed the emotion generated by such rituals as having the important function of binding together individuals in society and reinforcing the concept of society, as well as having important individual functions of catharsis. Such structured, collective, yet powerful emotional expression is noticeable by its absence in grief behavior in the United States. The cross-cultural research of Rosenblatt et al. (1976) appears to show that the working through of grief and the resumption of a normal life takes less time when such intense emotional expression is collectively displayed as part of funeral ceremonies. His finding that Americans experience grief longer and take longer to resume a normal pattern of life is not surprising in view of the relatively strong inhibitions on grief display in our society.

In considering the expression of grief in various cultures, it is relevant to consider the social position of the dying or dead person. Although most Americans would be quite reluctant to admit that the mourning of a person's death should, or does, correspond to their sex, age, or socioeconomic status, this does appear to be the case in all societies. In societies with high infant mortality, for example, a child's death does not occasion the extended ceremonies that take place for adults. In many societies a child is not considered a total social person until he or she has reached a certain age; dead children under that age are buried with hardly any ceremony. This seemingly casual attitude toward the death of children in some cultures is undoubtedly related to a high infant mortality rate. Where infant mortality is high, a relatively unemotional reaction to child deaths is probably adaptive. In India, for example, the infant mortality rate has always been high; even today, in a village very near the capital, New Delhi, Ruth and Stanley Freed report that death primarily strikes children under 4 years old (1980, p. 510). Popular Hinduism attributes the death of an infant to its bad actions in its last life. If a child dies, it is believed that its soul was overburdened by bad actions, and that it is better that such a child die so that it can be born again, shedding a bit of its bad actions in the process. These beliefs would appear to have some function in consoling the mother, particularly, who may find relief in the idea that the death was for the best. Among the Chinese, traditionally, the casualness with which the body of a dead child was disposed of—in a shallow grave—is explained by the Chinese belief that such children were not the genuine offspring of the stricken parents, but evil spirits, in the form of children, who sought to gain entrance into a household. Had they been received as proper children, they would bring disaster to the house, spreading disease and death to the other children.

Because a child is not considered a social person, its death often occasions less community response; the child has not yet taken on important social roles, and its loss to the community cannot be compared to that of an adult in the prime of life. Among the LoDagaa, whose customs are not atypical, no public grief is displayed for an unweaned child, and if a child dies within three or four months of its birth, even its parents may not mourn. Similarly, the death of a very old person does not occasion great public displays of grief, either. Such a person has usually ceased to maintain the affective relationships that would call forth the most important ritual expressions of grief, and has few surviving contemporaries to play the proper ritual roles. Even the political authority of such an old person as the head of the kinship group has often been taken over by another. Thus, like a child, such a person is not involved in a meaningful social network, and this tempers the communal expression of grief (Goody, 1962, p. 139).

The absence of public and ritualized grieving for children should not be taken to mean that their deaths do not cause intense emotions. A study of the impact of children's death on mothers among the Shona of Zimbabwe indicated that although few of the 124 women interviewed had public funerals for their very young children who had died, all but one reported experiencing grief over the death (Folta & Deck, 1988, p. 439). Furthermore, several of the mothers specifically mentioned the contradiction between the cultural taboo on public crying for a stillborn child, or an infant under six months, and their own personal, intense grief.

In addition to age, social status and relationship to the deceased account for intracultural variation in the expression of grief and in mourning behavior. In Chinese culture this is made explicit in the concept of mourning circles, the *wu fu,* or five degrees of mourning. The first of these was for one's parents and for a wife mourning her husband. In the second circle are grandparents and a husband mourning his wife. In the third circle are sisters and brothers; in the fourth circle, uncles and aunts; and in the fifth circle, remote relatives. For the death of a great-great-grandparent, however, joy, rather than grief, was expressed, because the person had lived to such a ripe old age (Fried & Fried, 1980, p. 174).

Although in our society, feelings of loss and sadness are considered the most appropriate ones to express at death, feelings of anger and aggression are frequently expressed in grief in other societies. Self-mutilation as described among the Warramunga of Australia is not uncommon; Rosenblatt et al. (1976) found that grief reactions involving aggression were described for 76 percent of a cross-cultural sample.

It is not difficult for professionals to understand why anger and aggression might accompany bereavement, perhaps even predominating over sorrow, when a very near and loved person has died. From a social point of view, the question is how to prevent the anger and aggression of the bereaved from damaging the social relations of the survivors and from inhibiting the reintegration of the group. Most societies try to channel the anger and aggression of grief along nondestructive paths. Here ritual activities and specialists play an important role by providing predictable and correct activities for the bereaved to engage in, minimizing the frustration that might come from not knowing what to do when death occurs. Ritual activities also keep the close survivors busy—often praying, singing, dancing, even engaging in sexual orgies that may divert aggressive energies into channels that do not result in harmful attacks on other persons. Ritual specialists are also useful in defining the often ambiguous feelings of bereaved persons as sorrow rather than anger; ritual itself may channel anger and aggression toward institutionalized targets; for example, out-groups, or, as we saw among the Warramunga, oneself.

In complex, socially stratified societies, where religious obligations in burial and mourning entail expense, anger toward one's poverty and toward established religious institutions may be a prominent emotion elicited by the death of a family member. In *A Death in the Sanchez Family,* Oscar Lewis (1970) exposes the wide range of emotions that come into play as a poor Mexican family tries to organize a decent burial for one of its members. As Lewis says in his introduction, "For the poor, death is almost as great a hardship as life itself." He goes on to describe that the difficulties the poor have in disposing of their dead are simply an extension of the difficulties they encounter in their powerless, impoverished lives: "Guadalupe died as she had lived, without medical care, in unrelieved pain, in hunger, worrying about how to pay the rent or raise money for the bus fare for a trip to the hospital" (p. x). Her survivors, being very poor themselves, had to spend a great deal of energy raising the money for her funeral; their anger at being exploited almost matches their grief at the death of their aunt. While in our culture, anger may be an individual's response to a death, anger is not an emotion culturally considered appropriate at death.

But in other societies, anger is not culturally suppressed, but rather culturally elicited as the appropriate, even honorable, expression of grief. Among the Kwakiutl tribes of the Northwest Coast of North America, the death of a close relative was experienced predominantly as an affront to one's dignity and status. The shame that was felt at a death had to be partly wiped out by holding a great feast (potlatch), at which great quantities of goods were distributed. Only by such feasts could the status lost by a death in the family be regained. A more aggressive way of handling a death was by head hunting, called "a killing to wipe one's eyes." This was a means of "getting even" by making another household mourn. When a chief's son died, the chief set out in his canoe to the village of a neigboring chief, who may have had nothing at all to do with the death. The bereaved chief would address his host, saying, "My prince has died today, and you go with him." Then he would kill the host chief. According to the Kwakiutl, this was a noble way to behave; a chief could not allow himself to suffer the humiliating degradation of status loss and struck back, not in revenge, but to wipe out the blemish on himself and his community. In death, as in life, the Kwakiutl were mainly concerned with their individual reputations and considerations of social status (Benedict, 1961, p. 216).

Another cultural context in which aggression is elaborated as a response to death is in those groups where either no deaths, or few deaths, are considered natural, and where the first question raised by the deceased's kin is "Who is to blame?" One of the societies where no death is blameless is that of Dobu, an island in the Western Pacific. The Dobuans live in perpetual distrust of everyone in their communities except for a very small group of trusted people. On Dobu every death is believed to be caused by "witchcraft, sorcery, poisoning, suicide, or by actual assault." Every person on the island has knowledge of some spells for causing specific diseases or death. Therefore, after a death, the kin of the dead use various divination techniques to find out whose grudge killed their kinsman. They watch the corpse as the mourners walk by, and when the guilty person passes, the corpse is believed to twitch in one place or another. Since sorcery is most effectively practiced when two persons are friends or kin, the most suspicion often falls on those who have been closest to the deceased in the months before death (Fortune, 1932). Although most societies are not as ridden with suspicion as the Dobu, the projection of blame on others for a death appears to be a widespread, culturally institutionalized practice. Such institutions undoubtedly elicit aggression while channeling it onto institutionalized targets.

Suicide

> In some (Eskimo) tribes, an old man wants his oldest son or favorite daughter to be the one to put the string around his neck and hoist him to his death. This was always done at the height of a party where good things were being eaten, where everyone—including the one who was about to die—felt happy and gay, and which would end with . . . dancing to chase out the evil spirits. At the end of his performance, he would give a special rope . . . to the "executioner," who then placed it over the beam of the roof of the house and fastened it around the neck of the old man. Then the two rubbed noses, and the young man pulled the rope. Everybody in the house either helped or sat on the end of the rope so as to have the honor of bringing the old suffering one to the Happy Hunting Grounds where there would always be light and plenty of game of all kinds. (Freuchen, 1961, p. 146)

As this description of the Inuit (Eskimo) suggests, the attitudes, frequencies, and methods of self-inflicted death are all influenced by culture. The few culturally comparative studies of suicide (Bohannan, 1967; Devereux, 1961; Hendin, 1964; Davies, 1989) show very clearly that suicide is a socially meaningful action, and that the meanings are different in different societies. Certainly, the almost universally negative reaction to suicide in the United States, which is related to our prolonging of life at any price as well as our "fear of death" syndromes, is not a reaction found in all cultures.

The Inuit present a dramatic contrast to traditional American culture in their attitudes toward at least some kinds of self-inflicted death. The Inuit traditionally are said not to fear death, and this appears to be true even today, where large-scale conversion to Christianity is typical. According to Freuchen (1961, p. 145), life is the central Inuit concern, yet suicides are numerous; when "life is heavier than death," then no man hesitates to end his torment. This happens in old age, when a man can no longer hunt and may feel that he is a burden to his kin in addition to feeling sadness at not being able to participate in the activities of the group.

Inuit suicide contrasts with suicide in our own society, where every type of control is brought to bear on keeping the attempted suicide alive. Cultural meanings are invoked ("Suicide is a sin"); familial pressures are applied ("How could you abandon your spouse and children?"); psychological and even legal forces—attempted suicide is a crime—are mobilized to prevent the individual from attempting suicide. An interesting point is that although active control and initiative are encouraged in almost every aspect of American life and culture, in death the individual has been expected to remain passive.

It should not be assumed that suicide is a prevalent pattern in all nonWestern, nonliterate societies; the meanings and practices vary enormously. Among the Zuni Indians of the Southwestern United States, for example, suicide is hardly known; to them, it is a rather exotic custom that occurs among white people (Benedict, 1961, p. 117). Among the Plains Indians, however, the theme of suicide was highly elaborated, notably in the custom of the "suicide pledge." A man undertaking this pledge tied himself to a stake by an eight-foot-long buckskin stole in the midst of one of the frequent battles involving the Plains Indians. He therefore could not retreat with his comrades if the battle was going against them. If he survived this death-courting experience, he was awarded the highest honors of the tribe. Plains Indians also understood suicide as a response to unrequited love; among the Mohave, on the other hand, for whom there were many categories of suicide, love suicide was associated with white people. The Mohave label many different types of death as suicide, most of which would not be recognized as such in our culture: stillbirths that are believed to be caused by the unwillingness of a future shaman to be born; the death of a suckling who has to be weaned because its mother is pregnant and who makes itself sick from spite; the death of twins at birth or before they get married; the pseudosuicide of a man who wishes to marry a kinswoman and permits a horse to be killed at his wedding in his place, thereby breaking the kinship bonds between himself and his bride; the victim of a witch who refuses to seek the help of a curer; an aging witch who incites his victim's relatives to kill him so that he can join the ghosts of his victims and thus retain his hold over them forever; a warrior who is tired of living and deliberately strays into enemy territory in order to be killed; the suicide attempts (which appear never to be successful) that occur as the closest kin of someone deceased attempts to jump on the funeral pyre; and finally active suicides, which—judging from case histories—appear to involve people who kill themselves after they are disappointed or rejected in love, friendship, or affection by someone close to them (Devereux, 1961, p. 324).

Viewing suicide from a different perspective, it appears that there are similar motives in different cultures. Bohannan's (1967) conclusion about suicide in various African societies is that it springs from motives similar to those most frequently found in the United States—that is, domestic strife and the loss or fear of the loss of social status. In addition, the African societies studied by Bohannan and his colleagues have motives largely unknown here—for example, the fear of ghosts or other supernatural figures who are believed to have the power to cause one's death.

This motive brings us to a consideration of voodoo death, or death by sorcery or witchcraft. In Cannon's (1942) classic article, he quotes a description of this phenomenon in Africa: "I have seen Kru-men and others die in spite of every effort that was made to save them, simply because they had made up their minds, not (as we thought at the time) to die, but that being in the clutch of malignant demons, they were *bound* to die" (p. 169). Although Cannon clearly accepts the view that this is therefore not suicide, Western observers might include this as subintentioned death—that is, a form of death in which the deceased plays an indirect, covert, partial, or unconscious role in his or her own demise.

The most vivid descriptions of this type of death come from Australian aboriginal societies in which the sorcerer is believed to work his magic by pointing a bone at the victim:

> The man who discovers that he is being boned . . . stands aghast, with his eyes staring at the treacherous pointer, and with his hands lifted as though to ward off the lethal medium, which he imagines is pouring into his body. His cheeks blanch and his eyes become glassy and the expression of his face becomes horribly distorted. . . . His body begins to tremble and the muscles twist involuntarily. He sways backwards and falls to the ground, and after a short time appears to be in a swoon; but soon after he writhes as if in mortal agony, and, covering his face with his hands, begins to moan. After a while he becomes very composed and crawls to his worley. From this time onwards he sickens and frets, refusing to eat and keeping aloof from the daily affairs of the tribe. Unless help is forthcoming in the shape of a countercharm . . . his death is only a matter of a comparatively short time. (Basedow; quoted in Cannon, 1942, p. 172)

After a man has been boned, his social life collapses; he is in a taboo state and is shunned by others out of fear. This state of social isolation is itself suggestive of death, and is one of the many suggestions incorporated by the victim who is in a highly suggestible state and who cooperates in withdrawing from life. Even before the victim dies, furthermore, the community holds a sacred ceremonial moving him from the land of the living to the otherworld of the totemic ancestors. In attempting to explain voodoo death, Cannon notes that a common element is that the victim, convinced that life is running out, refuses to eat or drink and succumbs to weakness and death in a matter of days. Cannon's view is that the extreme fear reaction causes a disastrous fall of blood pressure, which in turn damages the organs necessary for adequate circulation. This, combined with the lack of food and water, causes death. He thus sees voodoo death as similar to a true state of shock in the medical sense, being induced by a prolonged and tense emotion. Although later researchers (Lex, 1977) have suggested other medical explanations, there is no contradiction of Cannon's basic point that voodoo death is real, and that it is caused by repressed or obvious terror. Since little intensive interviewing has been done and few life histories taken for the few documented cases, it is difficult to know whether listing them as suicide reflects our own categories, based on our understandings of the workings of the unconscious, or native categories of victimology.

The Rituals of Death: Funerals and Mourning

In all cultures death raises a series of problems pertaining to the obligations imposed on the survivors: the corpse must be looked after; the deceased must be placed in a new status; the roles vacated by the deceased must be filled and their property disposed of; the solidarity of the group must be reaffirmed; and the bereaved must be comforted and reestablished in their relationships to others. In this section on the rituals of death, funeral rites are dealt with first, followed by rituals of mourning, with the focus on the mourning of spouses and especially that of widows.

Mortuary or funeral rites have many functions: they give meaning and sanction to the separation of the dead person from the living; they help effect the transition of the soul to another, otherworldly realm; they assist in the incorporation of the spirit to its new existence. In most societies, the kin and the entire community are prominent in these rituals. Through performing mortuary rituals, as well as through observing mourning behavior, community members have a vital role in realizing a communal goal—the removal of the dead person's spirit so that it will not menace the living. This is most frequently accomplished by the practice of secondary treatment of the corpse.

Secondary treatment is the regular and socially sanctioned removal of some or all of the relics of the person from the place of temporary storage to a permanent resting place. It is one of the most frequent elements in death rituals in other cultures. Among the Berawan of Borneo, for example, there are two major ceremonies, separated by a period of anywhere from eight months to five years. The first ceremony begins immediately after the death. The corpse is displayed for a day or two, until it has been viewed by all the close kin. It is then put into a coffin or a large jar. At the end of a week, this is removed for temporary storage and is placed either in the longhouse or on a platform in the graveyard. At the second ceremony, people come from all over. The coffin or jar is brought to a small shed on the longhouse veranda. Every evening for about a week there is a party near where the jar of bones is kept. The bones are then transferred to their final resting place, either in a wooden mausoleum or in the niche of a massive, carved wooden post (Huntington & Metcalf, 1979).

In societies like that of the Berawan, where secondary treatment is practiced, death is not seen as immediate. Rather, there is a period during which the individual is believed to be neither alive nor finally dead. During this period, the process of decomposition of the corpse may be said to represent the liminality, or transition period, of the soul. As the body decays and is in an impermanent and miserable state of rotting, so the soul too, is in its impermanent and restless position, wandering around the living, perhaps seeking to pull others after it. It is at this time that the corpse is most feared, and the fear of the corpse mirrors the fear of the spirit of the dead person. After the secondary treatment (burial or cremation of the bones), the soul of the deceased is considered to have reached and been integrated into the afterworld and is no longer feared. Secondary treatment rituals often are the official end to the mourning period and mark the point at which a surviving spouse may remarry.

The frequency of secondary treatment of the corpse corresponds to the widespread belief in the fear of ghosts. In fact, the United States stands almost alone of all the world's peoples in its cultural disapproval of perceptions and/or fear of ghosts (Rosenblatt et al. 1976). In other cultures, ghost fears may involve a fear of the dead coming back to extract revenge for past hurts or, more commonly, the fear that they may want to bring some of the living to join them. However these beliefs are phrased, they may be viewed as psychologically useful in helping break the ties with the dead, and thus lead societies to reintegrate more quickly. The rituals of secondary treatment are socially useful, as well as beneficial for the bereaved—particularly bereaved spouses, who in most societies are expected to remarry.

Another contrast between death rituals in our own society and in many others is the important role played by symbolic demonstrations of the themes of sexuality, fertility, and the continuation of life at funerals. These values are noticeable by their absence in America, where funerals are generally subdued, if not gloomy, affairs. In Madagascar, by contrast, among the Bara people, funerals involve "bawdy and drunken revelry enjoined upon the guests" (Huntington & Metcalf, 1979, p. 103). An important part of the funeral procession, during which the coffin is carried from the house to a cave in the hills, is a chase in which young girls run after the youths carrying the coffin, followed by adults and, finally, the family cattle. Only boys who have had sexual experience can participate in this, and it is viewed as essentially a sexual contest between boys and girls for possession of the corpse. About halfway up the mountain, the procession halts, the cattle are stampeded around the coffin, and the young men compete with each other in cattle wrestling. Then the procession begins again. Disorderly conduct of various kinds is essential at Bara funerals and secondary burial ceremonies. Toward this end, rum is served, and dancing, contests involving cattle, and sexual activities are part of the festivities.

This kind of behavior is not uncommon. Among the Cubeo of South America, simulated and actual ritual coitus is part of the mourning ritual. According to Goldman (1979) the dances, rituals, and dramatic performances, as well as the sexual license, have the purpose of transforming grief and anger at a death into joy. To understand sexual license as part of funeral and mourning ceremonies, we can view it as an introduction of the life principle into the fact of death. Given the trauma of death to the social fabric, it is not surprising that the aim of many death rituals is to restore a feeling of vitality and joy to the group. Rosenblatt et al. (1976) have also shown that attendance at funerals appears to be correlated with the distribution of food and drink, and with sexual license. Since they further demonstrate that attendance at funerals correlates with a relatively rapid working through of grief, it would appear that such festivities have important psychological and social functions related to resuming normal behavior.

Rituals surrounding death often have an elaborate hold on a culture, expressing as they do underlying beliefs about both life and death. While death rituals vary, as we have seen, according to the social status of the deceased, there is also an important underlying similarity or unity in death rituals across wide cultural and historical spaces. In China, for example, where the correct performance of death ritual was of concern to both commoners and elites, funeral practices throughout society consisted of many common elements: public notification of death; donning of mourning clothes by kin of the deceased; ritualized bathing of the corpse; the provision of food, goods, and money to the deceased; the preparation of a soul tablet for the domestic altar; music to accompany the corpse and settle the spirit; the sealing of the corpse into an airtight coffin; and the expulsion of the corpse from the community. Aided by the role of the Chinese state, which took the initiative in setting proper norms for death ritual, and the advent of printing, which permitted pamphlets on the correct ritual to be spread far and wide across the empire, a unity of death ritual has characterized China from late imperial to modern times, speaking of the strength of cultural elements in death beliefs and practices (Watson & Rawski, 1988).

Mourning

Mourning rituals function to reintegrate persons, particularly the spouse of the deceased, into society. Undoubtedly, one of the important functions of a mourning period is to limit the grief of the bereaved so that they may eventually return to more or less normal patterns of behavior. Just as funerary rites provide a passage in status for the deceased, so mourning rites provide a passage in status for the survivors. In all societies bereavement is not expected to be permanent. To the extent that a culturally defined mourning ritual exists, it both supports the expression of grief in a culturally approved way and limits the period of grief by limiting the period of mourning.

Two widespread mourning practices are marking and isolating the close survivors of the deceased. Isolation involves a limited time period during which close and specified kin of the deceased are kept apart from the rest of society. Isolation occurs more frequently for widows than for widowers, and more for spouses than for parents of a dead child or for adult children of aged parents. This suggests that grief may be less when the deceased is economically marginal. Where concepts of pollution or certain taboos must be observed involving isolation or marking, it is most frequently the spouse who is most subject to them. Among the Tlingit, for example, all those who participated in touching the corpse in preparation for its cremation were under taboos of various sorts; but the deceased's widow, in particular, "was the prisoner of taboo" (Fried & Fried, 1980, p. 158). She was not allowed to speak for 12 days after the death of her husband, nor allowed to do work of any kind. She was not allowed to use a knife or cup. It was believed that if she broke a cup, it could cause the death of her next husband. Her clothing and bedding were taken from her and burned along with the clippings of her hair, which she had cut for the cremation. A rock was placed on her bed, which was supposed to assure her next husband a long life. A rope was placed around her waist, and this was said to guarantee long life for her relatives. These customs clearly imply a responsibility in the widow for the life and well-being of her closest kin, as well as the expectation that she would remarry.

Among the Berawan, spouses were subjected to even severer restrictions. Widows and widowers had to stay for 10 days in a tiny cell made of mats, next to the corpse. They were not allowed to bathe and had to wear filthy clothes, eating only the poorest food, which was "shared" with the deceased. They could sit or sleep only with their legs tucked up in a cramped position. Huntington and Metcalf (1979) suggest that these restrictions are a way for the spouse to take on the burden for the whole community of appeasing the ghost of the deceased, by appearing to share the conditions of discomfort in which the deceased's soul resides. More general functions of isolation and restrictions may be to treat the bereaved with more consideration, or to help enlist aid for the bereaved, or to deflect aggression by putting distance between the most immediately affected by the death and the rest of the community.

In a cross-cultural survey of mourning behavior, Rosenblatt et al. (1976) found that the mourning of spouses for each other finds the most frequent ritual and emotional expression in most societies. The average time of mourning was found to be 305 days for widows, 215 days for widowers, and 198 days for adult children who had lost a parent. Clearly, the practice of sutee in India, where the widow was enjoined to throw herself on her husband's funeral pyre, was an extreme example of the asymmetry of mourning behavior. A widower was not expected to act in this way, and this was obviously related to his greater ability to remarry. Remarriage for widows was forbidden.

It is also true cross-culturally that women are permitted, and perhaps expected, to behave more emotionally than men when a death occurs. There are several possible explanations for this. Men may actually experience a loss less deeply, since women in their roles as wives and mothers may experience stronger attachments than men do in their roles. Another explanation may be that women are more strongly coerced than men by the normative requirements of mourning (and other) behavior. Still another explanation may be that women, being generally of lower status than men, are expected to take on the symbolic burden of distress and grief for the whole community. Finally, it should be pointed out that a lifetime of economic dependence on a man may lead women to experience the loss of a spouse more keenly than a man does. In the following lament from a widow among the Jivaro, the themes of dependency and loss are clearly mixed:

> O my dear husband, why have you left me alone, why have you abandoned me? . . . Who will hereafter fell the trees for me and clear the ground to make the manioc and banana plantations, or help me with cleaning and tending the fields? Who will hereafter make a red-striped *tarachi* for me for the feasts, who will bring me game from the forest or the gaily colored birds which you used to shoot with your blowgun and your poisoned arrows? All this you did for me, but now you lie there mute and lifeless. . . . O, dear me, what will become of me? (Karsten; quoted in Rosenblatt et al., 1976, p. 2)

As has already been suggested, in many societies remarriage is expected and encouraged after a suitable mourning period. In these societies, there are various mourning ceremonies that have the effect of breaking ties with the dead spouse and thus encouraging remarriage. The most common of these are destroying or giving away the deceased's personal property, observing a taboo on the name of the deceased, changing the residence of the survivor, and changing feelings about the spouse through ghost fears. All these practices may be viewed as moving the spouse of the deceased to undertake new personal commitments more readily. Such rituals also make it easier for others to relate to the deceased's spouse in terms of new relationships. Tie-breaking rituals appear to be particularly frequent in societies that have the levirate or the sororate—that is, where the deceased's spouse is expected to marry the brother or sister of the deceased (Rosenblatt et al., 1976).

The LoDagaa, previously mentioned, are such a group. Among the LoDagaa, the funeral ritual is, above all, a time at which the social roles that the dead man, especially, played throughout his life are reallocated. Funeral ceremonies provide institutionalized procedures for other persons to take over these roles. This is done through the mechanism of funeral orations, accompanied by gifts. A person in a particular relationship to the deceased makes a speech about him, telling of his good qualities that were important in that relationship. The speaker then produces gifts of food and beer, which are offered to the dead man, but also to the person who is prepared to fill his place in the relationship. In these ceremonies the dead man's roles as husband and father, as friend and even lover, are handed over to others. The persons who accept the gifts also accept the responsibility of the roles, and of filling them not merely perfunctorily but satisfactorily (Goody, 1962).

It seems appropriate to end this chapter with the preceding account of the funeral customs of the LoDagaa, which contrast so strongly with our own. In the United States, the absence of funeral or mourning rituals that satisfactorily reintegrate the closest survivors of the deceased, especially widows, into new statuses and new social networks appears to underlie many of the emotional problems that death causes us. Almost without exception, studies have shown that widows, particularly, suffer increased isolation and feelings of depression at their husbands' death. The LoDagaa, and other cultures like them, appear wiser than we in preparing for death and in developing their rituals, which—though they may seem outlandish and extreme to us—appear to be more than reasonably successful in meeting the needs of individuals and societies in their moments of greatest crisis.

SUMMARY ❧

Death is universally regarded as a significant event both for the individual and the social group. In every culture there are beliefs about death, rituals that are carried out at death, and emotions that are considered appropriate at death. Many cultures have beliefs and rituals that express the ideas of the continuity of society and the ongoing relationship between the living and the dead. In our own society, such beliefs are noticeable by their absence. The social and psychological functions of such beliefs are many: at an individual level such beliefs may comfort a person who is dying; at the social level these beliefs help society reorganize itself around the vacuum caused by the death of one of its members.

The emotions that surround dying and death in different cultures vary, although grief is one of the most common. Grief may be expressed in different ways, however: in some cultures it is accompanied by wailing and aggressive behavior, whereas in other cultures its expression is inhibited. In most cultures the expression of grief is tempered by the age, sex, social status, and social relationships of the deceased, all of which are reflected in the mourning ritual. The aim of culturally normative grief reactions is to console the persons closest to the deceased: mourning ritual in general is a useful social mechanism because it puts limits on grieving, and thereby aids in the reintegration of the survivors into normal social life. This appears to be particularly important for widows, who—in the absence of such meaningful rituals in our own society—appear to suffer particularly intense feelings of isolation and depression.

By examining cultural variation in death reactions and rituals, we can begin to think about alternative kinds of responses that might be useful in our society in aiding individuals to deal with death and dying more adequately.

LEARNING EXERCISES ❧

1. Sioux Chief Crazy Horse stated that a good day to die is one where "all things of my life are present." How might Americans identify a "good death" or a good day to die? Compare this to notions of a "good death" in other cultures.
2. Discuss what this chapter suggests about death and dying in other cultures that you think would be helpful for Americans to adopt. What cultural barriers stand in the way of the adoption of such practices?
3. Compare the attitudes toward assisted death in our own culture with those in other cultures. What are the major differences? How do these differences relate to a culture's attitudes about the meanings of life and death?
4. How do beliefs in ancestral spirits and ghosts affect practices toward the dead and dying in other cultures? How do you think American practices surrounding the dead and dying would be different if we held such beliefs?

AUDIOVISUAL MATERIAL ❧

Death Is Afraid of Us. 26 minutes/videocassette/1980. Granada Television International. 1221 Avenue of the Americas, Suite 3468, New York, NY 10020.
A beautifully produced documentary about the men and women who live in the mountains of Soviet Georgia who live to be over 100 years old, leading active lives.

Dreamspeaker. 75 minutes/film. Filmmakers Library, 124 East 40th Street, New York, NY 10016
A fine film about an aged Nootka Indian shaman, who when a white boy he befriends commits suicide, decides to die a noble death himself.

Good-bye Old Man. 70 minutes/film or videocassettee/1975. Extension Media Center, University of California at Berkeley, 2223 Fulton Street, Berkeley, CA 94720.
A filmed record of a burial and bereavement of the Tiwi, an aboriginal tribe of Australia, narrated by a member of that society.

The Spirit Possession of Alejandro Mami. 27 minutes/videocassette. Pennsylvania State University, Audio Visual Services, University Park, PA 16802.
A documentary of an old man's battle with aging and bereavement among the Aymara Indians of South America. At 81 years of age, feeling rejected, lonely, and possessed by evil spirits, Mami is drawn toward suicide.

REFERENCES ❧

Ablon, J. (1973). Reactions of Samoan burn patients and families to severe burns. *Social Science & Medicine. 7,* 167–178.

Achebe, C. (1959). *Things fall apart.* Greenwich, CT: Fawcett.

Benedict, R. (1961). *Patterns of culture.* Boston: Houghton Mifflin.

Bohannan, P. (Ed.) (1967). *African homicide and suicide.* New York: Atheneum.

Cannon, W. B. (1942). "Voodoo" death. *American Anthropologist. 44,* 169–181.

Davies, C. (1989). The ethics of certain death: Suicide, execution, and euthanasia. In A. Berger, P. Badham, A. Kutscher, J. Berger, M. Perry, and J. Beloff (Eds.), *Perspectives on death and dying: Cross-cultural and multi-disciplinary views.* Philadelphia: The Charles Press.

Devereux, G. (1961). *Mohave ethnopsychiatry and suicide: The psychiatric knowledge and the psychic disturbances of an Indian tribe.* Smithsonian Institution, U.S. Bureau of American Ethnology Bulletin #175. Washington, DC: United States Government Printing Office.

Elkin, A. P. (1964). *The Australian aborigines.* Garden City, NY: Doubleday.

Firth, R. (1967). *Tikopia ritual and belief.* London: Allen and Unwin.

Firth, S. (1989). The good death: Approaches to death, dying, and bereavement among British Hindus. In A. Berger, P. Badham, A. Kutscher, J. Berger, M. Perry, and J. Beloff (Eds.), *Perspectives on death and dying: Cross-cultural and multi-disciplinary views.* Philadelphia: The Charles Press.

Folta, J., & Deck, E. (1988). The impact of children's death on Shona mothers and families. *Journal of Comparative Family Studies. 19* (3), 431–451.

Fortune, R. (1932). *Sorcerers of Dobu: The social anthropology of the Dobu islanders of the Western Pacific.* New York: Dutton.

Freed, R., & Freed, S. (1979). The effects of urbanization in a village in North India. 3. Sickness and health. *Anthropological Papers of the American Museum of Natural History. 55* (part 5). New York: American Museum of Natural History.

Freed, R., & Freed, S. (1980). Rites of passage in Shanti Nagar. *Anthropological Papers of the American Museum of Natural History. 56* (part 3). New York: American Museum of Natural History.

Freuchen, P. (1961). *Book of the Eskimo.* Greenwich, CT: Fawcett.

Fried, M. N., & Fried, M. H. (1980). *Transitions: Four rituals in eight cultures.* New York: Norton.

Goldman, I. (1979). *The Cubeo: Indians of the Northwest Amazon.* Urbana, IL: University of Illinois Press.

Goody, J. (1962). *Death, property and the ancestors: A study of the mortuary customs of the LoDagaa of West Africa.* Stanford, CA: Stanford University Press.

Hendin, H. (1964). *Suicide in Scandinavia.* New York: Grune & Stratton.

Hertz, R. (1960). *Death and the right hand.* (R. & C. Needham, Trans.). New York: Free Press.

Humphreys, H. C., & King, H. (Eds.). (1981). *Mortality and immortality: The anthropology and archeology of death.* London: Academic.

Huntington, R., & Metcalf, P. (1979). *Celebrations of death: The anthropology of mortuary ritual.* Cambridge: University of Cambridge Press.

Kalish, R. A. (Ed.). (1980). *Death and dying: Views from many cultures.* Amityville, NY: Baywood.

Kenyatta, J. (1965). *Facing Mount Kenya.* New York: Random House.

Lewis, O. (1970). *A death in the Sanchez family.* New York: Random House.

Lex, B. (1977). Voodoo death: New thoughts on an old explanation. In D. Landy (Ed.), *Culture, disease and healing: Studies in medical anthropology.* New York: Macmillan.

Mauss, M. (1979). *Seasonal variation among the Eskimo: A study in social morphology.* (J. J. Fox, Trans.). Boston: Routledge & Kegan Paul.

Muwahidi, A. A. (1989). Islamic perspectives on death and dying. In A. Berger, P. Badham, A. Kutscher, J. Berger, M. Perry, and J. Beloff (Eds.), *Perspectives on death and dying: Cross-cultural and multi-disciplinary views.* Philadelphia: The Charles Press.

Palgi, P., & Abramovitch, H. (1984). Death: A cross-cultural perspective. *Annual Reviews in Anthropology. 13,* 385–417.

Rosenblatt, P., Walsh, R., & Jackson, D. (1976). *Grief and mourning in cultural perspective.* New Haven, CT: HRAF Press.

Sigerist, H. (1977). The special position of the sick. In D. Landy (Ed.), *Culture, disease and healing: Studies in medical anthropology.* New York: Macmillan.

Turnbull, C. (1961). *The Forest People: A study of the Pygmies of the Congo.* New York: Simon & Schuster.

van Gennep, A. (1960). *Rites of Passage.* (M. B. Vizedom & G. L. Coffee, Trans.). Chicago: University of Chicago Press.

Vatuk, S. (1990). "To be a burden on others": Dependency anxiety among the elderly in India. In Owen Lynch (Ed.), *Divine passions: The social construction of emotion in India.* Berkeley: University of California Press.

Watson, J. L., & Rawski, E. (Eds.). (1988). Death ritual in late imperial and modern China. Berkeley: University of California Press.

Wellenkamp, J. (1988). Notions of grief and catharsis among the Toraja. *American Ethnologist. 17* (3), 486–500.

Wolff, B. B., & Langley, S. (1977). Cultural factors and the response to pain. In D. Landy (Ed.), *Culture, disease and healing: Studies in medical anthropology.* New York: Macmillan.

Index

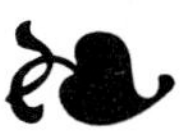

Tables and figures are designated by *tab* or *fig.*